PATIENT FINANCIAL SERVICES

Organizing and Managing
a Cost-Effective Patient
Financial Services Operation

PATIENT

FINANCIAL

SERVICES

Organizing and Managing

a Cost-Effective Patient

Financial Services Operation

ALLEN G. HERKIMER, JR.

Ed.D., FACHE, FHFMA, CMPA
Professor, Health Administration
Southwest Texas State University
San Marcos, Texas

PROBUS PUBLISHING COMPANY
Chicago, Illinois
Cambridge, England

To the
patient financial services managers
I've known—
and to those I've yet to meet

Permissions Acknowledgments

Grateful acknowledgment is made to the following for permission to reprint previously published material:

Excerpts, with permission of the publisher, have been taken from *No-Nonsense Delegation, Revised Edition,* by Dale D. McConkey, © 1986 AMACOM, a division of the American Management Association. All rights reserved.

References have been made, with permission, to material appearing in the 1993 *Accreditation Manual for Hospitals,* © 1992 by the Joint Commission on Accreditation of Healthcare Organizations, Oakbrook Terrace, IL.

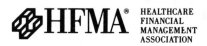 HEALTHCARE
FINANCIAL
MANAGEMENT
ASSOCIATION

ISBN 1-882198-14-X
Printed in the United States of America
BB
  2 3 4 5 6 7 8 9 0

Table of Contents

Foreword   xvii
Preface   xix
Author's Acknowledgments   xxiii

Chapter 1   Organizing the Patient Financial
              Services Department   1

              The Patient Financial Services Managers' Role   1
              Department Mission   4
              Missions, Goals, and Objectives   5
              Management Planning Defined   7
              Organizational Design   8
              Fundamental Rules of Organizational Design   10
              Operational Management Planning   11
              Delegation of Responsibility   16
              Job Analysis   19
              Job Description   20
              Summary   22

Chapter 2   Standard Plans and Their Use   25

              Policies   25
              Procedures   27
              Methods   29
              Standard Plans' Benefits   30
              The Department Operating Manual   30

Chapter 3   The Healthcare Accounting Process   33

              Principles of Accounting   33
                  Double-Entry Accounting   34
                  Accrual Accounting   36
                  Fund Accounting   39
              Prerequisites of an Accounting System   41
                  Organizational Structure   42
                  Chart of Accounts   42
                  Documented Proof   43

	Journals and Ledgers	43
	The Accounting Process	45
	Statement of Condition	46
	Statement of Operations	47
	Cash Flow Statement	48
	Statement of Changes in Financial Position	49
	Working Capital	56
	Application of the Accounting Process	58
	Incurred-but-Not-Reported Claims	62
	AICPA's Revised Reporting Requirements	66
	Patient Service Revenues	66
	Bad Debts	68
	Charity Care	68
	Net Patient Accounts Receivable	69
Chapter 4	**Managerial Accounting and Its Application**	**71**
	Managerial Accounting: An Overview	71
	Managerial Reporting	72
	Principles of Expense Behavior	74
	Operating Costs	75
	Opportunity Costs	75
	Social Costs	77
	Managing Operating Costs	78
	Global Expense Management	78
	Segmented Expense Management	79
	Expense Behavioral Patterns	80
	Fixed Expenses	80
	Variable Expenses	80
	Step-Variable Expenses	82
	Overhead and Other Expense Classifications	84
	Cost Analysis	85
	Application of Expense Behavior Principles	88
	Developing a Variable Budget	91
	Developing a Control Budget	95
	Variance Analysis	97
	Salary Variance Analysis	97
	Nonsalary Variance Analysis	99
Chapter 5	**Developing a Productivity Improvement Program**	**107**
	The Effective Productivity Improvement Program	107
	The Production Unit	109
	Macro Production Units	109
	Micro Production Units	110

Selecting Production Units   112
The Production Unit's Uses   114
   Staffing and Budgetary Control   115
   Evaluating Departmental Performance   118
   Evaluating Employee Performance   120
   Developing Employee Incentive Plans   122
   Allocating Costs   125
Developing Production Standards   125
   How to Develop Production Standards   126
The Need for Productivity Improvement   133

Chapter 6   **The Budgetary Control System**   **137**

The Budgetary Control System: An Overview   137
   The Importance of Staff Involvement   138
   Identifying and Quantifying Desired Results 139
   Multilateral vs. Unilateral Approaches to
     Budgeting   139
   Managing for Economic Results   140
   The Budget   140
The Patient Financial Services Managers' Role   141
Approaches to the Budgetary Control System   142
   Functional Accounting and Budgeting   142
   Responsibility Accounting and Budgeting   142
Budget Types   145
The Budgetary Control System's Typical Elements   148

Chapter 7   **Application of Variable Budgeting**   **153**

The Variable Budgeting Concept   153
The Purpose of Variable Budgeting   153
Relationship of Standard Costs to Variable Budgeting   154
Developing Standard Rates and Costs   155
Developing the Variable Budget   157
Developing the Variable Control Budget   166
Analyzing Salary Budget Variances   168
Analyzing Nonsalary Expense Variances   172
Analyzing Step-Variable Staffing and Expense
   Variances   173

Chapter 8   **The Cost-finding Process**   **181**

Why Cost Finding?   181
Cost-finding Applications   182
Cost-finding Objectives   184
Cost-finding Methods   185

	Direct Allocation	185
	Stepdown	186
	Double Apportionment	186
	Algebraic	188
	Keys to the Cost-finding Process	188
	A Cost-finding Case Study	190
Chapter 9	**Financial Requirements and Rate Setting**	**203**
	The Healthcare Organization as a Business	203
	Financial Requirements	204
	Third-Party Impact on Published Rates	206
	Case Study of Payment Procedures	207
	Reasonable-Cost Reimbursement	213
	Medicare Reimbursement Improvements	213
	Funds for Future Use	213
	Capital-related Costs	214
	Day-to-Day Expenses	215
	Medicare Bad Debts	215
	Addressing Provider Needs and Concerns	215
	Rate Setting	217
	The Per-Diem Rate	218
	The Per-Service Rate	219
	Sensitivity Testing	220
	Monitoring Product and Product-Line Profitability	222
Chapter 10	**Cash Forecasting and Management**	**227**
	Laying the Groundwork	227
	The Purposes of Cash Forecasting and Management	228
	Major Components	229
	Cash Inflows	229
	Cash Outflows	231
	Borrowings and Investments	232
	Float	233
	Cash Forecasting Methods	233
	Cash Receipts Analysis	233
	Cash Disbursement Analysis	239
	The Patient Financial Services Managers' Role	247
Chapter 11	**Analyzing the Financial Statements**	**251**
	Using Financial Ratios	251
	Ratio Analysis Types	254
	Liquidity Ratios	255
	Leverage Ratios	258

Activity Ratios	260
Profitability Ratios	263
Profit-planning Ratios	264
Measuring Liquidity of Patient Accounts Receivable	267
Accounts Receivable Turnover Rate	268
Patient Receivables to Charges	268
Patient Receivables to Current and Total Assets	269
Patient Receivables to Equity	269
Opportunity Costs	269
Other Performance Analyses	270
Statement of Condition (Balance Sheet)	270
Statement of Changes in Financial Position	272
Statement of Operations	272
Employee Turnover Rate	272

Chapter 12	Internal Audit and Control of Receivables	275
	Internal Audit	276
	Internal Control	277
	Financial vs. Operational Auditing	279
	External vs. Internal Auditing	279
	Patient Financial Services Audit Instrument	281
	Billing Audits	282
	Flowcharting	290
	Managing Accounts Receivable	299
	Payer Classifications	300
	Payment Systems	301
	Segmentation of Patient Accounts Receivable	301
	Monitoring Bad Debts and Accounts Out for Collection	303
	Implementing Electronic Data Interchange	306
	Summary	307

Chapter 13	Patient Financial Services' Impact on the Healthcare Organization's Marketing and Public Relations	309
	The Marketing Concept	309
	Healthcare Marketing's Mission	310
	Healthcare Marketing's Functions	310
	Patient Financial Services Managers'	
	Role in Marketing	312
	Preadmission	312
	Admission	314
	In-House	314
	Discharge	314

	Postdischarge	315
	Marketing to the Family Unit	315
Chapter 14	The Future for Patient Financial Services Managers	317
	The Healthcare Industry in Transition	317
	Patient Financial Services Managers' Expanding Responsibilities	318
	Patient Financial Services Management: an Overview	318
	Position Title	319
	Position Qualifications	319
	New Responsibilities	320
	Major Opportunity Areas	322
	Other Future Considerations	323
	Preparing for a Successful Career	325
	Glossary	329
	Index	349

List of Illustrations

Exhibit 1–1	Illustrative Structure of Departmental Goal and Supporting Objectives	6
Figure 1–1	Seven Steps to a Successful Management Planning Process	9
Figure 1–2	Traditional Organizational Design	12
Figure 1–3	Patient Service Representative (PSR) Organizational Design	13
Exhibit 1–2	Cost-Benefit Analysis	15
Figure 1–4	Sample Job Description Form	21
Figure 2–1	Flowchart of Preadmission Procedure	28
Figure 2–2	Example of a Color-coded Cash Receipt	29
Table 3–1	Double-Entry Accounting Impact Matrix	35
Table 3–2	Statement of Operations Using the Cash Accounting Method	37
Table 3–3	Cash Flow Statement	37
Table 3–4	Comparative Analysis of Cash and Accrual Methods	39
Exhibit 3–1	Consolidated Statement of Condition	41
Figure 3–1	Organizational Chart	44
Figure 3–2	The Accounting Process	47
Exhibit 3–2	Daily Cash Flow Analysis Form	49
Table 3–5	One-Year Cash Flow Projection	50
Table 3–6	Four-Year Cash Flow Forecast	51
Table 3–7	One-Year Statement of Operations Summary	52
Table 3–8	Four-Year Statement of Operations Summary	53
Table 3–9	Statement of Changes in Financial Position	54
Table 3–10	Comparative Statement of Condition	55
Table 3–11	Ratio Analysis of Patient Accounts Receivable	56
Table 3–12	General Ledger T Accounts	61
Table 3–13	General Ledger Trial Balance	63
Table 3–14	Statement of Condition	64
Table 3–15	Statement of Operations	65
Table 3–16	Cash Flow Statement	66
Figure 4–1	Comparative Line Graph	73
Figure 4–2	Flowing Line Graph with Minimum and Maximum	74
Figure 4–3	Single-shaded Line Graph	75
Figure 4–4	Levels of Expense Classifications	76

Figure 4–5	Methodologies Used to Control Departmental Expenses	79
Figure 4–6	Departmental Fixed Expense	81
Figure 4–7	Departmental Variable Expense	81
Figure 4–8	Total Departmental Expenses	82
Figure 4–9	Step-Variable Staffing Requirements	83
Figure 4–10	Total Departmental Direct Expenses	86
Figure 4–11	Total Departmental Variable Expenses	87
Figure 4–12	Total Departmental Production Unit Expenses	87
Table 4–1	Comparative Analysis of Actual Performance to Target Budget	89
Table 4–2	Comparative Analysis of Actual Performance to Control Budget	90
Table 4–3	Comparative Analysis of Actual Performance to Target and Control Budgets	90
Table 4–4	Comparative Analysis of Actual Performance to Fixed (Target) Budget	92
Table 4–5	Comparative Analysis of Actual Performance to Variable Control Budget	93
Table 4–6	Comparative Analysis of Performance to Step-Variable Control Budget	103
Table 4–7	Comparative Analysis of Actual Performance to Variable and Step-Variable Control Budgets	104
Exhibit 5–1	Job Description Form	114
Table 5–1	Variable Staffing Requirement	117
Figure 5–1	Relevant Ranges of Staffing Requirements	118
Table 5–2	Summary Salary Performance Analysis	119
Figure 5–2	Summary Performance Analysis of Volumes	121
Figure 5–3	Summary Performance Analysis of Salary Expenses	121
Figure 5–4	Employee Performance Record	123
Table 5–3	Departmental Task List	127
Exhibit 5–2	Daily Employee Self-logging Worksheet	128
Table 5–4	Standard Time Development Worksheet for Logging Inpatient Admissions	129
Table 5–5	Standard Time Development Worksheet	130
Table 5–6	Performance Factor Calculation Worksheet	132
Figure 5–5	Production Trend Chart	134
Figure 6–1	Functions of the Patient Financial Services Department	143
Figure 6–2	PSR-Patient Financial Services Department Organizational Structure	143
Figure 6–3	Traditional Patient Financial Services Department Organizational Structure	144
Figure 6–4	Budgeting Classification Tree	147

Figure 6–5	The Budgetary Control System	149
Figure 6–6	Budgetary Control Cycle	151
Table 7–1	Patient Financial Services Department's Chart of Accounts	158
Table 7–2	Cost Classification—Chart of Accounts	159
Table 7-3	Target of Fixed Budget	160
Table 7–4	Variable Budget Worksheet	162
Table 7–5	Comparative Analysis of Fixed Target Budget to Actual Performance	164
Table 7–6	Comparative Analysis of Volume to Variable Paid Hours	165
Table 7–7	Comparative Analysis of Variable Control Budget to Actual Performance	167
Table 7–8	Comparative Summary Analysis	168
Table 7–9	Computation and Analysis of Variances of Variable Salary and Wage Expenses	171
Table 7–10	Computation and Analysis of Variances of Variable Nonsalary Expenses	174
Figure 7–1	Step-Variable Cost Behavior	175
Figure 7–2	Variable Cost Behavior	175
Table 7–11	Computation of Step-Variable Adjustment to Actual Volume of Work	176
Table 7–12	Comparative Analysis of Step-Variable Budget to Actual Performance	177
Table 7–13	Comparative Summary Analysis	178
Exhibit 8–1	Cost-finding Spreadsheet	187
Table 8–1	General Fund Expense Summary	191
Table 8–2	Schedule of Depreciation	192
Table 8–3	Preliminary Direct Expense Apportionment	194
Table 8–4	Secondary Direct Expense Apportionment	196
Table 8–5	Summary of Revenue-producing Departments' Direct and Indirect Expenses	199
Table 8–6	Application of Short-Formula-1 Cost-finding Method	200
Figure 9–1	Memorial Medical Center's Financial Requirements per Patient Day for One Thousand Patients—Two-Party Payment System	208
Figure 9–2	Comparison of Memorial Medical Center's Average Charge per Patient Day with Its Cost-based Patients	210
Figure 9–3	Comparison of Memorial Medical Center's Average Charge per Patient Day (25 Percent) with Cost-based Patients (50 Percent) and 80%-of-Cost Patients (25 Percent)	212
Table 9–1	RCC Distribution of Gross Patient Charges by Managed-Care Contract	222

Table 9–2	RCC Analysis of Expense and Profitability of Managed-Care Contracts	224
Table 10–1	Master Cash Flow Forecast Statement	230
Table 10–2	Percentage Analysis of Gross Charges to Patients by Paying Agent	234
Table 10–3	Percentage Analysis of Cash Payment Schedules and Time-Lag Factors of Gross Charges to Patients by Paying Agent	235
Table 10–4	Percentage Analysis of Net Patient Charges by Paying Agent	236
Table 10–5	Analysis and Computation of Weighted Collection Percentage of Patient Charges Collected	236
Table 10–6	Weighted Average Cash Collection Schedule of Net Patient Charges	237
Table 10–7	Cash Inflow Analysis of Net Patient Charges	238
Table 10–8	Analysis of Monthly Cash Inflows from Other Operating Sources	239
Table 10–9	Analysis of Employee Payroll Check-cashing Process	240
Table 10–10	Analysis of Cash Outflow for Salaries, Wages, and Related Expenses	241
Table 10–11	Summary Analysis of Capital Expenditure Cash Flow Requirements	242
Table 10–12	Payment Priority Classification for Cash Outflows	242
Table 10–13	Schedule of Noncapital and Nonsalary Cash Outflow Requirements	243
Table 10–14	Analysis of Noncapital and Nonsalary Cash Outflows by Priority Classification	244
Table 10–15	Schedule of Noncapital and Nonsalary Cash Outflow Requirements	245
Exhibit 10–1	Daily Cash Report Form	248
Table 11–1	Five-Year Analysis of Patient Accounts Receivable and Revenue	252
Figure 11–1	Five-Year Graphic Analysis of Patient Accounts Receivable and Revenue	253
Table 11–2	Memorial Medical Center's Average Percentage of Gross Patient Accounts Receivable to Gross Patient Revenue Compared with the Regional Average	254
Figure 11–2	Memorial Medical Center's Average Percentage of Gross Patient Accounts Receivable to Gross Patient Revenue Compared with the Regional Average	255
Table 11–3	Comparative Statement of Condition	257
Table 11–4	Comparative Statement of Operations	261

Table 11–5	Statement of Changes in Financial Position	271
Exhibit 12–1	Patient Financial Services Audit Instrument Form	283
Figure 12–1	Symbols Used in Flowcharting	292
Figure 12–2	Flowchart of Patient Charge System	293
Table 12–1	PERT Network of Tasks for Implementation of Patient Courtesy Card System	295
Figure 12–3	PERT Network for Implementation of Patient Courtesy Card System	295
Figure 12–4	PERT Network for Earliest Starting Times for Patient Courtesy Card System	296
Figure 12–5	PERT Network for Latest Starting Times for Patient Courtesy Card System	298
Figure 12–6	Gantt Chart for Implementation of Patient Courtesy Card System	299
Exhibit 12–2	Segmentation Matrix of Patient Accounts Receivable	303
Figure 13–1	Marketing Organizational Structure	310
Figure 13–2	Five Control Points for Effective Patient Financial Services Marketing and Collections	313
Figure 13–3	Patient Financial Services Department's Target Markets	316
Exhibit 14–1	Sample of a Career Action Plan for the Patient Financial Services Professional	326

Foreword

With this book, Dr. Herkimer provides the blueprint by which individuals involved in or preparing for a career in patient financial services can anticipate the requirements and objectives pertinent to managing the patient account functions. Because today's patient financial services environment provides opportunities for managers to use their skills in a variety of daily situations, the author outlines the basics these managers need to consider in organizing the patient financial services department, as well as in formulating the functional units' policies and procedures.

The patient financial services managers' role continues to evolve from its beginnings in the early years of hospital credit management. The position's responsibilities now include financial and resource management, public relations and marketing, and bottom-line responsibility that directly affects the healthcare provider's fiscal viability. Indeed, this evolution in patient financial services moves the managers into a number of new areas, corresponding with the healthcare provider's involvement in new reimbursement procedures, intensified marketing programs, and third-party data and information requirements. Dr. Herkimer stresses the importance of the managers' understanding basic accounting principles to be active financial team members in the provider's budgeting, cost-finding, rate-setting, and cash-forecasting processes. The managers' ability to review financial statistics, track performance, and monitor managed-care contracts is especially critical.

Patient financial services managers must also be able to monitor key indicators that measure the effectiveness of their operations and the ability of their department(s) to meet established goals and objectives. Dr. Herkimer identifies specific auditing and control mechanisms that will assist the managers in meeting these responsibilities. In addition, the author reviews, at each functional level, the patient financial services operations' impact on the healthcare organization's marketing and public relations program; that department's intimate involvement in the success of these programs is outlined.

In looking toward the future, Dr. Herkimer describes the projected continued expansion of the patient financial services managers' role, as well as their potential opportunities and challenges.

Don Shinnick, CMPA

Preface

During the past several decades, a silent but steady evolution has been taking place in the healthcare industry, especially within hospitals and multifacility healthcare systems and, to a lesser extent, within the physicians' offices and managed-care organizations.

I entered the healthcare industry long before the advent of Medicare. Those of us who were in charge of handling and collecting the healthcare facilities' patient receivables were commonly called credit managers; however, the title was a misnomer because we did not grant credit. Each facility's governing board handled this particular function with the policy that no person would be refused patient care. As a result, this well-meaning group of community-minded individuals opened the door to mandated credit granting.

Some years ago, the title *patient account manager* replaced *credit manager* for identifying the person responsible for managing and collecting the patient accounts receivable. This title is prevalent in various healthcare delivery organizations and professional associations. For the purpose of this book, I have chosen the title of *patient financial services manager* for identifying the position whose primary responsibilities include

- establishing and managing a payoff procedure, whether it is total cash collection upon discharge or some method of systematically amortizing the patient's debt to the healthcare provider;

- establishing and managing a routine billing and follow-up collection procedure for all unpaid accounts;

- identifying and referring all uncollectible patient accounts to professional collection agencies;

- supporting the controller or vice president of finance, who represents the healthcare provider in all third-party payment and related contract negotiations; and

- assisting in the design and selection of every data processing system that aids in recording and managing patient account revenues and receivables operations.

Essentially, the position's chief function has not changed over the past few decades: convert all of the facility's patient accounts receivable into cash as efficiently and as quickly as possible to protect the institution's financial viability. What *is* different is the increased recognition and importance patient financial services managers have achieved on the healthcare provider's management team. Some of this status improvement stems from a decrease in philanthropic donations and public grants; most healthcare organizations have been forced to depend almost entirely on their own operations for needed cash.

Another contributing factor to the position's growth in stature is professional associations such the Healthcare Financial Management Association (HFMA) and the American Guild of Patient Account Management (AGPAM), which have developed and promoted certification status for the position. The initial certification programs were Certified Manager of Patient Accounts (CMPA) and Certified Patient Account Manager (CPAM). The latest certification program, Certified Clinic Account Manager (CCAM), has been initiated and promoted by AGPAM. Each of these programs has contributed greatly to patient financial services management's professionalism.

However, the greatest contribution to the position's prominence and professionalism has been, and will continue to be, the patient financial services managers themselves. Position titles will continue to come and go, but the positive and professional attitude that these managers bring to their work will ultimately determine its status within the healthcare industry.

Along with the title changes, patient financial services managers' areas of responsibility and authority have expanded dramatically. Today's and tomorrow's managers will be expected to perform the following duties:

- Recommend patient financial services policies to the healthcare organization's administrators and/or governing board, and design procedures that will assure compliance with those policies.

- Know all third-party payment systems and assist in managing communications with these systems to ensure maximum cash payments.

- Develop, organize, and manage appropriate admitting, discharge, billing, and collection procedures within board-approved policies.

- Assist in designing and selecting the facility's data processing system that will expedite the analysis and collection of patient accounts receivable.

- Assist in the negotiation, control, and evaluation of all managed-care contracts.

- Assist in cash-flow forecasting and management.

- Develop and monitor the department's and its employees' performance evaluation system and standards.

- Assist in routine patient accounting procedures.

- Develop a management information system that can identify any weaknesses within departmental responsibility areas.

- Serve as an active member of the healthcare facility's financial, marketing, and strategic planning teams.

- Represent the organization as one of its premier "salespersons" by creating a market-oriented department within the facility and in the community.

Over the past several years, I have received letters and comments from participants at seminars I've conducted and from university students who want to learn more about patient financial services management. This book is written in response to their stated need. It is dedicated to those individuals who have experienced the evolution of the credit manager and who have contributed to the growth and development of this exciting and demanding profession.

The reader will notice that throughout this book I use the words *healthcare organization* or *healthcare facility* instead of *hospital*. I feel that these words reflect more accurately the all-inclusive nature of today's healthcare delivery methods, whether they take the form of a one-hundred-bed rural hospital, a teaching and research facility, a hospice, a healthcare maintenance organization, or an extended-care facility. Also, one word of caution: This book is not intended to instruct the reader on billing and collecting any patient account. This task I leave to those who are more familiar with this ever-changing process. The book is intended only to introduce the fundamentals of the effective management of patient financial services.

Allen G. Herkimer Jr.
January 1992

Author's Acknowledgments

This book never could have been written had I not actually worked with and socialized with people responsible for managing healthcare organizations' patient financial services departments. With these colleagues and friends I have labored and learned for more than thirty-five years. Though they are too numerous to identify here, I owe these specialists a considerable amount of gratitude. Over the years, I have assimilated much knowledge from them and have used many of their management tools to administer the patient financial services of healthcare entities effectively and efficiently.

However, there are always a few key individuals whose constant encouragement and/or direct involvement in developing and writing a book make such an endeavor possible. First, I must thank Don Shinnick, Robert Rolfsen, and my wife, Fay, for suggesting that I develop a "get-acquainted" book about patient financial services for those who are thinking about entering the profession and for those who are closely or directly associated with it.

Second, I am grateful to Alice McCart and Ron Keener for understanding the need for such a book and for accepting the challenge and responsibility of publishing it. Their assistance and support has been invaluable.

Third, I want to thank David Canfield, Brendan Collins, George Colman, Newt Courtney, Peggy Arnaud Demming, Beth Newman, Dan Rode, Joe Walton, and Carey Weeks for assisting me in projecting the patient financial services managers' future. I also valued the assistance of Scott Davis of Ernst & Young in providing current information on Medicare payment policies and procedures.

Finally, I wish to acknowledge the patient financial services managers of the future. The financial viability of this nation's healthcare organizations, and their continued ability to deliver quality care at a reasonable cost, is in these manager's hands.

Patient financial services management is a dynamic profession containing many opportunities. Apart from solid knowledge of their profession's responsibilities, all that effective managers need is a positive attitude and a healthy amount of ambition, imagination, risk taking, and plain old common sense. To those who qualify and accept the challenge, the sky's the limit.

A.G.H.

CHAPTER 1

Organizing the Patient Financial Services Department

This chapter will address, step by step, the organization and management of the patient financial services department. Effective patient financial services managers establish the department's mission; identify goals that will carry out the mission; design the department's organizational structure; and prepare well-defined job descriptions and performance evaluations. In taking the time to devlop a sound management plan, patient financial services managers, in effect, help to ensure the healthcare organization's financial viability.

The Patient Financial Services Managers' Role

The patient financial services managers' most important role is to manage their department effectively—to mobilize and manipulate its human and material resources efficiently so that the department reaches its established mission, goals, and objectives. Most economic and social goals are reached through organized group effort; managing the patient financial services department, then, can be the key to meeting the healthcare organization's financial and social responsibilities.

Management involves designing an environment in which individuals, working together in groups, efficiently accomplish selected goals. As managers, people carry out the management functions of planning, organizing, staffing, leading, and controlling.[1]

This definition includes the following key words:

- creation

- environment

- working together

- efficiently

- goals

Patient financial services managers must create an environment that enhances working conditions and improves productivity. It must be the kind of environment that minimizes dissension and inefficiency and maximizes productivity and employee morale. Patient financial services managers, with the cooperation of their department supervisors, are responsible for maintaining these working conditions within the internal environment. This kind of team attitude must not be limited to intradepartmental activities but must extend to other departments and be exhibited attitudinally throughout the healthcare organization.

There are two important points to remember about managing effectively:

1. Department managers establish the mode and/or style of management and the department's working climate.

2. Managers must select a management style that is comfortable and workable for them.

Traditionally, most management styles are based on Douglas McGregor's Theory X and Theory Y or some combination of the two. According to McGregor,

-   Theory X managers assume that people are fundamentally lazy, irresponsible, and need to be watched constantly.[2]

-   Theory Y managers assume that people are fundamentally hardworking, responsible, and need only to be supported and encouraged.[3]

Another management technique has recently come into focus. Japan's Theory Z suggests that when an important decision needs to be made, everyone who will feel its impact must be involved in making that judgment, in a process sometimes called a quality circle. This management style recognizes the worker as not only a laborer, but also as a planner and engineer. Theory Z assumes that

-   More important than the decision itself is people's commitment.

-   Everyone must be well informed about the decision to be made.[4]

Whichever management style they select, patient financial services managers must keep their department's primary goal always in focus—to maintain the working capital required to finance their healthcare organization's accounts receivable at a realistic minimum. The effective management of patient accounts receivable is the single most important factor in the organization's financial success. An efficient patient financial services function can literally prevent bankruptcy.

Effective management of patient accounts receivable involves more than just collecting money. The patient financial services department performs many other functions, including

-   establishing a charge structure for patient services that appropriately covers the healthcare organization's total financial requirements;

- designing accounting and cost allocation systems and procedures that maximize cash flow;

- maintaining open communication with third-party payment agencies to improve the facility's financial position;

- assuring that the healthcare organization's medical records and social services functions are performed adequately to enable timely billing and patient referral;

- maintaining cooperation and communication with medical staff to assure timely completion of patient charts and the provision of adequate patient information;

- developing appropriate performance standards and adhering to them; and

- serving as the "front line" in the organization's marketing and public relations program.

These functions are the responsibility of patient financial services managers, making their job much more complex than it was a few years ago. Among other responsibilities, today's patient financial services managers perform the functions of the following:

- systems analyst

- systems designer

- personnel manager

- marketing and public relations advocate

- contract negotiator and analyst

- collection agent

- policy and procedure analyst

- quality assurance and utilization reviewer

Data processing, for example, is one function that increasingly demands patient financial services managers' time. Whether the data processing system is manual or electronic, effective performance of this function is a major key to the managers' success, as well as that of their department and the entire healthcare organization. Each organization's chief executive officer may assign other functions to its patient financial services manager depending on the facility's needs, the area of responsibility in which the patient financial services management function is placed, and the manager's abilities; but the organization's need for timely, accurate, and meaningful information is always present.

Department Mission

The healthcare industry is dynamic, and the patient financial sevices managers' position is no less dynamic. Today's patient financial services managers must be trailblazers in carrying out this ever-challenging healthcare administrative position. To succeed, they must establish a formal mission or purpose for their department.

Whether patient financial services managers select a traditional organizational structure for their department, choose the patient service representative (PSR) system, or opt for a combination of the two approaches, they must adopt and consciously pursue certain missions and ignore others that might derail them. The formally adopted mission defines the department's reasons for existing and determines the range of activities in which the department might engage; for example, patient counseling, third-party negotiations, public relations activities, cash management, data processing, and utilization review.

In addition, the department's mission will dictate to a large degree the kind of employee best suited to the department in terms of skills, experience, and education. The mission adopted by patient financial services management can also determine the complexity and formality of decision-making mechanisms as well as the type of internal systems and controls required.

Finally, the patient financial services department's mission determines how the department relates to the healthcare organization's external environment, including its patient population, community groups, other healthcare providers, government and regulatory agencies, and special-interest groups, all of which influence the mission's successful accomplishment, either directly or indirectly.

In establishing a departmental mission or revising an existing one, patient financial services managers should realize the wide range of possible missions—all of which have definite implications for the department's long-range philosophical and operational character. By confronting this issue at the outset, patient financial services managers can anticipate difficulties and create operational mechanisms for resolving them.

Missions typically address the following issues:

- patient convenience and economics

- organization convenience and economics

- organization development

- patient service

Each of these issues has a spectrum of mission possibilities. A department may pursue several missions simultaneously or sequentially. In addition, a department may assign priorities for subsets of missions. Patient financial services managers should routinely review, modify, and update their department's mission to assure that their organization is satisfying the needs of every segment of its market; for example, patients, physicians, employees, and community.

Missions, Goals, and Objectives

For illustration, let us examine the mission that Memorial Medical Center, Anytown, U.S.A., has developed for its patient financial services department:

> To render patient financial (nonmedical) services to Memorial Medical Center's patients and their third-party guarantors that will not only expedite the collection of cash for services rendered but also create an attitudinal environment that constantly enhances the center's image in the community and generates a sense of pride among the center's medical staff, nonmedical staff, and associated employees; to assure the community that the center will produce sufficient cash resources to guarantee the organization's financial viability and its readiness to meet the community's healthcare needs.

In this example, the patient financial services manager has identified the following six goals as essential in carrying out the department's mission:

1.0   elevate and improve the status, quality, and quantity of financial services to the organization's patients

2.0   be cost-effective, without sacrificing quality of service

3.0   assist and counsel patients in managing and meeting their financial obligations to the medical center

4.0   minimize the medical center's losses due to bad debts and uncollectible accounts

5.0   work with the other medical center departments and the medical staff to create an effective two-way communication system that will enhance and expedite reimbursement to the center and the physician

6.0   accomplish these objectives in an environment that is efficient and pleasant for patients, medical staff, and medical center employees

The manager has identified each goal with a whole number. For example, the first goal, "elevate and improve the status, quality, and quantity of financial services to the organization's patients," is labeled 1.0, the second goal's number is 2.0, and so on. In identifying each goal's supporting objectives and/or strategies designed to achieve these goals, the manager numbered each objective with the related goal's whole number and a supporting number sequentially assigned; i.e., 1.1, 1.2, 1.3, and 1.4. Those objectives supporting Goal Number 2.0 are identified as 2.1, 2.2, 2.3, etc.

Exhibit 1–1 is an example of how to format the department's goals and supporting objectives.

In analyzing this goal and its supporting objectives, we can see that the goal is nonquantitative, but the objectives establish the desired number of groups and standards. Each objective also identifies (1) the desired results, the criteria to be used in evaluating whether the objective has been completed; (2) the desired date for the objective's completion; (3) the person responsible for performing the work; and (4) the amount of funds the organization has appropriated for the objective.

In summary, goals tend to be nonquantitative, whereas objectives are usually quantified for easier and more meaningful performance evaluations.

A *performance evaluation* is the process of testing whether the department achieves its goals and consequently its mission. To make this evaluation possible, patient financial services managers should develop a formal management plan (frequently stored in a departmental loose-leaf operating manual) that includes, in addition to their department's mission, goals, and objectives, the following:

- organization policies

EXHIBIT 1–1

Illustrative Structure of Departmental Goal and Supporting Objectives

---

Memorial Medical Center
Patient Financial Services Department

Goal Number 1.0 and Supporting Objectives

Goal 1.0:   elevate and improve the status, quality, and quantity of financial services to the organization's patients

Objectives   **1.1:**   develop and operate two (2) focus groups of discharged patients by types of service for a period of three (3) months

Desired Results:	actual development of focus groups
Completion Date:	January 15, 19xx
Responsible Person:	Sarah Vaughan, Supervisor
Budgeted Cost:	$2,000

1.2:   develop production standards for each position in the department

Desired Results:	actual development of all standards
Completion Date:	March 31, 19xx
Responsible Person:	Stanley Kenton
Budgeted Cost:	$4,000

- operating procedures

- information systems

- required resources

- performance standards

- financial plan (budget)

The managers must ascertain that each of these components is directed toward and complementary to their department's overall mission. The first four components will be discussed later in this chapter, performance standards will be covered in chapter 5, and financial planning will be discussed in chapter 6.

Management Planning Defined

Before discussing the methodology of effective management planning, defining *management* and *planning* may be useful. *Merriam Webster's Collegiate Dictionary, Tenth Edition,* defines *manage* as "to handle or direct with a degree of skill or address; to alter by manipulation; to succeed in accomplishing; to direct the professional career of; to direct or carry on business or affairs; to achieve one's purpose."[5] The key words in this definition are

- handle

- manipulate

- succeed

- direct

- achieve

Planning is "the act or process of making or carrying out plans; the establishment of goals, policies, and procedures for a social or economic unit."[6] The key words in this definition are

- process

- carrying out

- goals, policies, and procedures

In conclusion, *management planning* is the process management uses to organize and to plan strategy to successfully achieve an identified mission and its set of objectives in an orderly and systematic way.

Organizational Design

Management planning begins with organizational design; a well-designed organizational structure is necessary to implement the management plan. It is also important that the management plan and organizational design fit the manager's leadership style.

To manage effectively, patient financial services managers must first organize themselves and their subordinates. Seven steps comprise the organizational design planning process (see figure 1–1):

Step 1.   *Self-evaluation.* During this step, which might take a week or two, the manager relates personal abilities and skills to the strategies, policies, and systems necessary to accomplish the department's mission.

Step 2.   *Initial Documentation.* With personal strengths and weaknesses in mind, the manager jots down ideas related to strategies, organizational design, resources, and systems. (Ideas should be randomly written down every day as they come to mind.)

Step 3.   *Organization.* The manager organizes ideas collected up to this point according to the tasks required to achieve the department's mission. This list should be in sequential order, similar to those identified in exhibit 1–1.

Step 4.   *Preview.* After developing the initial plan, the manager should review it with the supervisors and subordinates who will be actively involved in its implementation, execution, or evaluation.

Step 5.   *Formalization.* The manager incorporates all appropriate suggestions from Step 4 into a formal document that must be approved in writing by the organization's chief executive officer or another appropriate supervising officer.

Step 6.   *Implementation and Execution.* The manager and the supervisors implement the plan and manage the operations.

Step 7.   *Review and Evaluation.* The manager and other appropriate individuals evaluate operating results in terms of preestablished performance standards. Review and evaluation should take place at least once a month, depending on the importance of the function being evaluated.

To assure maximum creativity and results, managers should work alone during Steps 2 and 3. The results of these "quiet times" will have a substantial impact on the method and organization of the department's operations. In completing Steps 2 and 3, managers should try to be as open-minded, daring, and creative as possible, yet be realistic. It is also wise not to expect to

FIGURE 1–1

Seven Steps to a Successful Management Planning Process

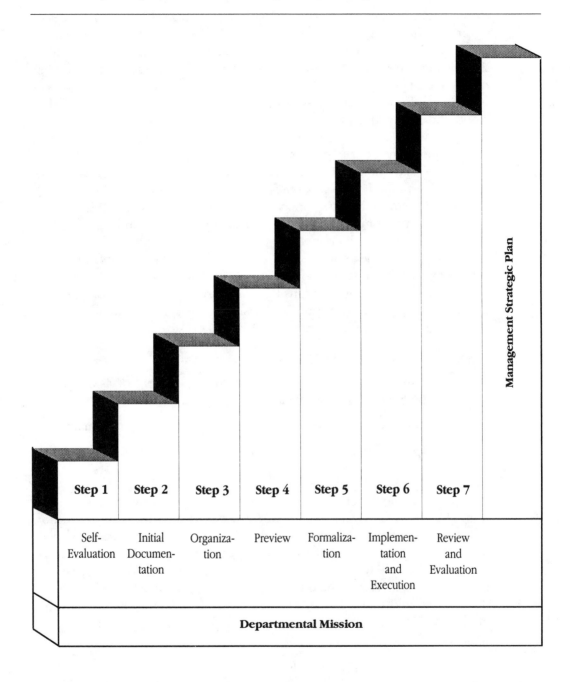

develop the ideal plan on the first attempt. Generally, many rewrites, additions, deletions, and revisions are needed to produce a preliminary organizational plan ready for previewing (Step 4).

Fundamental Rules of Organizational Design

Patient financial services managers must adhere to three fundamental rules of organizational design in preparing their department's organizational plan. The first rule is to identify primary responsibility centers (for example: admitting, billing, collections, counseling, etc.) and to *assign responsibility* for each center to one person. The individual's responsibility and standards of performance (production) must be well defined (in writing) and mutually understood and accepted. In addition, managers must delegate enough authority to the individual so as to provide sufficient latitude for effectively administering the area of responsibility.

The second rule entails *unity of command,* which stipulates that an employee report to only one supervisor. An employee should not be forced to choose between immediate supervisors. Frequently, someone in this awkward position becomes loyal to one supervisor at the expense of the other. At best, this person will be ineffectively loyal to both supervisors.

The third rule deals with *span of control,* or the maximum number of subordinates any one supervisor can effectively supervise. A supervisor managing too many subordinates runs the risk of either creating a bottleneck of indecision or making inappropriate decisions. The optimum number of subordinates reporting to one supervisor depends on several factors:

- the supervisor's ability to manage effectively;

- the financial or personnel impact of the supervisor's decisions on the department or the healthcare organization;

- the number or frequency of decisions the supervisor must make; and

- the subordinates' ability to manage themselves and allocate their time effectively.

Experts in the healthcare industry generally consider five to eight subordinates to be a manageable number for a department manager or section supervisor to supervise directly.[7] Individuals who perform routine and repetitious tasks generally require less direct supervision; consequently, a supervisor should be able to manage as many as twenty-five such employees.

Figure 1–2 illustrates the traditional design of a patient financial services department, and figure 1–3 is an example of an organizational design that incorporates the patient service representative (PSR) system. Both charts depict the rules of organizational design:

- delegation of responsibility

- unity of command

- span of control

Operational Management Planning

Once patient financial services managers have developed an organizational design for their department—keeping in mind that nothing is permanent at this point—the planning process continues. There are seven basic steps in the preliminary operational management planning process:

1. Identify specific goals and objectives that will achieve the department's mission.

2. Design the strategy to be used to attain specific goals and objectives.

3. Identify labor, nonlabor services and supplies, capital equipment, and financial resources required to implement the strategy.

4. Design an implementation plan that includes training and other start-up functions.

5. Develop an operational plan that includes policies, procedures, and methods.

6. Develop departmental and individual performance standards that can be used to monitor and evaluate operating results.

7. Develop a methodology and assign responsibility for giving feedback, evaluating actual operations in terms of performance standards, and taking necessary corrective measures.

Defining the department's specific objectives is one of the most important steps in the management planning process. There are two basic approaches to setting departmental objectives:

1. unilateral

2. multilateral

In the unilateral (Theory X) approach, managers do all of the planning and, specifically, objective setting, with little, if any, input from subordinates. The multilateral (Theory Y and/or Theory Z) approach, on the other hand, calls for the planning and establishment of objectives to be done by the people who have the ultimate responsibility for making the plan work. If planning time is limited and some stopgap decisions must be made, the unilateral approach will frequently effect desirable short-term results. However, multilateral planning's involvement approach generally improves employee morale and productivity over the long term; employees have a sense of ownership of the plan they helped to develop.

Once managers have identified their department's objectives (see exhibit 1–1) and established priorities, they must determine the strategy required to

FIGURE 1–2
Traditional Organizational Design

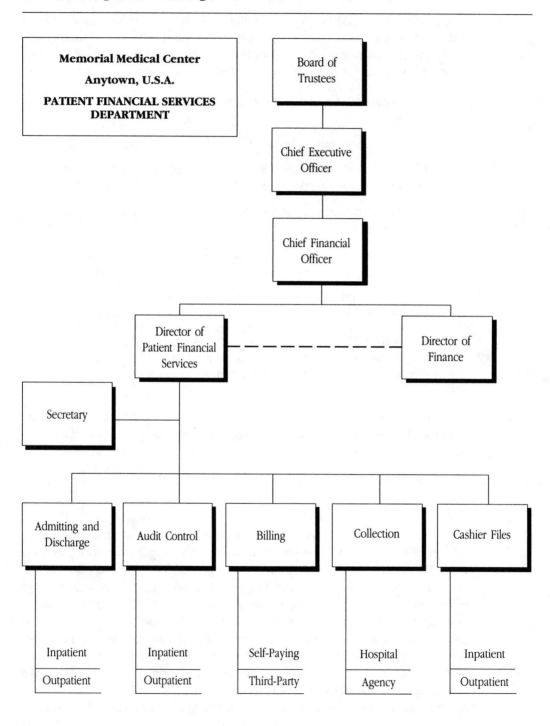

FIGURE 1–3

Patient Service Representative (PSR) Organizational Design

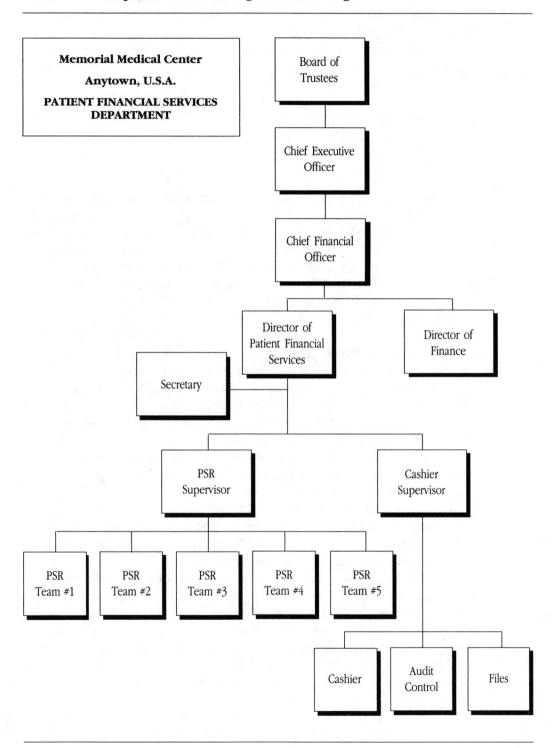

accomplish these objectives. Again, a multilateral approach generally produces the best long-term results because of its synergistic effect. Usually it requires more time than the unilateral method, but the long-term results tend to be worth the extra time required.

Identification of resources is the next step. These resources include the following:

- labor

- nonlabor supplies and services

- capital equipment and facilities

- financing

This step requires patient financial services managers to assess the resources their healthcare organization already possesses, as well as any additional resources needed to implement the strategic plan. A corresponding financial requirement plan (budget) is a critical management tool in this process; it will be discussed in chapter 6. Along with the financial plan, a cost-benefit analysis of every objective should be completed so that management can evaluate each program's economic and social feasibility. Exhibit 1–2 is an example of a cost-benefit analysis.

Managers can usually identify and estimate the total cost of any project with a reasonable degree of accuracy. In exhibit 1–2, the total cost of the Objective 1.1 project, $2,000, is recorded in the upper portion of the analysis. Some project benefits have a monetary value that can be easily calculated, while others may be difficult to appraise. On the other hand, managers will discover that they cannot easily identify social benefits, such as the value the community may receive from the project. Therefore, in many cost-benefit analyses, the benefits will be either monetary or nonmonetary. In this exhibit there is no identified nonmonetary benefit value, while $5,000 is the estimated value of the monetary benefits.

The managers' implementation and execution of their strategic plan is substantially easier if they give thoughtful consideration to the first five steps in the management planning process. A well-thought-out, formal plan makes their decision-making process almost automatic.

Actually, patient financial services managers should start reviewing and evaluating their department's strategic plan even before they implement it; they will have established performance standards as part of the preliminary operational management planning process. (Although people in the healthcare industry frequently use the terms *performance standard* and *production standard* interchangeably, this author prefers *performance standard*.) According to *Merriam Webster's Collegiate Dictionary, Tenth Edition, performance* is "the execution of an action; something accomplished; the fulfillment of a claim, promise, or request,"[8] whereas one of its definitions for *production* is "total output, especially of a commodity or an industry."[9]

EXHIBIT 1–2

Cost-Benefit Analysis

Memorial Medical Center

Cost-Benefit Analysis of Focus Groups (Objective 1.1) in the Patient Financial Services Department

Costs

1.	4 room rentals @ $50 each	=	$	200
2.	per-diem fees, 4 group meetings @ $25 x 10	=		1,000
3.	luncheon costs, 4 group meetings @ $10 x 10	=		400
4.	VCR rentals and tapes	=		200
5.	promotional supplies	=		200
	Total Costs	=		$ 2,000

Benefits

NONMONETARY

1. identify strengths of program(s)

2. identify weaknesses of program(s)

3. identify corrective measures

4. take corrective measures

MONETARY

1.	estimated increase in net patient revenue	=	$ 5,000
	Total Monetary Benefits	=	$ 5,000

Thus, a *performance standard* is a reasonable quantitative measurement or level of work that management expects to be accomplished over a specific period of time. Again, a multilateral approach to establishment of performance standards usually proves most effective. Management expectations must be realistic, attainable, and periodically reassessed to ensure that they are producing the desired results. Chapter 5 describes the development and use of performance standards in considerable detail.

As managers design their plan's review and evaluation process, they must make sure that it incorporates procedures that they can use to systematically and continually compare results with standards and take appropriate corrective measures.

Delegation of Responsibility

An adjunct function of the management planning process is the delegation of responsibility and authority. There are certain responsibilities patient financial services managers cannot delegate, including leadership, coordination, and evaluation. Staff assistants may help managers carry out these duties, but the managers are ultimately responsible. Thus, delegation means the assignment of only part of the managers' work.

Some managers are reluctant to delegate work because they believe they will lose control; other managers delegate work and forget about it. Both approaches are dangerous. In the first case, the manager is not developing a management team; in the second, the manager has abdicated a responsibility without providing for feedback or accountability. Managers need to remember when delegating responsibility that they must also delegate a corresponding amount of authority.

The process of delegation involves determining the results expected from a position, assigning tasks to a position, delegating authority for accomplishing these tasks, and holding the person in that position responsible for the accomplishment of the tasks. In practice, it is impossible to split this process; for example, it is unfair for managers to expect employees to accomplish goals without giving them the authority to achieve them.[10]

As Dale McConkey points out in his book *No-Nonsense Delegation,* managers also must remember to be on the lookout for delegation mistakes. Just as physical symptoms provide patients and doctors with guidance as to the nature and extent of illness, McConkey says that the following symptoms of weak delegation provide managers with the direction for corrective action:

- *Poor planning.* Lack of delegation is second only to untrained planners as the cause of weak planning. Plans that frequently go astray should be considered symptomatic of poor delegaton. Frequently, misguided managers were the plan developers, operating under the false premise that planning can be done only by those who are in a position high enough to see the overall picture. This premise is true when it comes to guiding and directing the organization. It fails to recognize, however, that the overall picture consists of smaller pieces and that the person in charge of the smaller operation knows that operation better than anyone else.

- *Too many orders.* The number of orders managers issue and the amount of detail they contain are valid indicators of how much delegation has taken place. The degree can vary from continually issuing detailed standard operating procedures to the subordinate to having that person manage under approved objectives with most of the "how to" left to the subordinate's discretion. The vital parts of delegation—discretion, initiative, and decision making—decrease as the frequency and detail of orders increase.

- *Overcontrol.* Even the best delegation can be destroyed by the manager's subsequent overcontrol. Symptoms of overcontrol include the daily staff meeting, frequent visits to the subordinate's unit, frequent interoffice telephone calls, requests for an excessive number of reports, a close check required of the financial department on components of the subordinate's operations, and encouraging the subordinate to check back with the boss excessively.

- *Undercontrol.* Undercontrol is detrimental to employees' motivation, because people tend to equate the importance of their jobs with the amount of interest others show in what they are trying to accomplish.

- *Fat briefcases.* The bulging briefcase carried home too often is a good indication that one or more of these conditions prevails: the manager doesn't have enough people to handle the work load; is overly cautious when making decisions; likes to revel in self-praise about output; is trying to impress others; or is a poor delegator.

- *Constant pressure.* Lack of delegation frequently manifests itself in a manager working under constant pressure. This unenviable position may have two different causes: the manager's boss has not delegated to the manager effectively; or the manager has not delegated to the subordinates.

- *Criticism of subordinates.* Managers who are always criticizing their subordinates, both directly and to their superior, probably have a delegation problem. Seldom, if ever, will one manager end up with all the poor performers in the organization. Managers must make sure that they provide subordinates with enough authority for them to accomplish their assigned tasks.

- *Lack of policy.* The lack of policy enunciation, communication, and feedback to subordinates can cause a delegation problem by design or by accident. Lack of policy is by design if the manager hasn't provided it as a means of forcing subordinates to check with the boss on all issues. If not by design, the checking back will occur anyway, simply because the subordinates do not have enough information to make a decision.

- *Too much policy.* An overabundance of policies, procedures, and administrative rules removes too much discretion from the subordinates' domain and often causes them to be more like policy administrators than managers of their responsibilities.

- *Lack of objectives.* Unless subordinates operate with clear-cut objectives, they don't know what their manager expects of them or what they should be doing at any time.

- *Slow decision making.* One of the requirements for prompt decision making is that employees know what they are supposed to accomplish and how much authority they have.

- *Misplaced decision making.* An outstanding example of a lack of clear-cut delegation occurs when a decision is made by the "wrong" manager, someone who is in a high position in the organization but lacks all the facts necessary for making the best judgment. Decisions should be made at the lowest possible level at which all of the information necessary for making the decision comes together.

- *Limited span of control.* The number of persons reporting to a manager is not, in itself, a valid indicator as to how much delegation has taken place—after all, a manager could have twenty-five subordinates without giving any of them any authority or accountability. Nonetheless, a limited span of control often indicates that the manager may be trying to centralize all operations and concentrate power in the hands of a few subordinates.

- *Ball carrying by subordinates.* One valid indication of poor delegation occurs when a manager does not permit subordinates to participate in many meetings and presentations or to make contacts with employees above their own level, even though they have the competence to participate in these relationships.

- *Penny-wise and pound-foolish.* Any delegation that isn't accompanied by the authority to spend the necessary money to carry it out—within preestablished limits—isn't a very extensive delegation.

- *Quoting the boss.* Whenever managers quote or use their boss's name to secure action, defer action, or sneak away from making a decision, one of three delegation components has broken down: the manager has not been delegated to, has not accepted the delegation, or is not competent to carry out the delegation.

- *Overly detailed job knowledge.* Managers, especially those who have a number of subordinates, cannot be expected to know the minor details of each employee's job. If they do, they may not be managing so much as they are getting too involved in the particulars of operations.

- *Lack of priorities.* Delegation requires establishing priorities. Managers who spend their time—no matter how conscientiously they apply themselves—on various matters without regard to the importance of each of them, probably has a delegation problem.

- *Everything's a secret.* Employees cannot carry out their accountability unless their managers regularly provide them with all the information and data that have an impact on their job. They should not be forced to seek out or request this information; it should flow to them naturally as a part of the system. By the same token, a lack of upward communications often results in the boss becoming isolated and acting on misinformation.

- *Disorganized effort.* Proper delegation should result in a smoothly running team, with each person contributing to the total effort. The only way employees can play their proper role is to have each person receive and accept a delegation of what must be done and when it must be done. Otherwise, the team will be replaced by an army of disorganized, uncoordinated individual efforts that work against accomplishing the overall goal.[11]

In summary, assembling, organizing, and developing an effective management team is undoubtedly one of the most important functions of patient financial services managers. When Andrew Carnegie was asked to what he attributed his success, he responded, "I hire the right people." The responsibility of developing an effective management team can be carried one step further: patient financial services managers have the additional responsibility of assisting their subordinates in expanding and developing their skills, capabilities, and horizons.

Job Analysis

An integral part of the management planning process is job analysis. This function requires patient financial services managers to analyze thoroughly the types of tasks delegated to each job or position in the organizational design and the personal qualities, experience, and education needed to perform these tasks.

For example, analyzing the patient service representative (PSR) position might yield a list of the following functions:

- Conduct preadmission and/or admission processing with inpatients being admitted to the healthcare facility or outpatients receiving services from the facility.

- Attempt to collect cash from patients according to the healthcare organization's policies.

- Initiate billing to either the patient and/or the third-party guarantor.

- Conduct follow-up billing on unpaid accounts.

- Prepare uncollectible accounts for referral to outside collection agents, and maintain a control file for these accounts.

- Serve as the patient's own healthcare organization representative and advisor on all issues concerning the patient's account receivable while he or she is in the facility and until the account is totally settled.

- Obtain a firm commitment from the patient or responsible party before or at discharge concerning the payment method and schedule for paying the account in full.

- Work with the patient, medical staff, and other healthcare organization personnel to assure prompt and full payment of the account receivable.

- Serve as the facility's goodwill ambassador and counselor to the patient and the community to enhance its image.

Some of the qualifications for this position might include the following:

- Education: high school graduate

- Experience: six months to one year

- Technical skills: ability to type at least forty words per minute and use calculator, telephone, word processor, and data entry terminal

- Personality traits: ability to meet and communicate with people easily; self-starter who can adjust quickly from one task to another; ability to keep information confidential

Job Description

Job analysis is the first step in writing a job description and developing performance standards (see chapter 5). The typical job description contains fourteen key pieces of information:

1. name of healthcare organization

2. job title

3. department

4. immediate supervisor

5. job code number

6. chart of accounts number

7. job or labor grade

8. primary job function

9. specific job functions

10. job qualifications

11. performance standards

12. date job description was written or revised

13. name and title of officer approving job description

14. date of approval

Figure 1–4 is an example of a job description format. This format is unique because it requires that each identified task have a performance standard. In this case, *performance standard* means that the employee must complete a certain number of activities properly and within a preestablished time period.

FIGURE 1–4

Sample Job Description Form

MEMORIAL MEDICAL CENTER
ANYTOWN, U.S.A.

JOB DESCRIPTION

Job Title _____ Job Code Number _____

Department _____ Job or Labor Grade _____

Immediate Supervisor _____ Chart of Accounts Number _____

Primary Function:

Specific Functions   Performance Standards

1.   1.

2.   2.

3.   3.

4.   4.

5.   5.

6.   6.

Job Qualifications

Education:

Experience:

Technical Skills:

Personality Traits:

Date Written/Revised: _____ 19 _____

Date Approved: _____ 19 _____

Approved by: _____ Title _____

A job description serves three purposes:

1. It assists managers or supervisors in identifying the basis or common ground upon which employees' performance can be evaluated.

2. It serves as a basis for evaluating the qualifications of prospective employees.

3. It assists employees in evaluating their own performance.

Job descriptions must be reviewed and approved by the appropriate supervisor. They should not be considered permanent but should be reviewed constantly to assure managers that they have delegated work appropriately according to the needs of the healthcare facility and the systems and procedures that management established. It is especially important for managers to review and evaluate performance standards continually. Each time the supervisor reviews and adjusts the job description, the approval date must be so noted.

Summary

The management planning process applied to the organization of the patient financial services department of a healthcare facility requires a considerable amount of patient financial services managers' time, forethought, and examination. As with any application of the management planning process, the managers must

- identify the mission and related goals and objectives;

- plan strategy to meet these goals and objectives;

- identify resources required to accomplish these goals and objectives;

- establish departmental and employee performance standards before operations begin;

- assign responsibility to monitor and evaluate actual performance in terms of established performance standards; and

- establish a feedback system and assign responsibility for taking corrective measures.

There is no single most effective management style to use; the approach that fits one manager's comfort level could be disastrous for another. To be effective, patient financial services managers should use the management planning approach and style that is the most comfortable and practicable for them.

NOTES

1. Harold Koontz and Heinz Weihrich, *Essentials of Management,* 5th ed. (New York: McGraw-Hill Book Company, 1990), 4.

2. Douglas McGregor, *The Human Side of Enterprise,* 25th anniversary ed. (New York: McGraw-Hill Book Company, 1985), 33–34.

3. McGregor, *The Human Side of Enterprise,* 47–48.

4. William G. Ouchi, *Theory Z: How American Business Can Meet the Japanese Challenge* (Reading, Mass.: Addison-Wesley Publishing Co., 1981), 43.

5. *Merriam Webster's Collegiate Dictionary, Tenth Edition* (Springfield, Mass.: Merriam-Webster Inc., 1993).

6. *Merriam Webster's Collegiate Dictionary, Tenth Edition.*

7. Allen G. Herkimer Jr., *Understanding Hospital Financial Management,* 2nd ed. (Rockville, Md.: Aspen Publishers, Inc., 1986), 29.

8. *Merriam Webster's Collegiate Dictionary, Tenth Edition.*

9. *Merriam Webster's Collegiate Dictionary, Tenth Edition.*

10. Koontz and Weihrich, *Essentials of Management,* 187.

11. Dale D. McConkey, *No-Nonsense Delegation,* rev. ed. (New York: AMACOM Division, American Management Association, 1986), 33–43.

CHAPTER 2

Standard Plans and Their Use

Patient financial services managers cannot manage well without clearly written, definitive standard plans governing each departmental function. The standard plan's distinctive characteristic is that it permits managers to reuse effective decisions and actions; the plan establishes a continuing pattern for dealing with everyday situations, thus enabling managers and their staffs to devote more time to unusual or difficult situations and to any procedural changes they wish to implement.

Standard plans can be divided into three major categories:

1. policies

2. procedures

3. methods

We will be examining these categories in detail to determine their use and benefits in the patient financial services department. Organizational structure, too, is a standard plan inasmuch as its assignment of tasks and the relationships established provide a continuing frame of reference to guide patient financial services managers and their staffs in their daily activities.

Policies

A *policy* provides a general plan of action that guides a healthcare facility's employees in their conduct and daily operations. The facility's governing board has the task of approving policies, while the organization's chief executive officer, chief financial officer, and patient financial services manager are in charge of implementing them. Management should review policies periodically to verify that each policy remains current and that the position or function to which a policy applies has not been altered or eliminated.

Within each policy's guidelines, managers must develop a procedure for the function it governs. Recognizing the difference between a policy and a procedure is important; a policy must be explicit in stating the healthcare organization's position regarding the function to which it refers. For example, management could formulate a collection policy based upon the following questions:

- Will the organization use a preadmission system?
- Will the organization require prepayment at admission?
- When and how is the patient's ability to pay established?
- When does the patient financial services department make the primary collection effort?
- When does the organization expect payment in full?
- Will the organization charge interest on unpaid balances?
- When is an account considered delinquent?
- When is an account considered uncollectible?
- When is an account referred to an outside collection agent?
- Will the organization permit the use of liens, attorneys, small-claims court, etc.?
- Will the organization give cash discounts?
- When is an account classified as a bad debt?

The answer to these and any other related questions should determine the healthcare organization's collection policy; the policy needs to be approved by the governing board before it is circulated to appropriate persons and implemented by the patient financial services manager and staff.

Although most policies require formal approval by the healthcare organization's governing board, the genesis of most policies generally originates from the facility's administrative staff. For example, assume that the patient financial services manager believes that the facility's policy for bad debts is inappropriate and ineffectual. This manager is therefore responsible for drafting a proposed revised policy for presentation at the next governing board meeting. Further, if a new policy would assist the organization in collecting its monies, the patient financial services manager is in charge of

- identifying the need for a new policy;
- drafting a proposed policy;
- reviewing the policy draft with the immediate supervisor, gaining his/her support; and
- soliciting support from the chief executive officer so that the proposed policy can be placed on the governing board's meeting agenda.

The important issue here is not who approves policies. The real question is, Who is responsible for recognizing ineffective policies and drafting others for handling the healthcare facility's patient accounts receivable? If any situation inhibits the prompt and efficient collection of the healthcare facility's cash, then it is the patient financial services manager's responsibility to implement corrective measures.

Procedures

Effective managers give appropriate and equal consideration to policies, procedures, and methods; distinguishing among them is necessary to the delegation process. In common usage, *procedure* and *method* are frequently used interchangeably. However, for this review, *procedure* will imply a method of carrying out activities; a set of instructions that reflects the organization's values and channels conduct to achieve the organization's purposes.[1] *Method*, on the other hand, will mean an orderly, logical, effective arrangement, usually in steps; the means taken in achieving an end.[2]

A standard procedure should ensure that appropriate, complete information flows to the appropriate individuals needing the data and that all people involved in the process understand what they are individually responsible for. When employees come to follow a standard procedure's regular order of steps as routine, the task of management is significantly simplified.

Written procedures usually follow one of two forms:

1. step-by-step narration

2. flowchart

Here is a sample step-by-step narration of a healthcare facility's preadmitting procedure.

Step 1. Physician's office notifies admitting office of pending admission.

Step 2. Preadmitting clerk obtains name, address, and telephone number of patient; also obtains admitting diagnosis.

Step 3. Preadmitting clerk telephones patient; obtains complete and accurate demographic and financial information.

Step 4. Preadmitting clerk (or insurance verifier) contacts payment guarantor to verify amount of insurance coverage.

Step 5. After verifying coverage, clerk telephones patient again. If insurance coverage is inadequate, clerk informs patient of healthcare facility's requirements for advance payment, or payment in full by discharge.

Step 6. Preadmitting clerk informs patient of time he or she is expected in admitting office.

The facility's management determined its policy governing the preadmitting procedure from answering questions arising from a collection policy and from questions that management resolved before drawing up an admitting policy. This step-by-step narrative procedure can be illustrated on a flow-chart, as depicted in figure 2–1.

Many procedures require transferring information to various persons or departments in written form. Whenever this is necessary, the design of the standard forms that will be used becomes an important part of the procedure. User confusion can be reduced if forms are uniform in size, with clearly defined lines and spaces for recording essential information. Properly de-signed forms facilitate accurate recording of information, permit rapid use

FIGURE 2–1

Flowchart of Preadmission Procedure

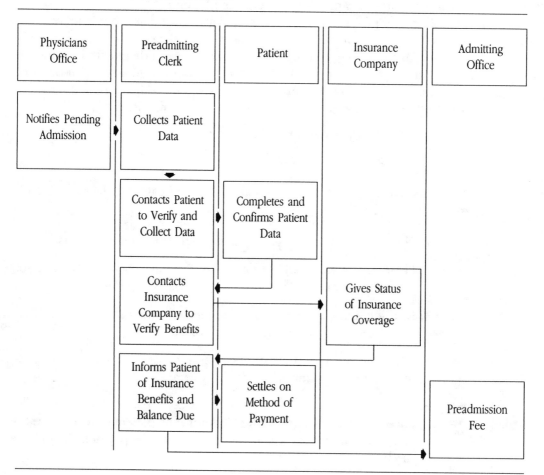

FIGURE 2–2
Example of a Color-coded Cash Receipt

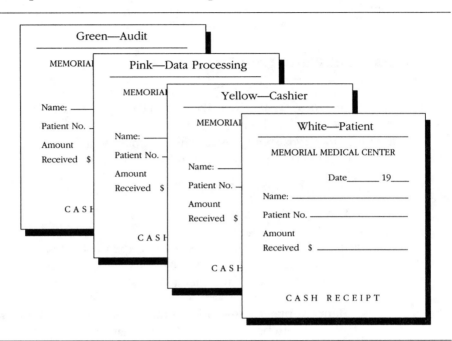

and verification, and standardize the record storage requirements. Color coding a multipart form helps to assure that all designated users will receive the correct copy. Figure 2–2 shows how four different colors can identify where each copy of a cash receipt is to be distributed.

Methods

A method differs from a procedure in that it deals with only one operation. Defining one specific method for use assumes that there is only one most efficient routine for a particular job or situation; managers must rely on testing and experience before determining the best method. Patient financial services managers are responsible for training their personnel and maintaining standard operating conditions within their department; within these conditions, they expect every employee to perform according to an approved method.

Standard methods contribute to the department's efficiency and to the maintenance of the desired level of work quality. Standard methods may be detailed or general to allow management to adjust for existing conditions.

A method patient financial services managers could specify for use in the preadmitting procedure might be a prepared set of questions and responses; another might be a prepared "script" for talking with discharged patients who are delinquent in payments. Standard methods that have been tested for effectiveness and that result in these procedures can assure collection of the complete, accurate data that the function demands.

Standard Plans' Benefits

The three types of standard plans—policies, procedures, and methods—guide patient financial services managers and their staffs in uniformly implementing and consistently maintaining departmental functions. Managers' development and use of these standards provoke some practical questions:

- When should they be used?

- How specific and detailed should they be?

The answers to these questions become apparent when the patient financial services managers recognize the benefits of using written standard operating policies, procedures, and methods:

- Standard plans result in less time spent in crisis management; decision making becomes virtually automatic.

- Standard plans facilitate the maintenance of performance and work quality because, theoretically, the patient financial services manager has identified the one most efficient method.

- Standard plans, together with a well-designed organizational structure, facilitate the delegation of authority and responsibility.

- Standard plans are the basis of patient financial services managers' evaluation of performance by an individual, a group, a system, or a subsystem in the department.

- Standard plans ensure that employees will conduct interdepartmental and intradepartmental activities consistently and efficiently.

The Department Operating Manual

After patient financial services managers have developed their department's standard plans, they need to complete one simple, yet critical task: organize all departmental policies, procedures, methods, forms, and other related documents into an operating manual that is readily accessible to all department personnel. A loose-leaf notebook is generally the best manual type because managers can update its contents easily.

The manual should contain, but not be limited to, the following eight sections:

1. institutional policies relating to patient financial services department operations

2. departmental operating policies

3. departmental operating procedures accompanied by illustrative flow-charts

4. patient financial services organizational chart

5. departmental job descriptions

6. budget forms and reports

7. billing and collection forms and related procedures

8. admitting and discharge policies and procedures

This manual should serve as a training device as well as a reference source. If at all feasible, all department employees should have their own copy of the manual to enhance continuity in the department's operations.

NOTES

1. David R. Hampton, *Management,* 3rd ed. (New York: McGraw-Hill Book Company, 1986), 198, 200.
2. *Merriam Webster's Collegiate Dictionary, Tenth Edition* (Springfield, Mass.: Merriam-Webster Inc., 1993).

CHAPTER 3

The Healthcare Accounting Process

The healthcare organization's chief financial officer and accounting staff are responsible for the quality and integrity of the financial and statistical information that the facility generates. The proper interpretation of this information, however, is the responsibility of patient financial services managers. This chapter will acquaint these managers with the basic concepts and principles of healthcare accounting for a better understanding of key financial reports and their generation. The chapter ends with a discussion of managed-care contracting, a potential liability account; and recent changes in financial reporting requirements issued by the American Institute of Certified Public Accountants.

Principles of Accounting

Seawell states that, unlike the natural laws governing the physical sciences, accounting's basic concepts and principles—which are sometimes called postulates, rules, conventions, or standards—are the result of a continuing evolutionary process, and are therefore subject to periodic reevaluation and possible change. These concepts and principles can be modified or even discarded in response to changes in economic or social conditions, technology, methods of conducting economic activity, or user demands for more serviceable information. According to Seawell, this absence of absolute permanency is not entirely undesirable. Describing accounting as an art, not a science, he points out that it must change as its environment and the needs of its users change.[1]

Healthcare accounting is based on three fundamental principles:

1. double-entry accounting

2. accrual accounting

3. fund accounting

One of these principles, fund accounting, seems to be used less now than previously, especially in the taxable healthcare organizations.

Double-Entry Accounting

The underlying theory of double-entry accounting is that the recording of every transaction requires a minimum of two entries or changes in the accounting records—hence, the name, *double entry*. The basic principle of double-entry accounting is that for every debit there must be an equal and offsetting credit.

Debit and *credit* (abbreviated as Dr. and Cr., respectively, derived from their Latin word equivalents) are the terms used to distinguish one side of the double entry from the other. Debits are recorded on the left side of the ledger, while credits are recorded on the right side, as illustrated in the T-account format below:

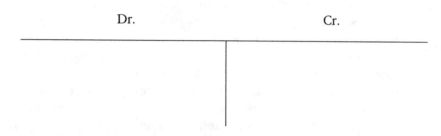

Named for its shape, the T account serves as the substitute for a formal ledger account. The informal tool appears on analysis sheets to assist the accountant in analyzing a transaction.[2]

Table 3–1 shows the basic principles for using debits and credits in key accounts. The important fact to remember is that there must be equal and offsetting debits and credits in every accounting transaction. This does not mean that the accountant can make only one debit and only one credit at a time; it does mean, however, that the debits' total dollar amount must equal the credits' total amount.

The two basic types of accounting entries or transactions are (1) single, and (2) compound. The single entry records transactions in only two accounts. For example, the accountant makes one debit entry and one credit entry in the journal, listing the debit first and indenting the credit:

Description	Account Number	Dr.	Cr.
Cash	100.0	$1,000	
Accounts Receivable	110.0		$1,000

To record cash received on accounts receivable from the cash receipts journal.

TABLE 3–1

Double-Entry Accounting Impact Matrix

Account Description	Debt Impact	Credit Impact
Asset	Increases Value	Decreases Value
Liability	Decreases Payable	Increases Payable
Capital or Equity	Decreases Worth	Increases Worth
Revenue	Decreases Income	Increases Income
Expense	Increases Costs	Decreases Costs

In T accounts, these entries would appear as follows:

100.0 Cash		110.0 Accounts Receivable	
$1,000			$1,000

The compound entry records transactions in more than two accounts, but the total dollar debits equal the total dollar credits, as illustrated below:

Description	Account Number	Dr.	Cr.
Accounts Receivable 110.0		$1,000	
Nursing Revenue 451.0			$600
Surgery Revenue 452.0			150
Laboratory Revenue 453.0			100
Radiology Revenue 454.0			100
Pharmacy Revenue 455.0			50

To record revenues generated from accounts receivable to the revenue journal.

These entries would appear in T accounts as follows:

110.0 Accounts Receivable		451.0 Nursing Revenue	
$1,000			$600

452.0 Surgery Revenue		453.0 Laboratory Revenue	
	$150		$100

454.0 Radiology Revenue		455.0 Pharmacy Revenue	
	$100		$50

These examples illustrate the use of double-entry accounting in the health-care accounting process. It is important to note that in both the single and compound transactions, debits always equal credits.

Accrual Accounting

The accrual concept of accounting requires that revenues, expenses, and other related transactions be recognized and recorded as they are incurred, regardless of the related cash flow. The accrual concept is exactly the opposite of the cash concept of accounting, under which revenues and expenses are recognized and recorded only when the cash is actually received or disbursed.

In the past, the healthcare organization typically used cash accounting, although the method does not accurately report the organization's true financial condition. In the cash accounting system, the accountant does not record revenues until the facility receives cash from the patient; therefore, revenues for a given accounting period may be overstated or understated. Similarly, the organization may not have enough cash to pay current obligations, so the accountant does not record expenses represented by the unpaid vendor invoices. As a result, operating expenses for the accounting period may be understated. Conversely, if all vendors are paid up-to-date, expenses could be overstated.

When the healthcare organization uses the cash accounting system, its statement of operations might report a break-even financial condition (see table 3–2) when the organization is actually operating at a loss because it is indebted to vendors and a considerable amount of accounts receivable are uncollected. In this case, the statement of operations would be more accurately described as a cash flow statement (see table 3–3).

The two missing elements or accounts in the cash accounting system are (1) accounts receivable, and (2) accounts payable. Incorporating these primary accounts into the accounting system in effect turns it into an accrual

TABLE 3–2

Statement of Operations Using the Cash Accounting Method

Memorial Medical Center
Anytown, U.S.A.

STATEMENT OF OPERATIONS

For the Three-Month Period Ending September 30, 19x1

This Month		Year to Date
$100,000	Revenue	$300,000
99,000	Less: Expense	299,000
$ 1,000	Profit (Loss)	$ 1,000

TABLE 3–3

Cash Flow Statement

Memorial Medical Center
Anytown, U.S.A.

CASH FLOW STATEMENT

For the Three-Month Period Ending September 30, 19x1

This Month		Year to Date
$100,000	Cash Received	$300,000
99,000	Less: Cash Disbursed	299,000
$ 1,000	Cash on Hand	$ 1,000

accounting system: revenues and expenses are recognized and recorded during the accounting period in which they are earned or incurred.

To illustrate the month's transactions in tables 3–2 and 3–3 using the accrual accounting system, the following account entries are made:

Journal Entry Number	Description	Account Number	Dr.	Cr.
1	Cash	100.0	$100,000	
	Accounts Receivable	110.0		$100,000

To record cash received on patient accounts receivable during the month from the cash receipts journal.

Journal Entry Number	Description	Account Number	Dr.	Cr.
2	Accounts Payable	210.0	$ 99,000	
	Cash	100.0		$ 99,000

To record cash disbursed on accounts payable during the month from the cash disbursements journal.

Journal Entry Number	Description	Account Number	Dr.	Cr.
3	Accounts Receivable	110.0	$150,000	
	Revenue	400.0		$150,000

To record revenue charged during the month from the revenue journal.

Journal Entry Number	Description	Account Number	Dr.	Cr.
4	Expenses	500.0	$125,000	
	Accounts Payable	210.0		$125,000

To record expenses incurred during the month from the purchase journal.

The T-account entries would appear as follows:

100.0 Cash	
(1) $100,000	(2) $99,000
Balance $1,000	

110.0 Accounts Receivable	
(3) $150,000	(1) $100,000
Balance $50,000	

210.0 Accounts Payable	
(2) $99,000	(4) $125,000
	Balance $26,000

400.0 Revenue	
	(3) $150,000
	Balance $150,000

500.0 Expenses	
(4) $125,000	
Balance $125,000	

To illustrate further the impact of the difference between the cash and accrual accounting systems, table 3–4 provides a comparative analysis of the month's activity. The supplemental information given in this table is usually reported in the organization's statement of condition, which is sometimes called a balance sheet.

TABLE 3–4

Comparative Analysis of Cash and Accrual Methods

Memorial Medical Center
Anytown, U.S.A.

STATEMENT OF OPERATIONS
For the Three-Month Period Ending September 30, 19x1

	Cash Method	**Accrual Method**
Revenue	$100,000	$150,000
Expense	99,000	125,000
Profit (Loss)	$ 1,000	$ 25,000
Supplemental Information		
Cash	$ 1,000	$ 1,000
Accounts Receivable	Not Recorded	50,000
Accounts Payable	Not Recorded	(26,000)
Total	$ 1,000	$ 25,000

The matching of revenue and expense is an integral function of the accrual accounting system. Not only must revenues and expenses associated with a specific accounting period be reported together, but deductions from gross revenue, such as contractual allowances, policy discounts, and other adjustments to generated revenues, must also be reported together to assure a true matching of revenues and expenses.

Fund Accounting

Fund accounting distinguishes traditional healthcare accounting from the accounting systems used in most other businesses. When the American Hospital Association originally recommended fund accounting in its publication *Chart of Accounts for Hospitals,* many healthcare organizations were receiving substantial amounts of money in the form of donations, grants, and other restricted monies. Therefore, it was imperative that healthcare organizations record and manage these funds in compliance with their individual legal and fiduciary restrictions. Hence, most of these organizations came to use fund accounting, especially the nontaxable facilities.

The principle of fund accounting requires that each fund be segregated into independent, "self-balancing" groups of accounts. In addition, each fund must have its own balance sheet accounts; that is, assets, liabilities, and fund balance. These funds are divided into two major groups: (1) unrestricted, and

(2) restricted. The unrestricted fund has no external restrictions on its use and purpose; the organization can use it for any purpose chosen by the governing board and/or administration. Restricted-fund donors limit the money's use to specific purposes. In some cases, such as endowment funds, the original donation is restricted, but its investment income can be used for operations or other purposes.

Healthcare organizations typically divide both the restricted and unrestricted fund categories into three parts, as follows:

- unrestricted fund

    1. current operating accounts

    2. board-designated accounts

    3. plant asset and related debt accounts

- restricted funds

    1. specific-purpose funds

    2. plant replacement and expansion funds

    3. endowment funds

Note the use of the singular and plural in the above outline. Although healthcare organizations frequently divide the unrestricted fund into three parts, Seawell stresses that these account divisions are for accounting purposes; for financial reporting purposes, the unrestricted fund must be viewed as a single fund. On the other hand, the restricted category generally contains several different funds, each of them a distinctive entity that the healthcare oganization must account for and report separately.[3]

Accounting procedures for funds can become complex because of the "due to" and "due from" accounts necessary to assure that each fund is always in balance. Another problem encountered in fund accounting is that the resulting financial statements may be misleading to the user. The user who does not look at all of a healthcare organization's statements of condition is aware of only part of the facility's total assets and liabilities. Therefore, it is imperative that the accountant report the facility's financial condition in a consolidated statement of condition similar to the one shown in exhibit 3–1.

Despite its usefulness in internal record keeping and managerial control,[4] is fund accounting necessary in the healthcare industry? While acknowledging that certain circumstances may require detailed records and reports for special purposes, the Principles and Practices Board of the Healthcare Financial Management Association recommends that institutional healthcare activities be reported in a manner comparable with other businesses; that is, all assets, liabilities, and equity should be presented in a single aggregated

EXHIBIT 3–1
Consolidated Statement of Condition

Memorial Medical Center
Anytown, U.S.A.

CONSOLIDATED STATEMENT OF CONDITION
As of September 30, 19x1

	Total	Operating Fund	Specific-Purpose Fund	Endowment Fund	Plant Fund
Assets					
Current Assets	$ xxx	$ xxx	$ xxx	$ xxx	$ xxx
Fixed Assets	xxx	xxx	xxx	xxx	xxx
Total Assets	$ xxx	$ xxx	$ xxx	$ xxx	$ xxx
Liabilities and Capital					
Current Liabilities	$ xxx	$ xxx	$ xxx	$ xxx	$ xxx
Fixed Liabilities	xxx	xxx	xxx	xxx	xxx
Total Liabilities	$ xxx	$ xxx	$ xxx	$ xxx	$ xxx
Capital	xxx	xxx	xxx	xxx	xxx
Total Liabilities and Capital	$ xxx	$ xxx	$ xxx	$ xxx	$ xxx

balance sheet without differentiation by fund. Single-fund reporting, it stresses, would reduce the diversity of practice and inconsistency in financial reporting among institutional healthcare providers.[5] The American Institute of Certified Public Accountants is another organization that has raised the question of the necessity of fund accounting.[6]

Prerequisites of an Accounting System

Certain key management tools are prerequisites for an accounting system's successful operation:

- organizational structure
- chart of accounts
- documented proof
- journals and ledgers

Organizational Structure

An effective organization is composed of a group of individuals who cooperate successfully to achieve a common objective.[7] In building an effective management team, one must consider

- the organizational structure, that is, the grouping of functions that most effectively promotes cooperation and determination of the optimal relationship among those groups;

- the proper delegation of responsibility and authority to all managers and supervisors; and

- the selection of the right people for every job.

The final test of the effectiveness of an organizational structure is its ability to

- provide the services required of it,

- provide those services at minimal cost without sacrificing quality, and

- develop competent personnel.

The organizational structure (chart) puts all of these factors together in a formal, easily understood format that identifies

- major operational functions, departments, or responsibility centers,

- lines of authority and communication, and

- delegation of responsibility.

In addition, the organizational structure serves as the basis for identifying and assigning departmental account numbers from the healthcare organization's chart of accounts; it also lays the groundwork for the organization's accounting and management control system.

The organizational structure approach assumes that the individual assigned to each responsibility center as department manager is responsible for the center's revenues, if any, and expenses. Accordingly, this person is authorized to manage the unit and its related functions and is held accountable for its total operations. This concept is called responsibility accounting, and it is the keystone of effective healthcare management.[8]

Chart of Accounts

Chart of Accounts for Hospitals, originally produced by the American Hospital Association and acquired in 1990 by the Healthcare Financial Management Association, defines the chart of accounts as a list of account titles (with numerical coding) designed for the compilation of financial data concerning an enterprise's assets, liabilities, equity, revenues, expenses, gains, and losses. Because the chart of accounts should accumulate information that is as useful as possible for managerial planning and control, classification of the healthcare organization's revenues and expenses in the chart of accounts should correspond to the division of authority and responsibility shown in the facility's organizational chart.[9]

Although the chart of accounts is designed primarily for management's informational needs, the requirements of investors, creditors, third-party payers, donors, taxing and regulatory agencies, oversight bodies, and other external parties may influence its design. In addition, because no two healthcare organizations are organized in precisely the same manner, no two organizations will employ identical charts of accounts unless mandated by state or federal statutes.[10]

Figure 3–1 shows how an organizational chart and a chart of accounts may be linked by expanding the traditional organizational design shown in figure 1–1 and using the *Chart of Accounts* numerical coding system for fiscal and administrative services.[11] Please keep in mind, however, that it is impossible to develop a chart of accounts that would meet all of the requirements of all healthcare organizations. For this reason, the use of the chart of accounts and the numerical coding system in this book is illustrative and representative, but it is not exhaustive.

Documented Proof

Before recording an accounting transaction, the accountant must have documented proof that supports this entry into the accounting system. Documented proof is necessary to protect the entry's integrity and to provide evidence for internal and external audits.

Many healthcare accounting experts have argued over what financial value should be entered in the healthcare organization's books of record, especially in the area of capital assets. Some experts advocate recording the replacement cost of capital assets, while others recommend using the amount paid for the asset plus operating expenses. Healthcare accounting authorities have established that the cost value concept is the most appropriate and reasonable financial value because it requires that something of value, that is, cash, be exchanged for an item or service before the transaction can be entered in the accounting system. Certainly, an important advantage of using the cost of an item or service as the financial value entered is that the accountant can obtain well-documented proof that the transaction actually occurred.

Journals and Ledgers

Seawell differentiates between accounting journals and ledgers in this manner:[12]

Journal: a "book of original entry" wherein transactions are recorded in chronological sequence.

Ledger: the groups of accounts used in recording the healthcare organization's transactions—a book of secondary entry.

FIGURE 3–1
Organizational Chart

Memorial Medical Center
Anytown, U.S.A.

ORGANIZATIONAL STRUCTURE

Fiscal and Administrative Services

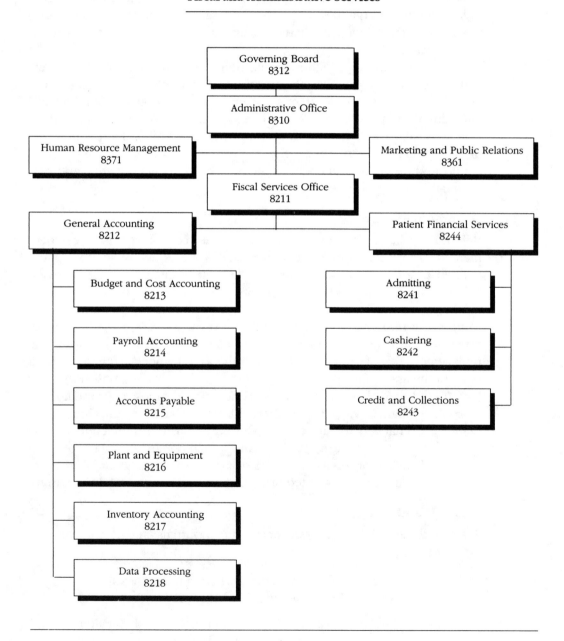

The healthcare organization's journal system might include such journals as the following:

- general journal
- cash receipts
- cash disbursements
- purchase
- revenue

Whereas journals are "books of original entry," ledgers are support documents that can include the accumulated financial activity in the following areas:

- general ledger
- patient accounts receivable
- plant equipment and depreciation
- payroll
- inventory
- accounts payable

Before electronic data processing, accountants maintained healthcare organizations' accounting journals manually on columnar paper sheets bound together in "post binders." They maintained ledgers using hard sheets of paper that they stored in filing trays. With the advent of automated data processing, journals and ledgers are printed and maintained by computer and stored according to the user's needs.

The Accounting Process

The accounting process consists of the systems and procedures required for recording and maintaining the accounting transactions during an accounting period—usually not shorter than one month nor longer than one year. Most healthcare organizations end each accounting period at the end of each month and develop annual statements based upon the operations of twelve months. An annual accounting period, usually called a fiscal year, need not begin on January 1 and end on December 31. Furthermore, there is an accounting system that divides a year into thirteen four-week accounting periods. This system eliminates the need to adjust accrual journal entries (for example: payroll) for the odd number of days in a month.

As illustrated in figure 3–2, the accounting process begins with the accountant gathering source documentation for services rendered to patients, services or items purchased for the organization, and cash received or disbursed by the organization. The process ends with the development of four principal financial statements:

1. statement of condition
2. statement of operations
3. cash flow statement
4. statement of changes in financial position

The accountant generates these financial statements from the general ledger, which is a consolidation of all the information contained in the journals.

In the accounting process, each asset, liability, equity, revenue, and expense account in the organization's chart of accounts has a separate journal card or record on which the accountant identifies each debit and credit transaction affecting both the account and the account balance. Together, all of these journal accounts are referred to as the healthcare facility's general ledger.

Statement of Condition

The statement of condition, which is occasionally referred to as the balance sheet, shows the financial position—that is, assets, liabilities, and equity—of the healthcare organization at a specific time; namely, when the accounting records are closed at the end of the accounting period. The healthcare organization's financial position will change as soon as the facility incurs an additional expense, such as wages or supplies, or renders a service through a revenue department. The formula for the balance sheet is

$$Assets = Liabilities + Equity$$

The healthcare organization's *equity* is the difference between the facility's total assets and its total liabilities. *Equity* has many synonyms, such as the following:

-   capital
-   net worth
-   surplus
-   retained earnings
-   fund balance

In reality, equity, or any other term used in its place, represents the organization's net assets, computed as follows:

$$Assets - Liabilities = Equity$$

FIGURE 3–2
The Accounting Process

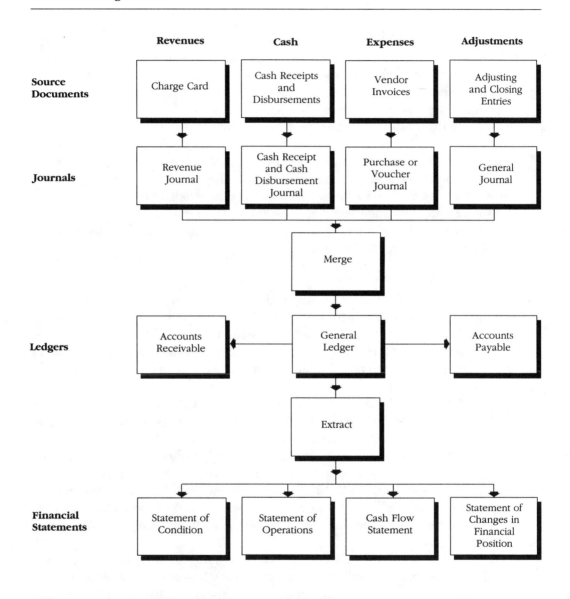

Statement of Operations

The statement of operations, also known as the income statement or profit and loss (P&L) statement, reports all of the facility's operating and non-operating revenue as well as the expenses it has incurred during the accounting period; the statement also shows the net profit (or loss) for the accounting or operating period. The formulas for the statement of operations are

Revenue = Expense + Profit (or Loss)

Profit (or Loss) = Revenue – Expenses

Time is the basic distinction between the statement of condition and the statement of operations. The statement of condition represents the healthcare organization's financial position or condition at one *specific* point in time; the statement of operations reflects the results of revenue and expense transactions over a *period* of time.

In this book, the author prefers the term *statement of condition* to *balance sheet* because the former term more accurately describes what the statement really is: the presentation of the healthcare organization's financial position at one *specific* point in time. Also, the author prefers the term *statement of operations* to *income and expense statement* because the first term more accurately indicates the actual information the statement contains: the net results, that is, revenue and expense and profit or loss, of the facility's operations over a *period* of time.

Cash Flow Statement

The *cash flow statement* is a supplemental or analytical statement that identifies actual and/or projected cash receipts (inflows) and cash disbursements (outflows) for a period of time. The cash flow statement can be developed for any period of time that management desires. For example, the organization's accounting staff can report cash flow on a daily, weekly, monthly, annual, or long-range basis.

Exhibit 3–2 is an example of a combination daily/monthly cash report. It starts with a beginning cash balance, which represents the cash on hand at the beginning of the period, and ends with the cash balance as of the day of the report. Tables 3–5 and 3–6 illustrate cash flow projections for a one-year period and a four-year period, respectively, based on income and expense summaries in tables 3–7 and 3–8. The one-year cash flow projection reports cash on a monthly basis, while the four-year cash flow forecast shows cash by quarter during the first year and in total annual amounts for the subsequent years.

It is imperative for a healthcare organization's financial viability not only for the accounting staff to maintain daily and monthly cash flow reports, but also for it to develop and maintain a long-range cash report; that is, one that shows cash flow projections for one to three years. These reports are especially essential because of all the changing payment regulations imposed by third-party payers such as Medicare, Medicaid, and managed-care contracts.

Patient financial services managers should play a key role in the cash flow reporting and analysis process because accounts receivable is the largest single source of cash flow from healthcare operations. In addition, these managers should participate in the process to give the cash flow analysis

EXHIBIT 3–2
Daily Cash Flow Analysis Form

Memorial Medical Center
Anytown, U.S.A.

DAILY CASH FLOW ANALYSIS

For the Month of _____ **19__**

Date:_____ 19__

	Today	Month to Date Actual	Budgeted
Beginning Cash Balance	$ _____	$ _____	$ _____
Cash Inflows			
Accounts Receivable	$ _____	$ _____	$ _____
Borrowings	_____	_____	_____
Other (Specify) _____			
	_____	_____	_____
Total Cash Inflows	$ _____	$ _____	$ _____
Total Cash on Hand	$ _____	$ _____	$ _____
Cash Outflows			
Payroll	$ _____	$ _____	$ _____
Accounts Payable	_____	_____	_____
Long-Term Liabilities	_____	_____	_____
Other (Specify) _____			
	_____	_____	_____
Total Cash Outflows	$ _____	$ _____	$ _____
Ending Cash Balance	$ _____	$ _____	$ _____

greater creditability and to ensure their self-development and professional survival.

Statement of Changes in Financial Position

The *statement of changes in financial position* is a comprehensive financial statement that identifies all the changes that have occurred from one balance sheet period to the next. This statement is sometimes referred to as the statement of sources and application of funds; differences in liability accounts reflect the sources of funds, and changes in asset values are classified as applications of funds. The statement of changes in financial position in table 3–9 was developed using the two statement of condition period changes as reported in the comparative statement of condition in table 3–10. Table 3–9's statement includes a subsection entitled "Changes in Working Capital" totaling $25,000, which is tied into the Funds Applied section.

TABLE 3–5
One-Year Cash Flow Projection

Memorial Medical Center
Anytown, U.S.A.

	Year One												
	1 Sept.	2 Oct.	3 Nov.	4 Dec.	5 Jan.	6 Feb.	7 Mar.	8 Apr.	9 May	10 June	11 July	12 Aug.	Total
Beginning Cash Balance	$ -0-	$ 23	$ 838	$ 653	$ 844	$ 473	$ 102	$ 775	$ 10	$ 41	$ 217	$ 166	$ -0-
Cash Inflows													
Accounts Receivable	$ -0-	$ -0-	$ -0-	$ -0-	$ -0-	$ -0-	$ 3,534	$ 7,980	$14,136	$17,100	$24,738	$30,780	$ 98,268
Borrowings/Investments	12,000	75,000	18,000	27,000	36,000	29,000	27,000	30,000	33,000	29,000	22,000	28,000	366,000
Total Cash Inflows	$12,000	$75,000	$18,000	$27,000	$36,000	$29,000	$30,534	$37,980	$47,136	$46,100	$46,738	$58,780	$464,268
Cash on Hand	$12,000	$75,023	$18,838	$27,653	$36,844	$29,473	$30,636	$38,755	$47,146	$46,141	$46,955	$58,946	$464,268
Cash Outflows													
Corporate Payroll and Benefits	$11,977	$17,185	$17,185	$17,185	$18,747	$18,747	$18,747	$18,747	$18,747	$24,476	$24,476	$27,288	$233,507
Unit Payroll and Benefits	-0-	-0-	-0-	7,874	7,874	7,874	7,874	15,748	15,748	15,748	15,748	23,622	118,110
Physicians	-0-	-0-	-0-	750	750	750	1,240	2,250	2,610	2,700	3,565	4,780	19,395
Corporate Accounts Payable	-0-	57,000	1,000	1,000	1,000	1,000	1,000	1,000	1,000	1,000	1,000	1,000	67,000
Unit Accounts Payable	-0-	-0-	-0-	-0-	8,000	1,000	1,000	1,000	9,000	2,000	2,000	2,000	26,000
Total Cash Outflows	$11,977	$74,185	$18,185	$26,809	$36,371	$29,371	$29,861	$38,745	$47,105	$45,924	$46,789	$58,690	$464,012
Ending Cash Balance	$ 23	$ 838	$ 653	$ 844	$ 473	$ 102	$ 775	$ 10	$ 41	$ 217	$ 166	$ 256	$ 256

TABLE 3–6
Four-Year Cash Flow Forecast

Memorial Medical Center
Anytown, U.S.A.

	Year One				Total			
	1st Quarter	2nd Quarter	3rd Quarter	4th Quarter	Year One	Year Two	Year Three	Year Four
Beginning Cash Balance	$ –0–	$ 653	$ 26	$ 435	$ 813	$ 2,574	$ 19,161	$ 11,859
Cash Inflows								
Accounts Receivable	$ –0–	$ –0–	$ 25,650	$ 72,618	$ 98,268	$ 948,081	$2,168,394	$3,287,416
Borrowings/Investments	105,000	66,000	45,000	13,000	230,000	(475,000)	(1,500,000)	(1,340,000)
Total Cash Inflows	$ 105,000	$ 66,000	$ 70,650	$ 85,618	$ 328,268	$ 473,081	$ 668,394	$1,947,416
Cash on Hand	$ 105,000	$ 66,653	$ 70,676	$ 86,053	$ 329,081	$ 475,655	$ 687,555	$1,959,275
Cash Outflows								
Corporate Payroll and Benefits	$ 46,347	$ 54,679	$ 56,241	$ 76,240	$ 233,507	$ 388,494	$ 416,196	$ 416,196
Unit Payroll and Benefits	–0–							
Physicians	–0–							
Corporate Accounts Payable	58,000	3,000	3,000	3,000	67,000	12,000	57,500	58,000
Unit Accounts Payable	–0–	9,000	11,000	6,000	26,000	56,000	105,000	164,000
Investment Accounts	–0–	–0–	–0–	–0–	–0–	–0–	97,000	1,313,000
Total Cash Outflows	$ 104,347	$ 66,679	$ 70,241	$ 85,240	$ 326,507	$ 456,494	$ 675,696	$1,951,196
Ending Cash Balance	$ 653	$ 26	$ 435	$ 813	$ 2,574	$ 19,161	$ 11,859	$ 8,079

TABLE 3–7

One-Year Statement of Operations Summary

Memorial Medical Center
Anytown, U.S.A.

							Year One						
	1 Sept.	2 Oct.	3 Nov.	4 Dec.	5 Jan.	6 Feb.	7 Mar.	8 Apr.	9 May	10 June	11 July	12 Aug.	Total
Volume													
Calendar Days	30	31	30	31	31	28	31	30	31	30	31	31	365
Units	0	0	0	0	1	1	1	1	2	2	2	2	2
Beds	0	0	0	0	18	18	18	18	36	36	36	36	36
Capacity	0	0	0	0	558	504	558	540	1,116	1,080	1,116	1,116	6,030
Patient Days	0	0	0	0	62	140	248	300	434	540	713	806	3,243
Percent Occupancy	0	0	0	0	11.1	27.8	44.4	55.6	38.9	50.0	63.9	72.2	53.8
Revenue													
Gross Charges	$ -0-	$ -0-	$ -0-	$ -0-	$ 3,534	$ 7,980	$14,136	$17,100	$24,738	$30,780	$40,641	$45,942	$184,851
Expense													
Corporate													
Staff and Benefits	$11,977	$17,185	$17,185	$17,185	$18,747	$18,747	$18,747	$18,747	$18,747	$24,476	$24,476	$27,288	$233,507
Public Relations	55,000	-0-	-0-	-0-	-0-	-0-	-0-	-0-	-0-	-0-	-0-	-0-	55,000
Miscellaneous Expenses	2,000	1,000	1,000	1,000	1,000	1,000	1,000	1,000	1,000	1,000	1,000	1,000	13,000
Total Corporate Expenses	$68,977	$18,185	$18,185	$18,185	$19,747	$19,747	$19,747	$19,747	$19,747	$25,476	$25,476	$28,288	$301,507
Units													
Staff and Benefits	$ -0-	$ -0-	$ -0-	$ 7,874	$ 7,874	$ 7,874	$ 7,874	$15,748	$15,748	$15,748	$15,748	$23,622	$118,110
Physicians	-0-	-0-	-0-	750	750	750	1,240	2,250	2,610	2,700	3,565	4,780	19,395
Training and Travel	-0-	-0-	-0-	8,000	-0-	-0-	-0-	8,000	-0-	-0-	-0-	8,000	24,000
Miscellaneous Expenses	-0-	-0-	-0-	-0-	1,000	1,000	1,000	1,000	2,000	2,000	2,000	2,000	12,000
Total Units Expenses	$ -0-	$ -0-	$ -0-	$16,624	$ 9,624	$ 9,624	$10,114	$26,998	$20,358	$20,448	$21,313	$38,402	$173,505
Total Expense	$68,977	$18,185	$18,185	$34,809	$29,371	$29,371	$29,861	$46,745	$40,105	$45,924	$46,789	$66,690	$475,012
Profit (Loss)	($68,977)	($18,185)	($18,185)	($34,809)	($25,837)	($21,391)	($15,725)	($29,645)	($15,367)	($15,144)	($ 6,148)	($20,748)	($290,161)

TABLE 3–8

Four-Year Statement of Operations Summary

Memorial Medical Center
Anytown, U.S.A.

	Year One				Total			
	1st Quarter	2nd Quarter	3rd Quarter	4th Quarter	Year One	Year Two	Year Three	Year Four
Volume								
Calendar Days	91	90	92	92	365	365	365	365
Units	-0-	1	2	2	2	6	11	11
Beds	-0-	18	36	36	36	108	198	198
Capacity	-0-	1,062	2,214	3,312	6,030	29,610	56,448*	72,270*
Patient Days	-0-	202	982	2,059	3,243	20,043	41,824	59,193
Percent Occupancy	-0-	19.0	44.3	62.1	53.8	67.7	74.0	81.9
Revenue								
Gross Charges	$ -0-	$11,514	$ 55,974	$117,363	$184,851	$1,142,451	$2,383,968	$3,374,001
Expense								
Corporate								
Staff and Benefits	$ 46,347	$54,679	$ 56,241	$ 76,240	$233,507	$ 388,494	$ 416,196	$ 416,196
Public Relations	55,000	-0-	-0-	-0-	55,000	-0-	40,000	40,000
Miscellaneous Expenses	4,000	3,000	3,000	3,000	13,000	12,000	18,000	18,000
Total Corporate Expenses	$105,347	$57,679	$ 59,241	$ 79,240	$301,507	$ 400,494	$ 474,196	$ 474,196
Units								
Staff and Benefits	-0-	$23,622	$ 39,370	$ 55,118	$118,110	$ 456,692	$ 842,518	$1,039,368
Physicians	-0-	2,250	6,100	11,045	19,395	104,992	214,320	295,965
Training and Travel	-0-	8,000	8,000	8,000	24,000	32,000	32,000	32,000
Miscellaneous Expenses	-0-	2,000	4,000	6,000	12,000	51,000	103,000	132,000
Total Units Expenses	$ -0-	$35,872	$ 57,470	$ 80,163	$173,505	$ 644,684	$1,191,838	$1,499,333
Total Expense	$105,347	$93,551	$116,711	$159,403	$475,012	$1,045,178	$1,666,034	$1,973,529
Profit (Loss), before Taxes	($105,347)	($82,037)	($ 60,737)	($ 42,040)	($290,161)	$ 97,273	$ 717,934	$1,400,472
Percent of Profit to Revenue					(156.9)	8.5	30.1	41.5

*Capacity differs due to scheduling of unit openings

TABLE 3–9

Statement of Changes in Financial Position

Memorial Medical Center
Anytown, U.S.A.

STATEMENT OF CHANGES IN FINANCIAL POSITION
From December 31, 19x1 to December 31, 19x2

Funds Provided by	
Net Operating Profit	$240,000
Depreciation	100,000
Total Funds Provided from Operations	$340,000
Funds Applied to	
Purchase of Plant and Equipment	$250,000
Reduction of Mortgage Payable	65,000
Increase in Working Capital (see below)	25,000
Total Funds Applied	$340,000

Changes in Working Capital

Increases (Decreases) in Current Assets	
Patient Accounts Receivable	$120,000
Inventories	(5,000)
Prepaid Expenses	5,000
Net Increase in Current Assets	$120,000
Increases (Decreases) in Current Liabilities	
Accounts Payable	$ 10,000
Payroll Taxes Payable	(5,000)
Short-Term Notes Payable	90,000
Net Increase in Current Liabilities	$ 95,000
Increase in Working Capital	$ 25,000

TABLE 3–10

Comparative Statement of Condition

Memorial Medical Center
Anytown, U.S.A.

COMPARATIVE STATEMENT OF CONDITION
As of December 31, 19x1 and December 31, 19x2

	19x1	19x2	Increase (Decrease)
Assets			
Cash on Hand	$ 40,000	$ 40,000	$ –0–
Short-Term Investments	30,000	30,000	–0–
Net Patient Accounts Receivable	700,000	820,000	120,000
Inventories	50,00	45,000	(5,000)
Prepaid Expenses	25,000	30,000	5,000
Total Current Assets	$ 845,000	$ 965,000	$120,000
Land, Plant, and Equipment	6,000,000	6,250,000	250,000
Less: Accumulative Depreciation	1,250,000	1,350,000	100,000 (B)
Net Land, Plant, and Equipment	$4,750,000	$4,900,000	$150,000
Total Assets	$5,595,000	$5,865,000	$270,000
Liabilities			
Accounts Payable	$ 60,000	$ 70,000	$ 10,000
Payroll Taxes Payable	55,000	50,000	(5,000)
Short-Term Notes Payable	75,000	165,000	90,000
Total Current Liabilities	$ 190,000	$ 285,000	$ 95,000
Mortgage Payable	3,510,000	3,445,000	(65,000)
Total Liabilities	$3,700,000	$3,730,000	$ 30,000
Equity	1,895,000	2,135,000	240,000 (A)
Total Liabilities and Equity	$5,595,000	$5,865,000	$270,000

(A) Net Operating Profit for 19x2 = $240,000
(B) Provision for Depreciation during 19x2 = $100,000

Working Capital

Working capital has a variety of definitions, depending on one's interpretation of the term and its related purpose. For example, a businessperson or an economist may consider a business' current assets to be working capital. In this book, working capital requirements mean the difference between the healthcare organization's total current assets and its total current liabilities:

Working Capital = Current Assets − Current Liabilities

Working capital could also be called net current assets. A number of factors affect the healthcare organization's working capital requirements; appraising these requirements can guide management in estimating the need for future corrective measures. For example, table 3–9 shows that the facility needed $120,000 to finance the increase in patient accounts receivable. Assuming net average daily charges to patients of $8,700 in 19x1 and $9,000 in 19x2, this would mean an increase of 10.6 days in the number of days of average daily charges uncollected (see table 3–11).

Further, assuming that the medical center could invest the $120,000 at 12 percent, the opportunity costs (which will be discussed in chapter 4) to the healthcare organization would be $14,400 per year. To put it another way, if the medical center had to borrow the $120,000 in the open market to finance its patient accounts receivable at 18 percent, the additional cost would be $21,600.

To examine working capital or working capital requirements further, assume that the current assets represent the *uses* of working capital and the current liabilities are *sources* of working capital. This may not make much

TABLE 3–11

Ratio Analysis of Patient Accounts Receivable

Memorial Medical Center
Anytown, U.S.A.

RATIO ANALYSIS OF PATIENT ACCOUNTS RECEIVABLE
As of December 31, 19x2

Days Uncollected	*19x1*	*19x2*
Net Average Daily Charges to Patients	$ 8,700	$ 9,000
Net Patient Accounts Receivable	700,000	820,000
Number of Days of Average Daily Charge Uncollected	80.5	91.1

sense at first, but consider what accounts are included in each of the major groups:

Current Assets

- patient accounts receivable
- inventories
- prepaid expenses
- cash and short-term investments
- petty cash

Each of these accounts requires a certain amount of cash or working capital to maintain and support it, but where do the funds come from to invest in these accounts? They come from the current liabilities, the source of funds:

Current Liabilities

- accounts payable
- payroll taxes payable
- short-term notes payable

One can easily recognize short-term notes payable as a source of funds. But, accounts and taxes payable? Upon further examination, it becomes clear that this means delayed payments to vendors, etc. Certainly, these accounts must be eventually paid, but in the meantime, the debtor has the opportunity to operate on "other peoples' money," making it a source of working capital. Therefore, the changes in working capital statement in table 3–9 could be recast as follows:

Sources of Working Capital		
Accounts Payable	$ 10,000	
Payroll Taxes Payable	(5,000)	
Short-Term Notes Payable	90,000	
Total Sources of Working Capital		$ 95,000
Uses of Working Capital		
Patient Accounts Receivable	$120,000	
Inventories	(5,000)	
Prepaid Expenses	5,000	
Total Uses of Working Capital		120,000
Total Working Capital Requirements		$ 25,000

Finally, since the patient accounts receivable is the primary use of working captial, it is imperative that patient financial services managers continually strive to obtain and maintain a minimum balance in this account.

Application of the Accounting Process

To illustrate the mechanics of the healthcare accounting process and the development of a facility's financial statements, we will assume that during June 19x1, a group of investors purchased the assets of Memorial Medical Center of Anytown, U.S.A., for $7,500,000, paying $3,000,000 in cash and financing the balance with a long-term 10-percent mortgage.

The accounting transactions the medical center incurred during the month of June 19x1 are recorded initially in the journal as follows:

Journal Entry Number	Description	Account Number	Dr.	Cr.
1	Plant Assets	150.0	$7,500,000	
	Owners' Equity	300.0		$3,000,000
	Mortgage Payable	250.0		4,500,000
	To record the purchase of Memorial Medical Center as of June 1, 19x1.			
2	Accounts Receivable	110.0	$1,500,000	
	Routine Services Revenue	400.0		$900,000
	Ancillary Services Revenue	450.0		600,000
	To record the patient revenue for the month of June 19x1 from the revenue journal.			
3	Inventory	120.0	$250,000	
	Accounts Payable	210.0		$250,000
	To record the supplies purchased and inventoried during the month of June 19x1 from the purchase journal.			
4	Salary Expense	500.0	$850,000	
	Cash	100.0		$800,000
	Payroll Taxes Payable	211.0		50,000
	To record the payroll expenses paid and payable for the month of June 19x1 from the payroll journal.			
5	Cash	100.0	$1,200,000	
	Accounts Receivable	110.0		$1,200,000
	To record the cash received during the month of June 19x1 from the cash receipts journal.			

Journal Entry Number	Description	Account Number	Dr.	Cr.
6	Depreciation	655.0	$70,000	
	Reserve for Depreciation	155.0		$70,000
	To record the provision for depreciation expense for the month of June 19x1 from the plant journal.			
7	Interest Expense	650.0	$37,500	
	Mortgage Payable	250.0	20,000	
	Cash	100.0		$57,500
	To record the mortgage payment and interest expense for the month of June 19x1 from the cash disbursements journal.			
8	Provision for Bad Debts	490.0	$75,000	
	Reserve for Bad Debts and Allowances	111.0		$75,000
	To record the provision for bad debts at the rate of 5 percent of gross patient revenue for the month of June 19x1 from the general journal.			
9	Accounts Payable	210.0	$200,000	
	Cash	100.0		$200,000
	To record the amount paid on accounts payable during the month of June 19x1 from the cash disbursements journal.			
10	Provision for Contractual Allowances	491.0	$90,000	
	Reserve for Bad Debts and Allowances	111.0		$90,000
	To record the provision for contractual allowances (Medicare, Blue Cross, and Medicaid) for the month of June 19x1 frgm the general journal.			
11	Prepaid Expenses	115.0	$42,500	
	Cash	100.0		$42,500
	To record the payment of the medical center's annual insurance premiums from the cash disbursements journal.			
12	Insurance Expense	651.0	$3,5000	
	Prepaid Expenses	115.0		$3,500
	To record the provision for insurance expense for the month of June 19x1 from the general journal.			
13	Supply Expense	625.0	$200,000	
	Inventory	120.0		$200,000
	To record the supplies requisitioned during the month of June 19x1 from the inventory journal.			

Journal Entry Number	Description	Account Number	Dr.	Cr.
14	Short-Term Investments	105.0	$90,000	
	Cash	100.0		$90,000
	To record the cash invested in short-term notes during the month of June 19x1 from the cash disbursements journal.			
15	Provision for Income Taxes	675.0	$87,000	
	Income Taxes Payable	212.0		$87,000
	To record the provision for income taxes payable from the general journal.			

These transactions are then transferred, or posted, to the general ledger T account as shown in table 3–12. After the accounting staff completes all the posting to the general ledger T accounts, a balance is computed for each account for the end of the accounting period and summarized in a general ledger trial balance, as shown in table 3–13. Total debits must equal total credits in this analysis regardless of the financial statement in which these accounts will ultimately appear.

As a general rule, accounts are listed in the general ledger trial balance in numerical order corresponding to the healthcare organization's chart of accounts. In other words, asset accounts appear first and are followed by liability, equity, revenue, and expense accounts.

The statement of condition (see table 3–14) was developed using all the asset, liability, and equity accounts; however, the statement of operations in table 3–15 was developed from only revenue and expense accounts. It is important to note that to have the total assets equal the total liabilities and equity in the statement of condition, it was necessary to add the net operating profit (or loss) to the medical center's equity. Thus, to complete the formula:

$$Assets = Liabilities + Equity,$$

or

$$\$7,754,000 = \$4,667,000 + \$3,087,000$$

The equity statement is as follows:

Beginning Equity Balance	$3,000,000
Plus: Accumulated Profit (Loss)	87,000
Ending Equity Balance	$3,087,000

The cash flow statement in table 3–16 was developed from the analysis of the transactions in the T-account activity in table 3–12's general ledger cash account. The ending cash balance of $10,000 also appears as a current asset in the medical center's statement of condition. In this example, the investors purchased only the fixed plant assets and not the other assets and liabilities; therefore, the accountants did not develop a statement of changes in financial position.

TABLE 3–12

General Ledger T Accounts

Memorial Medical Center
Anytown, U.S.A.

GENERAL LEDGER T ACCOUNTS

100.0　Cash		105.0　Short-Term Investments		110.0　Accounts Receivable	
(5) 1,200,000	(4) 800,000	(14) 90,000		(2) 1,500,000	(5) 1,200,000
	(7) 57,500	Bal. 90,000		Bal. 300,000	
	(9) 200,000				
	(11) 42,500				
	(14) 90,000				
Bal. 10,000					

111.0　Reserve for Bad Debts and Allowances		115.0　Prepaid Expenses		120.0　Inventory	
	(8) 75,000	(11) 42,500	(12) 3,500	(3) 250,000	(13) 200,000
	(10) 90,000	Bal. 39,000		Bal. 50,000	
	Bal. 165,000				

150.0　Plant Assets		155.0　Reserve for Depreciation		210.0　Accounts Payable	
(1) 7,500,000			(6) 70,000	(9) 200,000	(3) 250,000
Bal. 7,500,000			Bal. 70,000		Bal. 50,000

211.0　Payroll Taxes Payable		212.0　Income Taxes Payable		250.0　Mortgage Payable	
	(4) 50,000	(15) 87,000		(7) 20,000	(1) 4,500,000
	Bal. 50,000				Bal. 4,480,000

300.0　Owners' Equity		400.0　Routine Services Revenue		450.0　Ancillary Services Revenue	
	(1) 3,000,000		(2) 900,000		(2) 600,000
	Bal. 3,000,000				

490.0	Provision for Bad Debts		491.0	Provision for Contractual Allowances		500.0	Salary Expense	
(8)	75,000		(10)	90,000		(4)	850,000	

625.0	Supply Expense		650.0	Interest Expense		651.0	Insurance Expense	
(13)	200,000		(7)	37,500		(12)	3,500	

655.0	Depreciation		675.0	Provision for Income Taxes	
(6)	70,000		(15)	87,000	

In addition, Memorial Medical Center's accounting staff initially recorded plant assets in the journal's operating or general fund rather than establishing a separate plant fund because it is not necessary to use fund accounting if the accountants consolidate accounting funds into one general fund and maintain the appropriate asset and reserve accounts.

In conclusion, the transactions presented in this illustration have been individualized so the reader can interpret and analyze each transaction in terms of its own logic, regardless of the source journal. Balances are identified in the asset, liability, and equity accounts because most of the accounts have multiple entries. These permanent accounts are never "closed out"; balances are always brought forward for new accounting periods. Balances in the revenue and expense accounts are not singled out for identification because there is only one entry in each of these accounts. These temporary accounts are always "closed out" at the end of each fiscal year.

Incurred-but-Not-Reported Claims

Preferred provider organizations (PPOs) and health maintenance organizations (HMOs) are rapidly becoming a significant percentage of a healthcare organization's clientele. At some facilities, as much as 50 percent of the nongovernment gross revenue is represented by these alternative healthcare financing systems.[13]

This managed-care (risk-based) contracting has brought another type of liability account into the healthcare accounting process. This is the potential liability known as incurred-but-not-reported (IBNR) claims against the managed-care provider.[14]

IBNR claims represent services rendered for the managed-care provider (HMO–1) to a member subscriber (HMO–1a) by another provider (HMO–2)

TABLE 3–13
General Ledger Trial Balance

Memorial Medical Center
Anytown, U.S.A.

GENERAL LEDGER TRIAL BALANCE
As of June 30, 19x1

Account Number	Account Description	Debits	Credits
100.0	Cash	$ 10,000	$
105.0	Short-Term Investments	90,000	
110.0	Accounts Receivable	300,000	
111.0	Reserve for Bad Debts and Allowances		165,000
115.0	Prepaid Expenses	39,000	
120.0	Inventory	50,000	
150.0	Plant Assets	7,500,000	
155.0	Reserve for Depreciation		70,000
210.0	Accounts Payable		50,000
211.0	Payroll Taxes Payable		50,000
212.0	Income Taxes Payable		87,000
250.0	Mortgage Payable		4,480,000
300.0	Owners' Equity		3,000,000
400.0	Routine Services Revenue		900,000
450.0	Ancillary Services Revenue		600,000
490.0	Provision for Bad Debts	75,000	
491.0	Provision for Contractual Allowances	90,000	
500.0	Salary Expense	850,000	
625.0	Supply Expense	200,000	
650.0	Interest Expense	37,500	
651.0	Insurance Expense	3,500	
655.0	Depreciation Expense	70,000	
675.0	Provision for Income Tax	87,000	
	Total	$9,402,000	$9,402,000

TABLE 3–14
Statement of Condition

Memorial Medical Center
Anytown, U.S.A.

STATEMENT OF CONDITION
As of June 30, 19x1

Assets

Current Assets

Cash		$ 10,000
Accounts Receivable	$ 300,000	
Less: Reserve for Bad Debts and Allowances	165,000	135,000
Prepaid Expenses		39,000
Inventory		50,000
Short-Term Investments		90,000
Total Current Assets		$ 324,000

Fixed Assets

Plant and Equipment	$7,500,000	
Less: Reserve for Depreciation	70,000	
Net Plant and Equipment		7,430,000
Total Assets		$7,754,000

Liabilities and Equity

Current Liabilities

Accounts Payable	$ 50,000
Payroll Taxes Payable	50,000
Income Taxes Payable	87,000
Total Current Liabilities	$ 187,000

Fixed Liabilities

Mortgage Payable	4,480,000
Total Liabilities	$4,667,000

Equity

	$3,000,000
Plus: Net Operating Profit (Loss)	87,000
Total Equity	$3,087,000
Total Liabilities and Equity	$7,754,000

TABLE 3–15

Statement of Operations

Memorial Medical Center
Anytown, U.S.A.

STATEMENT OF OPERATIONS
For the Month Ending June 30, 19x1

Gross Revenue		
Routine Services		$ 900,000
Ancillary Services		600,000
Total Gross Revenue		$ 1,500,000
Deductions from Gross Revenue		
Provision for Bad Debts	$ 75,000	
Provision for Contractual Allowances	90,000	
Total Deductions from Gross Revenue		165,000
Net Revenue		$ 1,335,000
Operating Expense		
Salaries	$ 850,000	
Supplies	200,000	
Interest	37,500	
Insurance	3,500	
Depreciation	70,000	
Total Operating Expense		$ 1,161,000
Net Operating Profit (Loss) before Taxes		$ 174,000
Provision for Income Taxes		$ 87,000
Net Operating Profit (Loss) after Taxes		$ 87,000

that does not belong to the subscriber's network. Therefore, HMO–1 is liable for the services HMO–2 renders to HMO–1a. This type of liability is called IBNR. At the end of each month, HMO–1's accounting staff makes an adjusting journal entry in the accounting records to provide for such anticipated claims.

The managed-care provider's finance department is responsible for monitoring the IBNR account's integrity and assuring management of the adequacy of the month adjusting entry. Patient financial services managers should be intensely involved in this process as well.

TABLE 3–16

Cash Flow Statement

Memorial Medical Center
Anytown, U.S.A.

CASH FLOW STATEMENT
For the Month of June, 19x1

Beginning Balance		$ –0–
Cash Inflows		
Accounts Receivable	$1,200,000	
Other	–0–	
Total Cash Inflows		$ 1,200,000
Total Cash on Hand		$1,200,000
Cash Outflows		
Payroll	$ 800,000	
Interest Expense	37,500	
Payment on Mortgage Principal	20,000	
Short-Term Investment	90,000	
Accounts Payable	200,000	
Prepaid Insurance	42,500	
Total Cash Outflows		$ 1,190,000
Ending Cash Balance		$ 10,000

AICPA's Revised Reporting Requirements

The American Institute of Certified Public Accountants' (AICPA) 1990 document, *Audits of Providers of Health Care Services* (hereafter referred to as the Guide), established dramatic changes in the manner that the healthcare facility accounts for and reports its patient service revenues, charity care, and bad debts. Most importantly, AICPA also changed the methodology required to determine the facility's net patient accounts receivable.

Patient Service Revenues

Historically, healthcare organizations have reported patient service revenues on a gross basis—that is, before any provisions for charity care, contractual allowances, and bad debts—determined by the entity's published charges. The organizations displayed each of these items on their statement of condition as follows:

Gross Charges to Patients		$ xx,xxx,xxx
Less: Provisions for Charity Care	$ xxx,xxx	
Contractual Allowances	xxx,xxx	
Bad Debts, Less Recoveries	xxx,xxx	
Total Deductions from Revenue		x,xxx,xxx
Net Patient Revenue		$ xx,xxx,xxx

The Guide requires that for financial reporting purposes, the healthcare organization must present patient service revenues net of all deductions from revenue. Accordingly, the organization subtracts from gross revenue all contractually agreed-upon allowances and other allowances or deductions, reporting only the net amount on the face of the financial statements, as follows:

Gross Patient Service Revenue		$ xx,xxx,xxx
Less: Contractual Allowances	$ xxx,xxx	
Charity Care	xxx,xxx	
Other Discounts and Allowances	xxx,xxx	
Net Patient Service Revenue		xxx,xxx
Other Revenue (Specify)		xxx,xxx
Total Revenue		$ xx,xxx,xxx
Less: Expenses, Including Bad Debts		xxx,xxx
Income from Operations		$ xx,xxx,xxx

The healthcare organization may disclose deductions from gross patient service revenues in the notes to its financial statements.[15] It is important to note that bad debts are included as an expense item.

Some healthcare professionals argue that the concept of gross revenue is less meaningful today than it was in 1972, when AICPA published the *Hospital Audit Guide.* These professionals contend that Medicare and the other prospective payment systems, along with the emergence of managed-care or coordinated-care contracts, have contributed to the decline of gross patient revenue's significance. This situation is especially true for a healthcare entity that projects its cash inflows upon its net revenue rather than its gross revenue.

Other industry professionals, however, believe that AICPA's requirement to report only net revenue tends to obscure the healthcare organization's level of government-mandated charge reductions and its charity work. Some providers are considering alternative methods of reporting such deductions, such as using explanatory footnotes to the financial statements. Regardless, the Guide's net-revenue reporting requirement is consistent with other segments of the healthcare industry. For example, nursing homes historically have reported revenue on a net basis because of the proliferation of per-diem or negotiated payment rates.[16]

Although the Guide requires the reporting of patient service revenues on a net basis, this does not remove the healthcare organization's need to maintain accurate records of gross charge data for purposes such as filing third-party cost reports or other reports with regulatory agencies. Another reason the facility should continue to accumulate gross patient services by functional departments is that gross revenue can serve as the basis for allocating expenses to third-party service purchasers, such as HMOs and managed-care organizations. Using the ratio of charges to charges as applied to costs, the healthcare organization can determine the cost of rendering services to these third-party purchasers. The facility can even use this same ratio to estimate the cost of the individual diagnosis-related groups (DRGs) that are used by the Medicare program to establish reimbursement rates in its prospective payment system.

Bad Debts

In the past, healthcare organizations reported their provision for bad debts as a deduction from gross patient service revenue, as follows:

Provision for Bad Debts	$xxx,xxx
Less: Recoveries	xx,xxx
Net Provision for Bad Debts	$xxx,xxx

Under the new Guide, bad debts are classified as an operating expense. The Guide states that bad debts result from "services rendered for which payment is anticipated and credit is extended to patient. Expense is estimated and recognized when providing an allowance for such amounts to be written off at the time the accounts are deemed collectible."[17] Otherwise, bad debts are generally considered to be losses resulting from the extension of credit to a customer/patient who is able, but unwilling, to pay.

Charity Care

Unlike bad debts, AICPA continues to classify charity care as a deduction from gross patient service revenue. The Guide states that charity care results from services rendered for which the healthcare organization anticipates no payment.[18] In other words, charity care implies that the facility expects no payment for services it rendered. According to the Financial Accounting Standards Board's (FASB's) Concepts Statement No. 6, "Elements of Financial Statements," when a healthcare organization renders services without expecting a cash inflow, FASB does not consider revenues to have been generated. Accordingly, the healthcare organization should consider charges related to charity care patients as gross revenue.

The Guide requires that each provider establish and disclose its policy regarding charity care along with the amount of charity care provided. Disclosure of the levels of charity care may be based on cost or the provider's established rates, or provided in the form of a statistic that indicates the portion of the provider's services given to charity care. Whichever policy the provider adopts should be consistently applied.[19]

Healthcare industry literature makes the basic distinction between bad debts and charity service in the healthcare setting by differentiating between the patient's unwillingness to pay and the patient's demonstrated inability to pay.[20]

In assessing each patient's ability to pay, the healthcare organization needs to follow certain guidelines at the time of the patient's admission, especially if this person is uninsured:

- number of dependents

- employment

- income

- marital status

- assets and liabilities

- estimated medical bill(s)

- other known hardships

Net Patient Accounts Receivable

The healthcare facility's accounting staff should report patient accounts receivable at their net realization value in the facility's statement of condition. This means that accountants should reduce the *gross* amount of receivables recorded at established service charges in the patient accounts to the *net* amount that can be reasonably estimated to be actually collectible in cash. Further, all anticipated allowances for contractual adjustments, charity, administrative policies, bad debts, and other discounts should be deducted from the facility's gross receivables.[21]

For a detailed understanding of these financial reporting changes, the author encourages the reader to obtain a copy of the Guide and read it thoroughly. If you still have questions concerning these changes, discuss the issues with your external auditors.

NOTES

1. L. Vann Seawell, *Hospital Financial Accounting: Theory and Practice,* 2nd ed. (Westchester, Ill.: Healthcare Financial Management Association, 1987), 19.

2. Allen G. Herkimer Jr., *Understanding Health Care Accounting* (Rockville, Md.: Aspen Publishers, Inc., 1989), 48.

3. Seawell, *Hospital Financial Accounting,* 82.

4. Herkimer, *Understanding Health Care Accounting,* 227.

5. Healthcare Financial Management Association Principles and Practices Board, *A Compilation of Statements 1–9* (Westchester, Ill.: Healthcare Financial Management Association, 1987), 63, 70.

6. Howard J. Berman, Lewis E. Weeks, and Steven F. Kukla, *The Financial Management of Hospitals,* 7th ed. (Ann Arbor, Mich.: Health Administration Press Division of the Foundation of the American College of Healthcare Executives, 1990), 39.

7. Allen G. Herkimer Jr., *Understanding Hospital Financial Management,* 2nd ed. (Rockville, Md.: Aspen Publishers, Inc., 1986), 24.

8. Herkimer, *Understanding Health Care Accounting,* 21.

9. L. Vann Seawell, ed., *Chart of Accounts for Hospitals* (Westchester, Ill.: Healthcare Financial Management Association, in press), paragraph 4.1.

10. Seawell, *Chart of Accounts,* paragraphs 4.2, 4.3.

11. Seawell, *Chart of Accounts,* p. 4.20.

12. Seawell, *Hospital Financial Accounting,* 693.

13. Jeffrey A. Gottlieb, *Healthcare Cost Accounting: Practice and Applications* (Westchester, Ill.: Healthcare Financial Management Association, 1989), 44.

14. Herkimer, *Understanding Health Care Accounting,* 82–84.

15. Ernst & Young, *Implementing the New Health Care Audit Guide* (Cleveland: Ernst & Young, 1990), SCORE Retrieval File No. J58783.

16. Ernst & Young, *Implementing the New Health Care Audit Guide,* 5.

17. Ernst & Young, *Implementing the New Health Care Audit Guide,* 8.

18. Ernst & Young, *Implementing the New Health Care Audit Guide,* 8.

19. Ernst & Young, *Implementing the New Health Care Audit Guide,* 1.

20. *"Definition of and Payment for Uncompensated Services"* and *"Special Problems of a Disproportionate Share,"* a monograph series ed. (Westchester, Ill.: Healthcare Financial Management Association, 1987), 2.

21. L. Vann Seawell, *Introduction to Hospital Accounting,* 3rd ed. (Westchester, Ill.: Healthcare Financial Management Association, 1992), 343.

Managerial Accounting
and Its Application

Managerial accounting gathers valuable information on a healthcare organization's activities, both in dollar amounts and in statistical terms. All levels of the facility's management need this information for effective decision making, and managers also need to track this information, especially revenues and expenses, under changing conditions. This chapter will address the development of a capable managerial accounting and reporting system. Next, it will describe the nature of different expense categories and their impact on the patient financial services department and the entire healthcare organization. The chapter closes with an explanation of variable and control budgets and variance analysis, key tools in cost analysis and control.

Managerial Accounting: An Overview

The healthcare organization's accounting system is its major quantitative information collection, processing, and reporting mechanism. An effective healthcare accounting system should provide information for the following three purposes:

1. internal reporting to managers for use in planning and controlling current operations

2. internal reporting to managers for use in making special tactical decisions and formulating long-range strategic plans

3. external reporting to third-party purchasers of health services, stockholders, governmental agencies, and the community

Information derived from the accounting system is typically classified as either financial (general) accounting or managerial accounting. *Financial accounting* is concerned with reporting an organization's activities to outside groups, so its information takes the form of financial statements that summarize the activities of the entire organization. Because the organization presents its financial accounting to outside parties having little or no power in determining how this information is prepared, the reports' contents must conform to a code of rules known as generally accepted accounting principles (GAAP). This code allows people who rely on the information to make meaningful comparisons of the organization's activities with other organizations, especially those in the same industry. GAAP, in other words, provides the creditability needed when reporting financial accounting information.[1]

Managerial accounting is concerned with the accumulation of financial information for an organization's internal users, such as the officers, managers, and supervisors, who in turn apply the information in running the organization's business more efficiently. Unlike financial accounting, which summarizes events for the entire organization, managerial accounting also summarizes the organization's various components, such as divisions, branches, or departments; further, it reports events both in dollar amounts and statistical terms, such as total employee hours worked in a given month.[2]

To summarize, financial accounting is "compliance work," and managerial accounting is "thinking work."[3] Both forms of accounting are essential to a healthcare organization's information system. The precise historical information generated by the facility's financial accounting system lays the foundation for its managerial accounting system. Financial accounting deals with basic operating revenues and expenses, while managerial accounting concentrates on providing all levels of management with the information necessary for decision making. A key part of this information is behavior patterns for revenues and expenses under changing conditions; these patterns will be discussed later in this chapter.

Managerial Reporting

Key to an effective managerial accounting and information system is the presentation of data in a way that allows users to obtain information they need to know. The challenge to patient financial services managers is to develop, with the cooperation of the accounting and data processing department managers, an information system that will assist in

- carrying out the patient financial services department's mission, goals, and objectives;

- analyzing patient accounts receivable in a timely and accurate manner;

- managing and controlling patient financial services department expenses;

- managing and controlling departmental and employee productivity;

- achieving timely and accurate patient billings; and

- monitoring each managed-care contract's costs and profitability.

Managerial accounting and reporting are meant to be working tools for the department's employees as well as its manager. Some patient financial services personnel may not be accounting-oriented or numbers-oriented individuals; therefore, managerial reports should not be limited to columns of numbers. Experience has shown that the best method of developing a managerial report is for its preparer to work with its users in designing it; the objective is to communicate in the simplest language possible. Also, the managerial reporting system should be flexible enough to supply one-time or single-purpose reports in addition to routine ones, such as monthly reports.

Figures 4–1, 4–2, and 4–3 show how patient financial services managers can use line graphs to represent statistical and financial data and to assist in analyzing trends in key indexes, such as

- gross accounts receivable,

- average daily gross charges,

- number of days of average gross charges uncollected,

- cash flow requirements and projections, and

- actual cash flow.

FIGURE 4–1

Comparative Line Graph

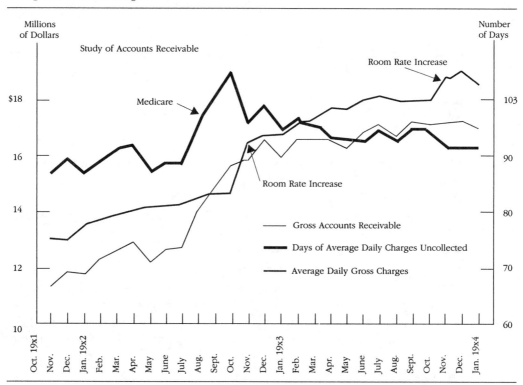

FIGURE 4–2

Flowing Line Graph with Minimum and Maximum

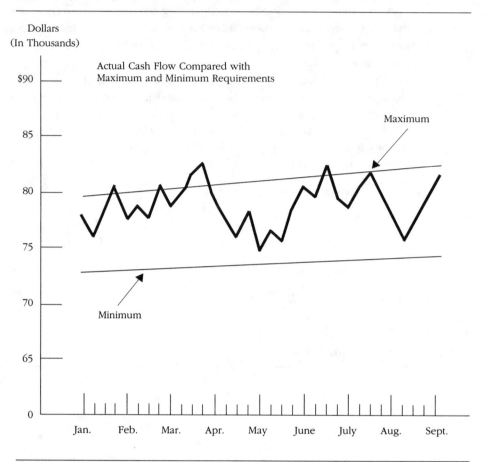

The design of the charts or graphs and the indexes to be depicted in these graphs must be determined by the patient financial services managers and the users of the information.

Principles of Expense Behavior

One unique feature of managerial accounting is that it classifies expenses according to the manner in which they interact under changing conditions—a situation known as volume variances. To make effective management decisions, patient financial services managers must understand expense characteristics, their behavior, and their impact on the department and on the entire healthcare facility's operation.

FIGURE 4–3
Single-Shaded Line Graph

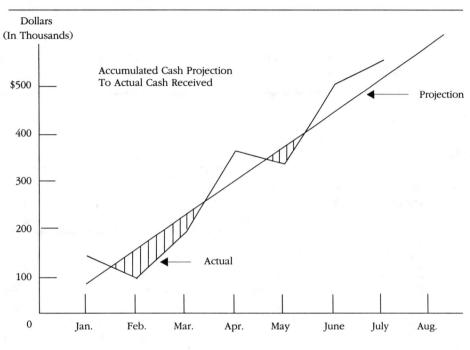

The expenses that patient financial services managers need to monitor can be divided into three major categories (see figure 4–4):

1. operating

2. opportunity

3. social

Operating Costs

Operating costs are the actual expenses a healthcare facility incurs to generate patient services. In other words, operating costs are those expenses incurred during the normal course of carrying out the facility's day-to-day responsibilities and functions: salaries and related employee benefits, supplies, depreciation, and other associated costs. The depreciation of capital expenditures are also included in operating costs.

Opportunity Costs

Opportunity costs are defined as the benefits relinquished when choosing an alternative use of resources.[4] To illustrate opportunity costs, assume that the total alternatives under consideration are described as Choices A–1, A–2, A–3, and A–4, and related costs and revenues are as illustrated:

FIGURE 4–4
Levels of Expense Classifications

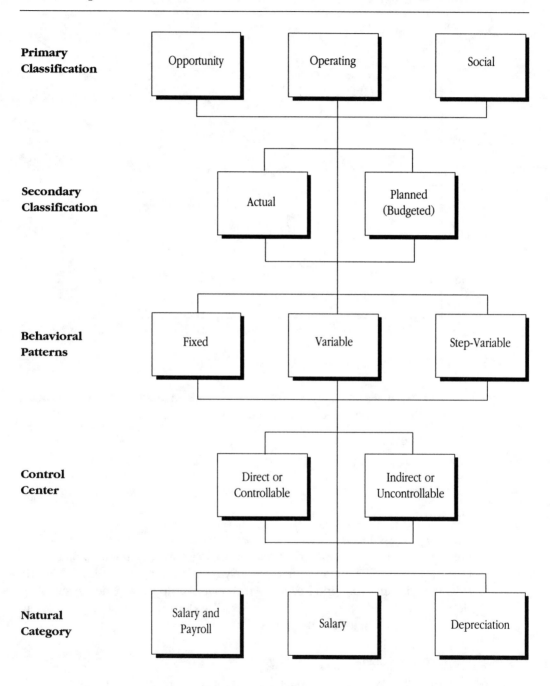

	Alternatives (In Thousands)			
	A-1	A-2	A-3	A-4
Revenue	$320	$280	$410	$360
Relevant Expenses	350	280	365	290
Profit (Loss)	$(30)	$ 0	$ 45	$ 70

According to this analysis, Alternative A–4 offers the most rewarding opportunity, a profit of $70,000. However, if management chose A–3, there would be an opportunity cost of $25,000, as calculated below:

OC	=	Opportunity Costs
A–4	=	Best Alternative
A–3	=	Selected Alternative

OC	=	A–4 – A–3
OC	=	$70,000 – $45,000
OC	=	$25,000

Theoretically, healthcare department managers accept only projects or capital expenditures yielding more that their actual operating and capital costs. By so doing, managers increase their department's contribution to the institution's net profit. However, all enlightened and appropriate decisions must be based on more than financial and statistical information; for example, managers need to consider customer service, historical experience, maintenance costs, and other factors.

Financial accounting systems usually confine their reporting to those facts that ultimately involve the actual exchanges of assets. Opportunity costs are not customarily included in financial accounting systems, but management must take them into serious consideration when making decisions such as choosing a data processing system, hiring a new employee, etc.[5]

Social Costs

Social costs are those costs that management knowingly or unknowingly imposes upon society or a specific segment of society as a result of its decisions. For example, assume a healthcare facility's management installs a new sewage system that drains directly into a nearby river. This system will eventually cause a health and/or environmental hazard requiring a cleanup campaign. The related costs of this cleanup campaign plus the costs of any sickness imposed upon the residents would be classified as social costs.

Occasionally, the "best" or most profitable alternative (A–4 in the above illustration) may result in substantial social costs. Perhaps this was the reason management selected Alternative A–3. In short, management decisions that impose costs, automatically or eventually, upon the general public are classified as social costs.[6]

Managing Operating Costs

Operating costs can be classified as either of the following:

- actual
- planned or budgeted

Actual costs are incurred expenses that can be supported by documentation. *Planned* or *budgeted expenses*, on the other hand, are those expenses that management predicts through the budgeting process or by estimates.

These types of expense, especially the actual costs, can be managed using one of two methodologies:

1. global
2. segmented

Global Expense Management

Global managers try to control a department's and/or a facility's expenses by surveying the organization's total expenses, making little or no attempt to categorize them other than by salary and nonsalary costs. For example, assume that Memorial Medical Center's patient financial services department has budgeted $750,000 for its expenses. The global manager would periodically compare the department's total actual expenses with its budgeted expenses, or compare the total actual salary and nonsalary expenses with the related budgeted expenses, as illustrated:

	Actual	*Budgeted*
Total Salary Expenses	$500,000	$475,000
Total Nonsalary Expenses	300,000	275,000
Total Operating Expenses	$800,000	$750,000

This global type of expense management is sometimes called the "bushel basket" method: it assumes that the department has $750,000 to spend and control as one large quantity. The global manager is looking only at the bottom-line total of $750,000, making little or no attempt to manage each expense at the most appropriate time for evaluating and/or justifying the costs incurred.

Segmented Expense Management

The segmented method of cost control takes the "bushel basket" of budgeted costs (see figure 4–5) and separates the total costs into manageable portions, as follows:

Step 1. The manager analyzes the department's total expenses by separating the salary, wage, and employee benefit expenses from the nonsalary and nonwage expenses.

Step 2. The manager divides each of the above two expense segments into either fixed or variable subsegments.

Using this approach, the patient financial services manager is no longer concentrating upon the bottom-line total, analyzing instead each of the four expense segments.

FIGURE 4–5
Methodologies Used to Control Departmental Expenses

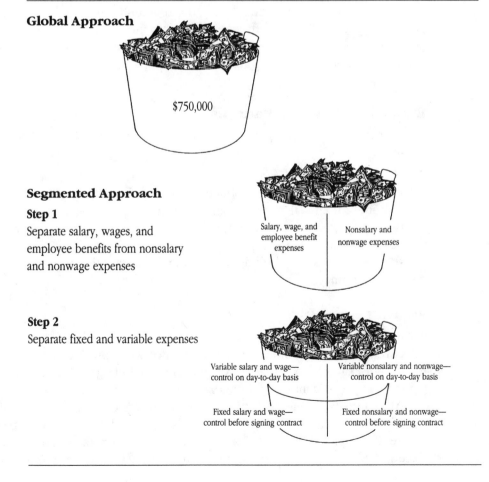

Global Approach

$750,000

Segmented Approach

Step 1
Separate salary, wages, and employee benefits from nonsalary and nonwage expenses

Salary, wage, and employee benefit expenses | Nonsalary and nonwage expenses

Step 2
Separate fixed and variable expenses

Variable salary and wage—control on day-to-day basis | Variable nonsalary and nonwage—control on day-to-day basis

Fixed salary and wage—control before signing contract | Fixed nonsalary and nonwage—control before signing contract

The key to the segmented method's success lies in the manager selecting the appropriate time to control each of these expense types. The time to control *any* fixed expense is before the manager signs a contract; for example, before hiring a new employee, purchasing a new insurance policy, or leasing a new data processing system. Once the manager has signed the contract for the lease, hired a new employee, or made a long-term commitment to use a different machine, the point of cost control has passed. The manager now must live with this decision for a relatively lengthy period of time. Consequently, managers who utilize the segmented management approach have adopted the philosophy that they will live with this fixed expense at least until the time for contract renewal and/or employee performance evaluation.

On the other hand, the time to control variable expenses is daily. Ideally, total departmental variable expenses should increase or decrease in direct relationship to the facility's volume of activity (work load). If the patient census goes down, the department will certainly need fewer office supplies, and perhaps the manager can reduce some employee paid hours.

In summary, patient financial services managers can manage department expenses much more efficiently using the segmented methodology than the global approach. The department budget's bottom line will eventually be evaluated, but the segmented approach, illustrated in figure 4–5, helps managers systematically evaluate and control expenses.

Expense Behavioral Patterns

Fixed Expenses

Fixed expenses tend to remain relatively constant regardless of volume or amount of work required to produce something (see figure 4–6). The salary of the patient financial services manager is an excellent example of a fixed salary expense, and depreciation, liability insurance, and rent are good examples of nonsalary fixed expenses. As stated earlier, management can control fixed expenses only before committing to expend them, such as at contract-signing time.

Variable Expenses

Total departmental variable expenses, on the other hand, tend to change in direct relationship to volume or the amount of work produced, as shown in figure 4–7. Examples of variable expenses include billing and admitting forms. Management can control variable expenses on a day-to-day basis.

After consolidating the information in figures 4–6 and 4–7, we can compute the total costs represented by the fixed and variable expenses. Figure 4–8 depicts the result. For example, assume that the department produced 10,000 units. The total expense for producing these units would be

FIGURE 4–6
Departmental Fixed Expense

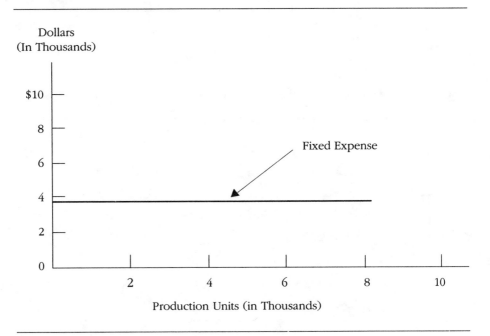

FIGURE 4–7
Departmental Variable Expense

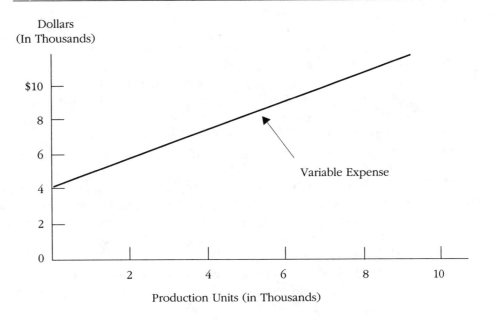

FIGURE 4-8

Total Departmental Expenses

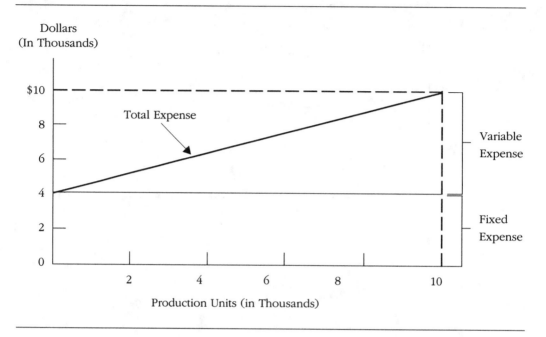

$10,000. Of that total, fixed expenses represent $4,000, and variable expenses account for $6,000.

Step-Variable Expenses

The most difficult expense classification to recognize and calculate is the step-variable expense. Its behavior combines the behavior of fixed and variable expenses. A step-variable expense may change abruptly at intervals according to relevant ranges of activity that can be measured in discrete segments. Salaries of billing and admitting clerks and most other nonadministrative personnel tend to be step-variable expenses because a staffing level will usually stay within a relevant range of volume or activity. Most staffing patterns have a certain amount of elasticity; a staff of a given size can handle a suddenly lower volume of activity (negative elasticity) or a suddenly higher volume of activity (positive elasticity). As with variable expenses, management can control step-variable expenses on a day-to-day operating basis by adjusting to trends in work-load volume.

For example, suppose that management has determined that three billing clerks can adequately process up to 4,000 bills per billing period. Salaries of the three billing clerks are a step-variable expense because once the billing volume reaches and consistently remains at 5,000, the reasonable elasticity of this staffing pattern has been exceeded, and management must increase the staff by one step (in this case, by adding one billing clerk). The additional clerk automatically establishes a higher range of volume or activity—4,000 to 8,000 bills (as illustrated in figure 4–9). The new staffing level, four billing clerks, remains fixed as long as billing activity remains within the 4,000-to-8,000 range. When volume reaches 8,000 to 12,000, the department will require five and one-half billing clerks: 5.5 full-time equivalents × 40 hours = 2,200 weekly hours. Staffing requirements are based on predetermined production standards, which will be discussed in chapter 5.

In addition to managing salary and other operating expenses, patient financial services managers should consider the impact of their decisions on opportunity and social expenses. They must ask questions such as

- What working capital expense is incurred by the healthcare organization at the present level of uncollected average daily revenue?

- How much are the healthcare organization's service area residents willing to pay for a new, automated billing system?

FIGURE 4–9
Step-Variable Staffing Requirements

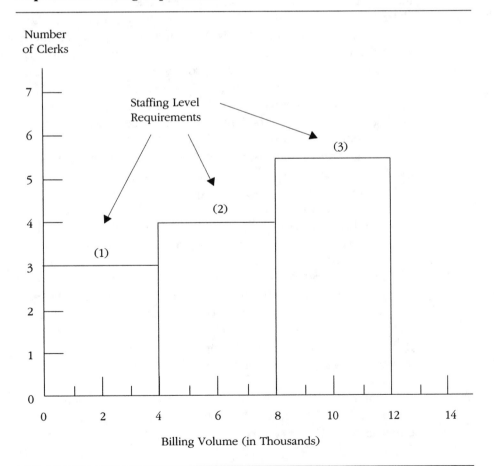

Billing Volume (in Thousands)

Managers need to realize that almost every decision they make affects not only the healthcare facility's operating expense budget but also the operating expenses of society. For this reason, they must weigh all aspects of each decision carefully.

Since patient financial services managers are concerned primarily with operating expenses, the balance of this discussion will be directed toward the management of operating expenses. Levels of expense classification are illustrated in figure 4–4.

Overhead and Other Expense Classifications

To evaluate the patient financial services department's total operating expenses, management must consider the department's indirect or noncontrollable expenses as well as its direct or controllable expenses, such as salaries, supplies, and depreciation. The noncontrollable expenses, sometimes referred to as overhead (see figure 4–4), are expenses that the department must share because it uses the services these expenses represent, such as housekeeping, computers, and utilities. Meeting these expenses is the responsibility of the managers of the departments from which they originate, such as environmental services and data processing; using a cost-finding process, management usually allocates the expenses proportionately to all departments using these services. Therefore, when evaluating the total cost of operating their department, patient financial services managers must keep these overhead expenses in mind.

As with fixed expenses, patient financial services managers must control overhead expenses before committing to the purchase of new equipment, the expansion of the department's square footage, or any other change. Once management approves and implements a change, using it increases the department's total cost. Effective patient financial services managers must weigh every proposed change's costs and/or benefits before committing to additional costs.

Inflation expense could be the most significant cost in the "other expense" classification with which the patient financial services manager must contend. Management generally budgets for this expense, but the inflation factor has been highly unpredictable due to general economic conditions. Because inflation can result in the need for an increase in the healthcare facility's working capital,[7] management must monitor its effects as carefully as possible.

Replacement expense is the actual or estimated expense of replacing a healthcare facility's present tangible assets. Generally, the term refers to the expense of replacing or renovating a building or office or replacing a piece of equipment such as a computer, word processor, typewriter, or desk. Unlike inflation expense, replacement expense can be computed relatively accurately. Although replacement expense is not usually recorded as an actual operating expense in the accounting system, some healthcare organizations provide for replacement expense by systematically depositing cash in a special capital replacement and depreciation investment fund that can be used to replace obsolete assets. This procedure is sometimes referred to as funded depreciation.

Committed expenses, sometimes called capacity expenses, include all fixed expenses that are incurred in the operation of the plant, equipment, and basic or core staff. Examples are depreciation, utilities, taxes, insurance, and salaries for key or core personnel. As stated earlier, management can control fixed or committed expenses only before making a commitment. Once management has made the decision to buy and has signed a contract, it has passed the cost control point and must be content to amortize the expense over a period of time.

Programmed expense is a fixed expense that arises periodically from management decisions regarding policies. Examples of programmed expenses include insurance premiums, auditing fees, and training programs. Programmed expenses, as committed expenses, have no relationship to volume or work load; management must control them before signing a contract.

To summarize, there are innumerable classifications managers can use to segregate expenses. The degree to which management classifies expenses and its terms for these expenses depend on the department's need to isolate and control specific costs. Frequently, management will select key or major expenses—travel in Administration, drugs in Pharmacy, utilities in Plant, or films in Radiology—for closer surveillance and control. Patient financial services managers must identify their own key or major expense need-to-know items and manage accordingly.

Cost Analysis

In analyzing the patient financial services department expenses, the total department fixed or capacity expenses, such as billings and admissions, remain constant within a relevant work volume range. Total variable department expenses, on the other hand, usually increase in direct proportion to increases in work volume. This phenomenon is illustrated in figure 4–10.

The following is a cost analysis of the patient financial services department's total direct expenses based on the three volume activity points in figure 4–10. The department's total variable expenses—sixty cents ($0.60) per unit of service—are shown in figure 4–11.

FIGURE 4–10

Total Departmental Direct Expenses

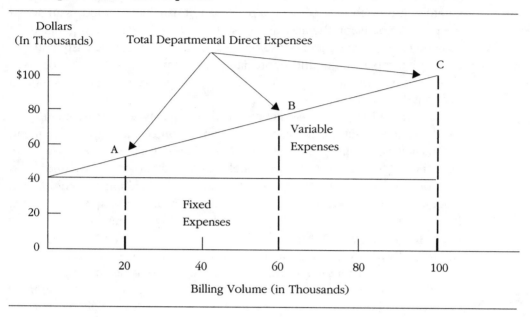

	Volume Activity Points		
Expense Description	*20-A*	*60-B*	*100-C*
Fixed Expense	$40,000	$40,000	$40,000
Variable Expense	12,000	36,000	60,000
Total Department Expense	$52,000	$76,000	$100,000

Although the total departmental direct expense curve increases as volume increases, as figure 4–10 shows, the total production unit cost curve declines as volume increases (see figure 4–12). For our purposes, a *production unit* is a quantitative measurement of work performed, i.e., billing, admission, etc.

The following is a cost analysis of the patient financial services department's total production unit expenses (as shown in figure 4–12), with billings being the production unit.

	Volume of Billing Activity				
Expense Description	*20,000*	*40,000*	*60,000*	*80,000*	*100,000*
Fixed Expense	$2.00	$1.00	$0.67	$0.50	$0.40
Variable Expense	0.60	0.60	0.60	0.60	0.60
Total Expense per Production Unit	$2.60	$1.60	$1.27	$1.10	$1.00

FIGURE 4–11
Total Departmental Variable Expenses

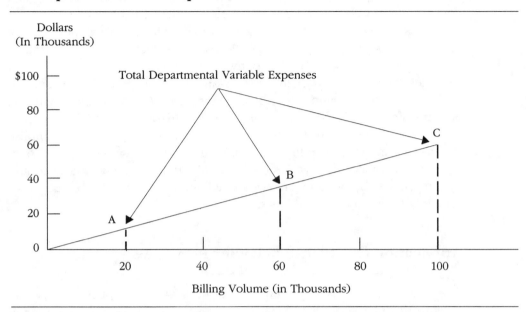

FIGURE 4–12
Total Departmental Production Unit Expenses

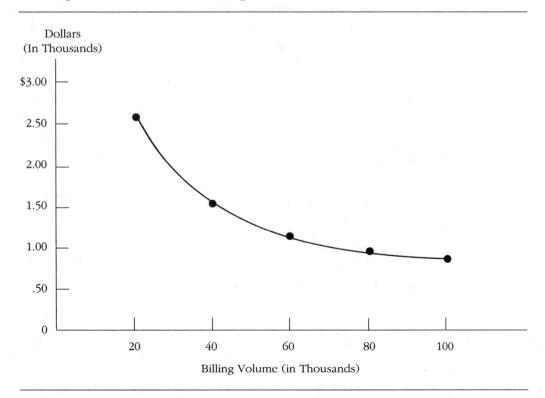

Using this analysis, the expense for each billing is $2.60 if the patient financial services department produces 20,000 billings, whereas total billing unit cost drops to $1.00 when the department produces 100,000 billings.

The knowledge of expenses and their related behavior will help patient financial services managers control the cost of operating their department. Fixed expenses are probably one of the most difficult expense categories for managers to control, especially after making the initial commitment, such as hiring an additional billing clerk. In such instances, management's challenge is to transform the fixed expense into a step-variable or a variable expense category to reduce total departmental expenses. Managers can accomplish this task by reducing the number of full-time employees and using more part-time or temporary employees as needed. In summary, the key is to control fixed expenses before they are committed and to control variable expenses on a day-to-day operational basis.[8]

Application of Expense Behavior Principles

The variable budget is an expense control system that applies expense behavior principles superbly. This system uses the standard variable cost concept, which establishes a standard rate or expected expense per production unit. The standard rate is computed by dividing the total annual variable expense by the budgeted or expected total annual number of units to be produced by the expense category.

To illustrate, assume that Memorial Medical Center's patient financial services manager has determined that an acceptable and reasonable performance standard per billing clerk is 1,000 bills per month. During the month ending September 30, 19x1, six clerks, each earning $1,000 per month, processed 5,400 bills. From this information, we extract the following relevant data:

Line	Description	Value
A.	Number of full-time clerks	6
B.	Monthly performance standard per clerk	1,000 billings
C.	Monthly capacity: A × B = C	6,000 billings
D.	Monthly salary expense per clerk	$1,000
E.	Total monthly salary expense: A × D = E	$6,000
F.	Standard salary expense per billing: E ÷ C = F	$1.00

Tables 4–1 and 4–2 illustrate the impact that volume changes and the use of standard expense rates have on a department's productivity and efficiency. In comparing the target budget with actual performance, as shown in table 4–1, we find no variance in salary expense; however, there is an unfavorable volume variance of 600 billings. This unfavorable volume variance becomes an unfavorable salary expense variance of $600 in table 4–2, where performance is compared with the control budget, whose volume has been adjusted to actual volume (thus eliminating the volume variance) and whose salary expense has been adjusted accordingly, using the standard salary rate per billing. Table 4–3 shows the impact of a 2,000-billing increase over the budgeted billing volume of 6,000.

TABLE 4–1
Comparative Analysis of Actual Performance to Target Budget

Memorial Medical Center
Anytown, U.S.A.

Patient Financial Services Department
COMPARATIVE ANALYSIS OF ACTUAL PERFORMANCE TO TARGET BUDGET
For the Month Ending September 30, 19x1

	Target Budget	*Actual Performance*	*Variance to Budget*
Volume (Billings)	6,000	5,400	(600) Unfavorable
Salary Expense	$6,000	$6,000	None

In summary, the variable budget methodology allows patient financial services managers to adjust the budget plan to actual performance volume. Using this methodology, the managers generate a standard rate for each classification of variable expense. They then multiply that rate by actual volume to develop a control budget; the control budget is then compared with actual performance. This process eliminates variances due to volume differences.

TABLE 4–2

Comparative Analysis of Actual Performance to Control Budget

Memorial Medical Center
Anytown, U.S.A.

Patient Financial Services Department
COMPARATIVE ANALYSIS OF ACTUAL PERFORMANCE TO CONTROL BUDGET
For the Month Ending September 30, 19x1

	Control Budget	Actual Performance	Variance to Budget
Volume (Billings)	5,400*	5,400	None
Salary Expense	$5,400	$6,000	($600)
			Unfavorable

*Adjusted to actual volume
Standard Rate $1.00 × Actual Volume 5,400 = $5,400

TABLE 4–3

Comparative Analysis of Actual Performance to Target and Control Budgets

Memorial Medical Center
Anytown, U.S.A.

Patient Financial Services Department
COMPARATIVE ANALYSIS OF ACTUAL PERFORMANCE
TO TARGET AND CONTROL BUDGETS
For the Month Ending September 30, 19x1

	Target Budget	Control Budget	Actual Performance	Variance
Volume (Billings)	6,000	NA	8,000	2,000
				Favorable
Volume Adjusted to Actual	NA	8,000	8,000	None
Salary Expense	$6,000	$8,000*	$6,000	$2,000
				Favorable

*Adjusted to Actual Volume × Standard Rate $1.00

Developing a Variable Budget

To develop a variable budget, management must classify each chart of accounts expense item in one of three categories:

1. *fixed expenses:* expenses that remain essentially constant in the short run regardless of changes in output volume

2. *variable expenses:* expenses that tend to vary directly in proportion to changes in output volume

3. *step-variable expenses:* expenses that are neither fixed nor variable (optional)[9]

To illustrate the use of variable expense for budgeting and control, assume that the fixed budget in table 4–4 is based on a volume of 100,000 billings and 12,000 admissions. Actual billings, however, were 90,000, and actual admissions were 11,250.

The following are the target production standards and rates that Memorial Medical Center's patient financial services manager developed for the admitting and billing clerks, along with the nonsalary variable expenses:

					Target Production	Total Expense	
(a)	*(b)*	*(c)*	*(d)*	*(e)*	*(f)*	*(g)*	*(h)*
Position	*Production Units*	*Total FTEs**	*Hours Paid*	*Total Volume*	*Volume per Hour (Paid) (e÷d=f)*	*Total Expense*	*Rate/ Hour Paid (Unit) (g÷d=h)*
Admitting Clerk	Number of Admissions	3	3,120	12,000	3.8	$18,000	$5.77
Billing Clerk	Number of Billings	6	6,240	100,000	16.03	$36,000	$5.77
Admitting Supplies	Number of Admissions	NA	NA	12,000	NA	$12,000	$1.00
Billing Supplies	Number of Billings	NA	NA	100,000	NA	$50,000	$ .50

*FTE = Full-Time Equivalent
In this illustration only: 26 weeks × 40 hrs = 1,040 hrs

TABLE 4–4

Comparative Analysis of Actual Performance to Fixed (Target) Budget

Memorial Medical Center
Anytown, U.S.A.

Patient Financial Services Department
COMPARATIVE ANALYSIS OF ACTUAL PERFORMANCE
TO FIXED (TARGET) BUDGET
For the Six-Month Period Ending June 30, 19x1

	Target Budget	Actual	Variance: Fav./(Unfav.)
Volume			
Admissions	12,000	11,250	(750)
Billings	100,000	90,000	(10,000)
Salary Expense			
Management and Supervision	$ 60,000	$ 59,000	$ 1,000
Executive Secretary	9,000	9,000	–0–
Billing Clerks	36,000	40,000	(4,000)
Admitting Clerks	18,000	15,000	3,000
Total Salary Expense	$123,000	$123,000	$ –0–
Nonsalary Expense			
Office Supplies, General	$ 24,000	$ 22,000	$ 2,000
Travel and Meetings	6,000	7,500	(1,500)
Dues and Subscriptions	1,000	1,000	–0–
Admitting Supplies	12,000	11,500	500
Billing Supplies	50,000	51,000	(1,000)
Depreciation	12,000	12,000	–0–
Total Nonsalary Expense	$105,000	$105,000	$ –0–
Total Expense	$228,000	$228,000	$ –0–

Table 4–5 compares a control budget based on the actual billing volume with actual performance. The key in this approach is to determine in advance which expense classification, fixed or variable, is appropriate.

TABLE 4–5

Comparative Analysis of Actual Performance to Variable Control Budget

Memorial Medical Center
Anytown, U.S.A.

Patient Financial Services Department
COMPARATIVE ANALYSIS OF ACTUAL PERFORMANCE
TO VARIABLE CONTROL BUDGET
For the Six-Month Period Ending June 30, 19x1

	Standard Rate	*Control Budget*	*Actual*	*Variance Fav./(Unfav.)*
Volume				
Admissions		11,250	11,250	–0–
Billings		90,000	90,000	–0–
Variable Expense				
Salary Expense				
Billing Clerks	$ 0.36	$ 32,400	$ 40,000	$ (7,600)
Admitting Clerks	$ 1.50	16,875	15,000	1,875
Total				
Variable Salary Expense		$ 49,275	$55,000	$ (5,725)
Nonsalary Expense				
Office Supplies, General	$132.60	$ 24,000	$ 22,000	$ 2,000
Admitting Supplies	1.00	11,250	11,500	(250)
Billing Supplies	0.50	45,000	51,000	(6,000)
Total				
Variable Nonsalary Expense		$ 80,250	$ 84,500	$ (4,250)
Total				
Variable Expense		$129,525	$139,500	$ (9,975)
Fixed Expense				
Salary Expense				
Management and Supervision		$ 60,000	$ 59,000	$ 1,000
Executive Secretary		9,000	9,000	–0–
Total				
Fixed Salary Expense		$ 69,000	$ 68,000	$ 1,000
Nonsalary Expense				
Travel and Meetings		$ 6,000	$ 7,500	$ (1,500)
Dues and Subscriptions		1,000	1,000	–0–
Depreciation		12,000	12,000	–0–
Total				
Fixed Nonsalary Expense		$ 19,000	$ 20,500	$ (1,500)
Total				
Fixed Expense		$ 88,000	$ 88,500	$ (500)
Total				
Fixed and Variable Expense		$217,525	$228,000	$(10,475)

After the appropriate production unit(s) has been identified, the following is a step-by-step methodology for developing a variable budget; it uses the data in table 4–4's target budget.

Step 1. Identify appropriate production unit, i.e., billing, admission, etc.

Step 2. Separate the fixed and variable salary expenses in the target fixed volume budget as follows:

Fixed Salary Expense		*Variable Salary Expense*	
Management and Supervision	$60,000	Billing Clerks	$36,000
Executive Secretary	9,000	Admitting Clerks	18,000
Total		Total	
Fixed Salary Expense	$69,000	Variable Salary Expense	$54,000

Step 3. Establish a standard variable salary rate for each position based on its production units using the following formula:

$$\frac{\text{Total Variable Salary Expense}}{\text{Total Relevant Production Units}} = \begin{array}{c}\text{Standard Variable Salary Rate} \\ \text{per Production Unit}\end{array}$$

For billing clerks, where total projected billings is the production unit:

$$\frac{\$36,000}{100,000} = \$0.36 \text{ (Standard Variable Salary Rate per Production Unit)}$$

For admitting clerks, where total projected admissions is the production unit:

$$\frac{\$18,000}{12,000} = \$1.50 \text{ (Standard Variable Salary Rate per Production Unit)}$$

Step 4. Separate the fixed and variable nonsalary expenses in the fixed or target budget as follows:

Fixed Nonsalary Expense		*Variable Nonsalary Expense*	
Travel and Meetings	$ 6,000	Office Supplies, General	$24,000
Dues and Subscriptions	1,000	Admitting Supplies	12,000
Depreciation	12,000	Billing Supplies	50,000
Total		Total	
Fixed Nonsalary Expense	$19,000	Variable Nonsalary Expense	$86,000

Step 5. Establish a standard variable nonsalary rate for each distinct nonsalary expense using the following formula:

$$\frac{\text{Total Variable Salary Expense}}{\text{Total Relevant Production Units}} = \frac{\text{Standard Variable Nonsalary Rate per}}{\text{Production Unit}}$$

Office Supplies, General

Since there is no distinct production unit for general office supplies, the number of calendar days will be used as the production unit in the example:

$$\frac{\$24,000}{181} = \$132.60 \quad \text{(Standard variable expense rate for general office supplies per calendar day)}$$

Admitting Supplies (Total projected admissions is the production unit):

$$\frac{\$12,000}{12,000} = \$\ 1.00 \quad \text{(Standard variable expense rate for admitting supplies per admission)}$$

Billing Supplies (Total projected billings is the production unit):

$$\frac{\$50,000}{100,000} = \$\ 0.50 \quad \text{(Standard variable expense rate for billing supplies per billing)}$$

Developing a Control Budget

The following is a step-by-step methodology for developing a control budget using the standard rates computed in the aforementioned variable budget process:

Step 1. The control budget volume is always the same as the actual volume; hence, there are no volume variances. In this case, the production unit volumes were 11,250 admissions and 90,000 billings.

Step 2. Compute variable salary expense as follows:

Actual Volume × Standard Rate = Total Expenses

For billing clerks, where total actual billings is the production unit:

$$90,000 \times \$0.36 = \$32,400$$

For admitting clerks, where total actual admissions is the production unit:

$$11,250 \times \$1.50 = \$16,875$$

Step 3. Compute variable nonsalary expense as follows:

$$\text{Actual Volume} \times \text{Standard Rate} = \text{Total Expenses}$$

For office supplies, where total calendar days is the production unit:

$$181 \times \$132.60 = \$24,000$$

For admitting supplies, where total actual admissions is the production unit:

$$11,250 \times \$1.00 = \$11,250$$

For billing supplies, where total actual billings is the production unit:

$$90,000 \times \$0.50 = \$45,000$$

Step 4. Fixed expenses in the control budget are identical to those in the original target budget, as follows:

Salary Expense		*Nonsalary Expense*	
Management and Supervision	$60,000	Travel and Meetings	$ 6,000
Executive Secretary	9,000	Dues and Subscriptions	1,000
		Depreciation	12,000

Step 5. To compare the accounting period's control budget, plot the corresponding actual expenses in the Actual column alongside of the relevant control budget expenses, as illustrated in table 4–5.

The total expense (bottom-line) result in the fixed budget (table 4–4) identifies no dollar variance. The variable control budget (table 4–5), on the other hand, identifies a $10,475 negative variance due to the following overspending:

Variable Salary Expenses	$ 5,725
Variable Nonsalary Expenses	4,250
Fixed Salary Expenses	(1,000)
Fixed Nonsalary Expenses	1,500
Total Variance	$10,475

Variance Analysis

Once management identifies the variances in the control budget, the next step is to determine why both the favorable and unfavorable variances occurred. Was the variance due to a change in the hourly rate? Was it due to employee inefficiency or to a production volume variance? These questions can be answered through a process known as variance analysis.

Salary Variance Analysis

Basically, there are two types of salary variance analysis:

1. efficiency

2. rate

The following process is a step-by-step computation of the salary variances that occurred during one six-month accounting period.

		Admitting Clerks	*Billing Clerks*
Step 1:	*Standard or Target*		
1.	Standard hourly rate	$5.77	$5.77
2.	Standard hours	3,120	6,240
3.	Total standard salary expense (line 1 × line 2 = line 3)	$18,002	$36,005
Step 2:	*Control Standard*		
4.	Standard hourly rate	$5.77	$5.77
5.	Actual hours paid (from Payroll)	2,542	7,272
6.	Control standard (line 4 × line 5 = line 6)	$14,667	$41,959
Step 3:	*Actual Performance*		
7.	Actual hourly rate (from Payroll)	$5.90	$5.50
8.	Actual hours paid	2,542	7,272
9.	Actual salary expense	$14,997	$39,996

	Admitting Clerks	Billing Clerks
Step 4: *Efficiency Variance*		
10. Standard hours	3,120	6,240
11. Actual hours paid	2,542	7,272
12. Hourly variance		
(line 10 − line 11 = line 12)	578	(1,032)
	Favorable	Unfavorable
13. Standard hourly rate	$5.77	$5.77
14. Efficiency variance		
(line 12 × line 13 = line 14)	$3,335	($5,955)
	Favorable	Unfavorable
Step 5: *Rate Variance*		
15. Actual hours paid	2,542	7,272
16. Actual hourly rate		
(from Payroll)	$5.90	$5.50
17. Standard hourly rate	$5.77	$5.77
18. Hourly rate variance		
(line 16 − line 17 = line 18)	($0.13)	$0.27
	Unfavorable	Favorable
19. Rate variance		
(line 15 × line 18 = line 19)	($330)	$1,963
	Unfavorable	Favorable
Step 6: *Summary of Salary Variances*		
A. Efficiency	$3,335	($5,955)
	Favorable	Unfavorable
B. Rate	($330)	$1,963
	Unfavorable	Favorable
Total salary expense		
variances	$3,005	($3,991)
	Favorable	Unfavorable
Net salary variance		($ 986)
		Unfavorable

Proof—Compare difference between standard salary expense and actual salary expense:

	Admitting Clerks	Billing Clerks
Standard salary expense (line 1.3)	$18,002	$ 36,005
Actual salary expense (line 3.9)	14,997	39,996
Total variance	$ 3,005	($ 3,991)
	Favorable	Unfavorable
Net salary variance		($ 986)
		Unfavorable

Nonsalary Variance Analysis

Nonsalary expenses also have two major types of variance analysis:

1. volume

2. rate

The following procedures comprise a step-by-step approach to computing these variances.

		Admitting Supplies	Billing Supplies
Step 1:	*Standard or Target*		
1.	Target volume	12,000	100,000
2.	Standard expense per unit	$1.00	$0.50
3.	Total standard expense (line 1 × line 2 = line 3)	$12,000	$50,000
Step 2:	*Control Standard*		
4.	Actual volume	11,250	90,000
5.	Standard unit expense	$1.00	$0.50
6.	Total control expense (line 4 × line 5 = line 6)	$11,250	$45,000
Step 3:	*Actual Unit Expense*		
7.	Total actual expense	$11,500	$51,000
8.	Total actual volume	11,250	90,000
9.	Actual unit expense (line 7 ÷ line 8 = line 10)	$ 1.022	$ 0.566

	Admitting Supplies	Billing Supplies
Step 4: *Actual Performance*		
10. Actual volume	11,250	90,000
11. Actual unit expense	$1.022	$0.566
12. Actual total expense (line 10 × line 11 = line 12)	$11,498	$50,940
Step 5: *Volume Variance*		
13. Target volume	12,000	100,000
14. Actual volume	11,250	90,000
15. Volume variance (line 13 − line 14 = line 15)	750 Favorable	10,000 Favorable
16. Standard unit expense	$1.00	$0.50
17. Volume expense variance (line 15 × line 16 = line 17)	$750 Favorable	$5,000 Favorable
Step 6: *Rate Variance*		
18. Standard unit expense	$1.00	$0.50
19. Actual unit expense	$1.022	$0.566
20. Unit expense variance (line 18 − line 19 = line 20)	($0.022) Unfavorable	($0.066) Unfavorable
21. Actual volume	11,250	90,000
22. Rate variance (line 20 × line 21 = line 22)	($248) Unfavorable	($5,940) Unfavorable
Step 7: *Summary of Nonsalary Expense Variances*		
A. Volume	$750 Favorable	$5,000 Favorable
B. Rate	($248) Unfavorable	($5,940) Unfavorable
Total nonsalary expense variances	$502 Favorable	($940) Unfavorable
Net nonsalary variance		($438) Unfavorable

	Admitting Supplies	Billing Supplies
Proof—Compare difference between standard nonsalary expense and actual nonsalary expenses:		
Standard nonsalary expense (line 1.3)	$12,000	$50,000
Actual nonsalary expense (line 3.9)	11,498	50,940
Total variance	$502	(940)
	Favorable	Unfavorable
Net nonsalary variance		(438)
		Unfavorable

The process outlined above illustrates an application of the variable budgetary control concept, which adjusts the variable expenses in direct proportion to the actual production volume. Some may say, justifiably, that variable salary expenses cannot be adjusted in direct proportion to the volume of work. They would argue that patient financial services managers cannot automatically hire a new admitting clerk just because admissions increase by 50 or 100. Conversely, patient financial services managers cannot automatically release an admitting clerk when admissions drop by 50 or 100. Most staffing patterns contain a certain amount of elasticity during a reasonable period of time; thus, elasticity tends to create plateaus in a patient financial services department's staffing requirements. Implementing a step-variable control creates a "lag factor" that allows the department to adjust to volume variance fluctuations.

We can use the following method to adjust for step-variable components in the situation of the admitting and billing clerks in the above case study:

		Expense Classification	
Step No.	Description	Admitting Clerks	Billing Clerks
1.	Standard or target volume	12,000	100,000
2.	Standard or target hours paid	3,120	6,240
3.	Standard units per paid hour (line 1 ÷ line 2 = line 3)	3.8	16.0
4.	Average hours per week	40	40
5.	Weeks per period	26	26
6.	Average paid hours per period	1,040	1,040

Step No.	Description	Expense Classification Admitting Clerks	Billing Clerks
7.	Average standard production per period (line 3 × line 6 = line 7)	3,952	16,640
8.	Standard or target volume	12,000	100,000
9.	Actual volume	11,250	90,000
10.	Volume variance (line 8 – line 9 = line 10)	750	10,000
11.	Average standard production per period (line 7)	3,952	16,640
12.	Average number of step variance (to the nearest whole number) (line 10 ÷ line 11 = line 12)	0	1 Unfavorable
13.	Average standard hourly rate	$5.77	$5.77
14.	Average expense per step (line 6 × line 13 = line 14)	$6,000	$6,000
15.	Step-variable adjustment (line 12 × line 14 = line 15)	None	$6,000 Unfavorable

Once the step-variable adjustment has been made, we can incorporate it into the control budget and compare it with actual performance, as shown in table 4–6.

Table 4–7 is a comparative analysis of the variable and step-variable approaches to adjusting variable expenses to match the actual volume of work.

In summary, developing and using a variable budgetary control system provides patient financial services managers with the flexibility to design an accounting system that best fits the needs of their own department and institution. Patient financial services managers and their superiors should work together to classify expenses into the appropriate categories—fixed, variable, and step-variable. Once that is done, the patient financial services managers can work with their facility's financial staff to design management reports that produce the desired results. Variable budgetary control is only one application of expense behavior analysis that can help patient financial services managers manage their department more effectively. Its potential uses are limited only by the imagination.

TABLE 4–6

Comparative Analysis of Actual Performance to Step-Variable Control Budget

Memorial Medical Center
Anytown, U.S.A.

Patient Financial Services Department
COMPARATIVE ANALYSIS OF ACTUAL PERFORMANCE
TO STEP-VARIABLE CONTROL BUDGET
For the Six-Month Period Ending June 30, 19x1

	Control Budget	Actual	Variance: Favorable/ (Unfavorable)
Volume			
Admissions	11,250	11,250	none
Billings	90,000	90,000	none
Variable Salary Expense			
Standard or Target Salary Expense:			
Admitting Clerks	$ 18,000	$ 15,000	
Billing Clerks	36,000	40,000	
Target Variable Salary Expense	$ 54,000	$ 55,000	
Less: Unfavorable Step-Variable Adjustment (line 15)	$ 6,000		
Total Variable Salary Expense	$ 48,000	$ 55,000	$ (7,000)
Variable Nonsalary Expense			
Admitting Supplies	$ 11,250	$ 11,500	$ (250)
Billing Supplies	45,000	51,000	(6,000)
Office Supplies, General	24,000	22,000	2,000
Total Variable Nonsalary Expense	$ 80,250	$ 85,000	$ (4,250)
Total Step-Variable Expense	$128,250	$139,500	$(11,500)
Fixed Expense			
Salary Expense	$ 69,000	$ 68,000	$ 1,000
Nonsalary Expense	19,000	20,500	(2,500)
Total Fixed Expense	$ 88,000	$ 88,500	$ (1,500)
Total Fixed and Variable Expense*	$216,250	$229,000	$(12,750)

* With adjustment for step-variable adjustment

TABLE 4–7

Comparative Analysis of Actual Performance to Variable and Step-Variable Control Budgets

Memorial Medical Center
Anytown, U.S.A.

Patient Financial Services Department
COMPARATIVE ANALYSIS OF ACTUAL PERFORMANCE
TO VARIABLE AND STEP-VARIABLE CONTROL BUDGETS
For the Six-Month Period Ending June 30, 19x1

	Actual Performance (Table 4–4)	*Variable Control Budget (Table 4–5)*	*Step-Variable Control Budget (Table 4–6)*
Volume			
Admissions	11,250	11,250	11,250
Billings	90,000	90,000	90,000
Fixed Expense			
Salary	$ 68,000	$ 69,000	$ 69,000
Nonsalary	20,500	19,000	19,000
Total Fixed Expense	$ 88,500	$ 88,000	$ 88,000
Variable Expense			
Salary	$ 55,000	$ 49,275	$ 48,000
Admitting Supplies	11,500	11,250	11,250
Billing Supplies	51,000	45,000	45,000
Office Supplies, General	22,000	24,000	24,000
Total Variable Expense	$139,500	$129,525	$128,250
Total Fixed and Variable Expense	$228,000	$217,525	$216,250

NOTES

1. Nathan S. Slavin, *Cost Accounting* (New York: John Wiley & Sons, Inc., 1986), 5–6.

2. Slavin, *Cost Accounting,* 6.

3. Allen G. Herkimer Jr., *Understanding Health Care Accounting* (Rockville, Md.: Aspen Publishers, Inc., 1989), 3.

4. Jeffrey A. Gottlieb, *Healthcare Cost Accounting: Practice and Applications* (Westchester, Ill.: Healthcare Financial Management Association, 1989), 16.

5. Allen G. Herkimer Jr., *Understanding Hospital Financial Management,* 2nd ed. (Rockville, Md.: Aspen Publishers, Inc., 1986), 46–47.

6. Herkimer, *Understanding Hospital Financial Management,* 46–47.

7. Healthcare Financial Management Association Principles and Practices Board, *A Compilation of Statements 1–9* (Westchester, Ill.: Healthcare Financial Management Association, 1987), 19.

8. Herkimer, *Understanding Hospital Financial Management,* 61.

9. Herkimer, *Understanding Hospital Financial Management,* 153–54.

CHAPTER 5

Developing a Productivity Improvement Program

Effective managers strive for the optimal use of resources available to them, such as personnel, supplies, and equipment. With this in mind, executives need to make their staff their top priority because employees determine an organization's performance capacity.[1] As it stands, however, most healthcare facilities are financially troubled due to substandard white-collar productivity, according to the chief executive officer of a successful healthcare chain.[2]

Employee productivity should increase steadily; otherwise, it soon declines. Productivity growth calls for a structured program and the means to monitor progress toward the program's goals.[3] This chapter will outline the elements of the successful productivity improvement program, chief among them the selection of appropriate production units to measure and evaluate department output and individual performance. For the purposes of this discussion, *productivity* is the ratio of outputs (the department's services) to the amount of inputs (resources) required to generate the outputs over a specific period of time.[4] Outputs will be represented as *production units,* quantitative measurements of work performed; for example, admissions, accounts billed, discharges, and items handled. Inputs will be represented as employee time (e.g., days, hours, and minutes), capital resources, and supplies.

The Effective Productivity Improvement Program

An effective productivity improvement program has two major components:

1. work measurement, and

2. performance evaluation.

Historically, healthcare organizations' chief financial officers evaluated their patient financial services department in terms of whether dollars actually spent by the department exceeded dollars budgeted. If the amount of dollars spent was less than dollars budgeted, management considered the patient financial services manager's performance to be favorable. On the other hand, the patient financial services manager's performance was considered to be unfavorable if the department's expenditures exceeded its budget. There are two fallacies inherent in this rationale. First, it does not allow for volume variances, and second, it does not take into account the performance of individual employees in the department. Precise performance evaluation requires that all departmental functions be separated into like tasks for like employees. In addition, evaluators should not use the dollar as their only performance yardstick; a production unit that reflects changes in work volume is preferable.

Nonetheless, many healthcare critics, especially from the governmental sector, have been comparing costs of healthcare facilities and departments in terms of dollars spent by the facilities to determine cost per patient day, for example. What is so wrong about comparing costs in this manner? Basically nothing, if each service studied is the same. But comparisons of service costs usually do not consider such variables as

- functional variations of the method used to perform the service;

- technological differences—i.e., the type of equipment used to generate the service;

- wage rate variances paid to personnel;

- skill level differences used in the staffing patterns; and

- intensity of services rendered to the patient.

Another important variable that distorts cost comparisons from one accounting period to another is the inflation factor.[5]

If healthcare managers were to depend solely upon the dollar cost to evaluate managerial and departmental performance, they would have to make adjustments for each of the above-mentioned variables, a time-consuming process. In all probability, they would have to make additional adjustments to assure comparability among departments and/or sections.[6]

In addition, because dollar comparisons yield only an unreliable gross figure that raises more questions than it answers, this evaluation system does not permit an appropriate and fair assessment of department managers' productivity, nor does it stimulate greater productivity. Worse, only pure rationalization can answer the questions this system raises.[7]

This is not to say that dollar cost comparisons are worthless; rather, managers should supplement them with other quantitative measurements that will remain relatively constant over an extended period of time and will reasonably reflect the resources required to produce a specific service or group of services. Production units, or units of service, are the needed additional quantitative measurements. Selecting specific production units will be discussed later in this chapter.

Through effective use of production units, patient financial services managers can identify and determine

- productivity per employee and/or department,
- cost per production unit, and
- charge (rate) per production unit.

Using production units will assist patient financial services managers in assigning responsibility for evaluating the effectiveness of the dollars spent to the employees who spent them. Production units also give managers a means of measuring their department's effectiveness. Although patient financial services managers will eventually assign a dollar value to the production unit, the dollar should not be the only measure of the patient financial services department's productivity or effectiveness.

Production units' importance lies in their enabling patient financial services managers to compare actual performance with a planned (budgeted) performance standard. Thus, the first step in developing a productivity improvement program is to identify appropriate production units. At the same time, however, patient financial services managers need to keep in mind that their people are a resource, not a cost; employees have to be managed to be responsible for their own as well as for their department's objectives and productivity.[8]

The Production Unit

As stated earlier, the production unit is a quantitative measurement of work performed. Since a department's efficiency frequently depends on its productivity, selecting appropriate production units is critical for proper budgetary planning and control.[9] In other words, it is important for patient financial services managers to remember that each production unit they select must accurately identify and reflect the service or commodity produced and the amount of resources used to produce the individual unit. For the purposes of this discussion, production units are divided into two major classes:

1. macro or gross
2. micro or weighted

Macro Production Units

Macro production units are the production units most commonly used in the healthcare industry because they require no special studies to determine a weighted value. They are also relatively easy to identify, collect, and audit. Macro production units in the patient financial services department include the following:

- inpatient preadmissions
- inpatient admissions

- inpatient discharges

- inpatient billings

- outpatient admissions

- outpatient discharges

- outpatient billings

- outpatient visits

Generally, macro production units do not reflect the amount of resources required to produce a service, nor do they segment a function into separate tasks such as interviewing patients, typing letters, completing admission forms, processing computer bills, or responding to telephone inquiries. Although macro production units are better than no measurement at all, they do not accurately reflect the amount of work or resources required to perform a given service. Therefore, patient financial services managers should employ them cautiously and only when there are no alternatives.[10]

Micro Production Units

Most macro production units can be divided into a number of micro production units. For example, we can divide inpatient admissions into the following micro production units:

- number of preadmission forms completed

- number of patients processed in admitting office *with* preadmission

- number of patients processed in admitting office *without* preadmission

- number of patients interviewed in their rooms

- number of patients escorted or transported to their rooms

- number of contacts with physician's office personnel

- number of physician contacts

- number of Medicare inpatient billings

- number of Medicare outpatient billings

As this example shows, the micro production unit reduces the macro production unit to the measurement that most accurately reflects the amount of resources, such as labor, supplies, equipment, and overhead, required to produce the service.

The micro unit can be employed as a relative value unit (RVU) to weigh the relevant relationship among macro production units that are employed in the same service department. This task is accomplished by establishing a basis from which to measure the amount of resources required to produce the macro units.[11]

For example, assume that a series of time and motion studies determined that the number of minutes of clerical time required to generate the following macro units is as shown:

Macro Unit	Clerical Time
Unit A	10
Unit B	50
Unit C	75

Further, assume that the following data represents the volume of macro production units generated by two patient financial services clerks:[12]

Macro Unit	Clerk A (Number Produced)	Clerk B (Number Produced)
Unit A	130	50
Unit B	50	55
Unit C	10	35
Total Units	190	140

At first glance it would appear that Clerk A has a greater volume of productivity than Clerk B, because A's total macro production units exceed B's by 50. The fallacy in making this conclusion is that we did not assign weighted values to these production units. By assigning clerical time as the relative value to the appropriate macro units, they assume a common relativity; we can then classify them as micro units or RVUs.[13]

A comparative analysis of Clerk A's and Clerk B's productivity follows:

Micro Unit	Value	Clerk A Macro	Clerk A Micro	Clerk B Macro	Clerk B Micro
Unit A	10	130	1,300	50	500
Unit B	50	50	2,500	55	2,750
Unit C	75	10	750	35	2,625
Total Units		190	4,550	140	5,875
Average Micro Units per Macro Unit		23.95		41.96	

If the macro unit is used to measure productivity, Clerk A appears to be more productive than Clerk B by 50 units; when the micro production unit methodology is used, however, Clerk B has 1,325 micro units of greater production efficiency. It can be concluded from this analysis that Clerk B is producing, on the average, a more complicated type of service, because B's average number of micro units per macro unit is 41.96, exceeding Clerk A's average of 23.95 by 18.01.[14]

In summary, using the micro unit as a relative value unit establishes measurements of relativity between macro units according to the amount of resources required to produce the units. This method eliminates much of the distortion inherent in production ratios, thereby laying the groundwork for accurate rate setting,[15] which is covered in chapter 9.

Currently, there is no micro production unit for the patient financial services department that is generally accepted in the healthcare industry. For that matter, there is no clear-cut, universally recognized list of functions performed by the department. It is important, therefore, that patient financial services managers and their employees select an appropriate macro and/or micro production unit(s) for each departmental position and use them consistently.

Selecting Production Units

The single most common and workable ratio for evaluating the patient financial services department is the number of days of average daily revenue uncollected. However, it is not appropriate to use only this index to evaluate department employee performance. In fact, there is no single production unit or ratio that effectively measures the productivity of patient financial services personnel. The department has many unique positions with exclusive tasks; consequently, most of the positions should have their own production units or sets of units.

Managers should use the following criteria for selecting any production unit:

- can relate to both fixed and variable behavior of the resources used (see next paragraph)

- has minimal susceptibility to variables other than volume of work performed

- is easily understood by employees and management

- incurs minimal clerical cost; i.e., easy to identify, record, and collect

- is easily audited and verified for accuracy

- is relatively inexpensive to compute and process

When patient financial services managers begin to select production units, they may find it necessary to select more than one unit for certain positions in the department to account for the fixed and variable components of the functions that make up those positions. Here is an example:

Position: executive secretary

Fixed Functions	*Production Units*
reception duties	number of days worked
secretarial and clerical duties	number of days worked
ordering and storing supplies	number of days worked
messenger duties	number of days worked
maintaining work and reception area	number of days worked
placing and answering telephone calls	number of days worked

Variable Functions	*Production Units*
dictation	number of times performed (frequency)
typing and transcribing letters	number of times performed (frequency)
typing, transcribing, and distributing memos	number of times performed (frequency)
filing	number of times performed (frequency)

Other production units might include the following:

Position	*Production Units*
inpatient admitting clerk	number of inpatient admissions processed
outpatient admitting clerk	number of outpatients processed
billing clerk	number of bills processed by payer; i.e., Medicare, Medicaid, commercial insurance, etc.
cashier	number of cash receipts processed
collection clerk	number of patient account guarantors contacted by (1) mail, and (2) telephone

Managers must remember to establish a standard of acceptable performance for each production unit they identify. For example:

Production Units	*Performance Standard*
number of letters typed	no typographical errors
number of bills processed	98 percent require no resubmission
number of cash receipts processed	maximum of $100 surplus or shortage per year

Every job description form should list the functions the position includes and the acceptable standards of performance for each of those functions (see exhibit 5–1).

EXHIBIT 5–1
Job Description Form

Memorial Medical Center
Anytown, U.S.A.

JOB DESCRIPTION

Job Title _____   Job Code Number _____

Immediate Supervisor _____   Job or Labor Grade _____

Department _____   Chart of Accounts Number _____

Primary Functions   *Standards of Performance*

1.   1.
2.   2.
3.   3.
4.   4.
5.   5.

Secondary Functions   *Standards of Performance*

1.   1.
2.   2.
3.   3.
4.   4.

Job Qualifications

1.   3.
2.   4.

Approved by: _____   Reviewed with employee: _____

Title: _____   Date: _____ 19_____

Date: _____ 19_____

Employee's signature: _____

Reviewer's signature: _____

The Production Unit's Uses

The production unit has five primary uses in the patient financial services department:

>   1.   establishing departmental staffing requirements and data for budgetary control

2. monitoring and evaluating departmental and employee performance

3. creating the basis for employee incentive payment plans

4. allocating costs to user departments

5. as a relative value unit, creating the basis for determining cost per production unit for rate setting (see chapter 9)

In selecting each production unit, managers and the affected employees must be satisfied that the unit is capable of the functions listed above and meets all the criteria mentioned earlier. Employee involvement in selecting and approving the production units is critical to the productivity improvement program.

Staffing and Budgetary Control

In establishing staffing requirements, patient financial services managers must determine the minimum number of positions that must be filled to start doing business. These positions, which form the fixed or core component of the department staff, might include the following:

Core Positions	Number Required
patient financial services manager	1.0
executive secretary	1.0
inpatient admitting supervisor	1.0
outpatient admitting supervisor	1.0
head cashier	1.0
billing and collection supervisor	1.0
total core positions	6.0

The number of core positions should not change when departmental work volume varies until that volume variance becomes substantial enough to warrant a step-variable or part-time employee (see chapter 4).

The department's variable positions accommodate most increases in work volume (for example, the number of patient admissions). These positions might include the following:

- billing clerks

- admitting clerks

- collection clerks

- cashiers

- file clerks

Managers determine the required number of variable positions the department needs by using the volume of work or production units to be produced as they relate to the positions' production standards. For example, assume that the following production standards have been established:

Variable Positions	Production Standards
billing clerk	1,000 accounts billed per month
admitting clerk	30 inpatient and outpatient admissions per day
collection clerk	500 accounts followed per month
cashier	50 inpatient and outpatient discharges processed per day
file clerk	100 inpatient and outpatient discharges processed per day

Further, assume that the medical center has the following volumes of production units during an average month:

- number of accounts: 9,000

- number of admissions: 3,000

- number of inpatient and outpatient discharges: 3,100

Table 5–1 depicts the staffing requirement that the above data would produce. To summarize the data presented in the table, the staffing requirement to cope with the hypothetical volume would be as follows:

(a) Positions	(b) Number of Positions	(c) Average Weekly Hours	(d) Number of Hours (b×c=d)	(e) Average Hourly Wage	(f) Total Monthly Budget Expense (d×e=f)
Fixed	6.0	40	240.0	$17.55	$4,212.00
Variable	21.3	40	852.0	5.15	4,393.60
Total	27.3		1,092.0		$8,605.60

Another approach managers can use in determining the staffing requirements of the patient financial services department is the volume-range method illustrated in figure 5–1. This method establishes relevant ranges of activity and identifies a fixed number of staff members to serve this range. For example:

Relevant Range of Activity (Number of Accounts)	Number of Billing Clerks Required
0–3,000	5
3,001–5,000	6
5,001–7,000	7
7,001–8,500	8
8,501–9,500	9
9,501–11,000	10
11,001–13,000	11

TABLE 5–2
Summary Salary Performance Analysis

Memorial Medical Center
Anytown, U.S.A.

Patient Financial Services Department
SUMMARY SALARY PERFORMANCE ANALYSIS
For the Month of June 19x1

	Standard Rate	Target Budget	Control Budget	Actual Performance	Control/Actual Variance: Fav. (Unfav.) $	%
Volume						
Accounts		9,000	8,750	8,750	–0–	–0–
Admissions		3,000	2,875	2,875	–0–	–0–
Discharges		3,100	2,950	2,950	–0–	–0–
Fixed Salaries						
Patient Financial Services Manager		$ 2,500	$ 2,500	$ 2,500	–0–	–0–
Executive Secretary		1,000	1,000	1,100	$(100)	(10.0)
Inpatient Admitting Supervisor		1,200	1,200	1,200	–0–	–0–
Outpatient Admitting Supervisor		1,200	1,200	1,100	100	8.3
Head Cashier		1,000	1,000	1,000	–0–	–0–
Billing/Collection Supervisor		1,200	1,200	1,200	–0–	–0–
Total Fixed Salaries		$ 8,100	$ 8,100	$ 8,100	–0–	(1.7)
Variable Salaries						
Billing Clerks	$.200	$ 1,800	$ 1,750	$ 1,850	$(100)	(5.7)
Admitting Clerks	.211	634	607	650	(43)	(7.1)
Collection Clerks	.147	1,320	1,286	1,250	36	2.8
Cashier	.155	480	457	480	(23)	(5.0)
File Clerks	.052	160	153	175	(22)	(14.4)
Total Variable Salaries		$ 4,394	$ 4,253	$ 4,405	$(152)	(3.6)
Total Fixed and Variable Salaries		$12,494	$12,353	$12,505	$(152)	(1.2)%

	Target	Actual	Variance Number	Variance Percent
Accounts	9,000	8,750	(250)	(2.7)
Admissions	3,000	2,875	(125)	(4.2)
Discharges	3,100	2,950	(150)	(4.8)

An unfavorable volume variance exists for each of the three production units used in the example. To adjust the target budget to compensate for these volume variances, a control budget* must be established that indicates the actual work volumes experienced; thus, there are never any volume variances between the control budget and the actual volumes.

Comparing fixed salary expenses is the second step of the departmental performance evaluation process. Because these expenses do not change with volume variances, management can simply transfer the target budget expenses to the control budget. Since most of these employees receive a fixed salary instead of an hourly wage, variances in this expense category should be minimal.

The third step in performance evaluation is comparing the actual variable salary expense with the control budget. The control budget uses a standard salary rate. The formula for the rate is

$$\frac{\text{Total Variable Salary Expense}}{\text{Total Relevant Production Units}} = \text{Standard Variable Salary Rate}$$

Graphs are an effective and clear method of communicating performance analysis information; they are also useful for displaying trends, projections, and forecasts. Figures 5–2 and 5–3 exemplify the use of bar graphs to illustrate the differences between the target budget, the control budget, and actual performance in volumes and salary expenses based on the information given in table 5–2.

Evaluating Employee Performance

The production unit enables patient financial services managers to evaluate each employee objectively. Since the production unit is a quantitative measurement of an employee's production or work, management can compare the actual units readily and objectively with a predetermined employee performance level.

Management's first step in this application of production units is to work with the employee to be evaluated. Both the employee and the patient finan-

---

* A control budget adjusts the standard rates in a fixed budget to the actual volume of work. As a result, it eliminates variances caused by volume fluctuations (see chapter 4).

FIGURE 5–2
Summary Performance Analysis of Volumes

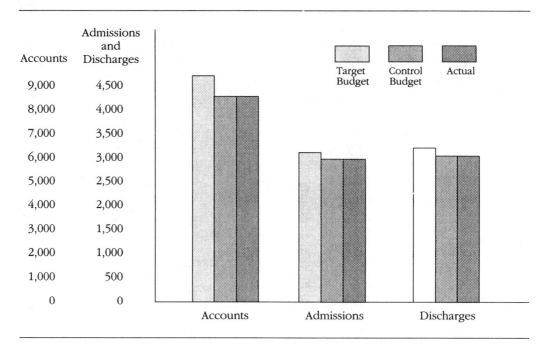

FIGURE 5–3
Summary Performance Analysis of Salary Expenses

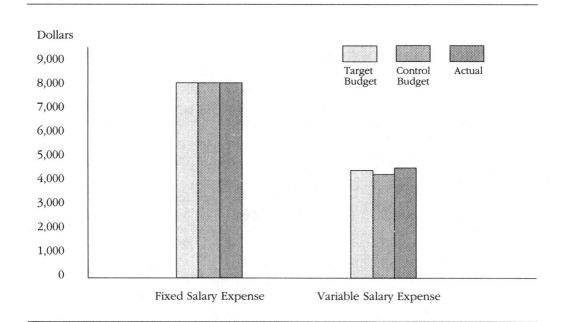

cial services manager must identify the production unit or units that best measure the tasks the employee performs. Once they select these units, the manager and subordinate must mutually accept these units as the basis for performance evaluation.

For illustrative purposes, assume that the billing clerks have agreed that the production unit to be used in evaluating their performance should be number of accounts billed. Also assume that both the clerical staff and management have accepted 300 accounts per eight-hour workday as a reasonable production standard. (Specific methods used to develop production standards will be discussed later in this chapter.)

On a document similar to the one shown in figure 5–4, the patient financial services manager records and monitors the predetermined production standard and the actual performance for each billing clerk. In this example, the manager computed the average number of accounts billed per week so that actual performance could be evaluated even before the month ended. The average weekly actual performances were as follows:

	Accounts Billed		
	1st Week	*2nd Week*	*3rd Week*
Monday	250	350	300
Tuesday	275	325	325
Wednesday	265	275	300
Thursday	285	250	275
Friday	315	275	325
Total	1,390	1,475	1,525
Average	278	295	305

By computing the weekly average actual performance, patient financial services managers can readily recognize problem employees and help them improve their performance. Management should review the employee performance record at least once a month and preferably once a week; each review period should include constructive suggestions for the employee's productivity improvement. This discussion should not be limited to the manager giving suggestions; rather, these review sessions should be two-way exchanges of ideas on how to improve productivity.

Developing Employee Incentive Plans

Because legislatively controlled healthcare programs, such as Medicare and Medicaid, frequently add to healthcare providers' struggles with increased accounts receivable, slowed cash flow, and reimbursement based more upon government budgetary constraints than on the services' economic costs,[17] it is becoming increasingly obvious that only the efficient healthcare organizations will survive. Healthcare systems whose managers can improve productivity, motivate employees, and reward efficiency will be the ones that con-

FIGURE 5–4
Employee Performance Record

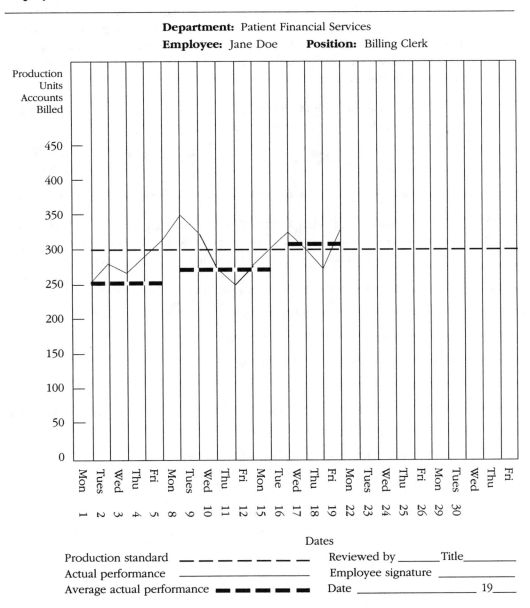

Department: Patient Financial Services
Employee: Jane Doe　　**Position:** Billing Clerk

Production standard ⎯ ⎯ ⎯ ⎯ ⎯ ⎯ ⎯　Reviewed by _____Title_____
Actual performance ⎯⎯⎯⎯⎯⎯⎯⎯　Employee signature _____
Average actual performance ▬ ▬ ▬ ▬ ▬　Date _____ 19____

tinue to operate. For this reason, it is imperative that patient financial services managers seriously consider implementing an employee incentive plan that rewards the efficient employee and motivates the less-efficient employee.

The healthcare industry uses a variety of employee incentive plans: some reward only the department manager, some reward the entire department staff, and others reward individual high performers. Ideally, the cornerstone of employee incentive plans should be some method of rewarding the high performer. Managers need to remember, however, that rewards based solely on individual performance reinforce the employee's view of the healthcare organization as a series of unrelated parts. To combat this perception, management should gear rewards (wages, benefits, vacations, promotions, etc.) and penalties (disciplinary actions) as much as possible to reinforce those human activities that

- increase the individual's awareness of and responsibility for as much of the total organization as possible;

- enlarge the experience of interdependence with others and with the whole; and

- increase the control that the whole has over its destiny.[18]

After establishing what they believe constitutes routine and incentive reward levels of performance, managers typically express these levels in terms of production units per person per workday or paid hour. For example:

- admitting—weighted admissions per paid hour

- credit—weighted admissions per paid hour

- cashier—weighted discharges and receipts per workday

- billing—accounts billed per workday

To illustrate the use of the production unit in an employee incentive plan, assume that management established the following production levels for the billing clerks:

- routine level—285 accounts billed per workday

- incentive reward level—300 accounts billed per workday

Using the actual average performance data given earlier, patient financial services managers can compute employee compensation in the following manner:

(a) Week	(b) Actual Performances	(c) Routine Performance Level	(d) Performance Factor (b ÷ c = d)	(e) Regular Hourly Wage	(f) Incentive Hourly Wage (d × e = f)
1st	278	285	97.5%	$5.00	$4.88
2nd	295	285	103.5%	$5.00	$5.18
3rd	305	285	107.0%	$5.00	$5.35

Managers can design employee incentive plans in numerous ways. However, no matter how sophisticated they may be, these plans cannot substitute for effective leadership.

Allocating Costs

Managers can use the production unit to allocate costs in the healthcare organization's cost-finding process. *Cost finding,* which is discussed in chapter 8, is the estimate, based upon statistical data, of the total cost of each revenue-producing department, including its proportionate share of the overhead expenses. This total cost is then divided by the total number of departmental outputs, or production units, to calculate the cost of a single departmental service.[19] The accuracy of cost finding results depends to a great degree on the selection of the production unit and the order of distribution. Although no general consensus exists in the healthcare industry as to which production unit is the most appropriate base for cost allocation, each healthcare organization should strive for the degree of sophistication it can justify economically in view of its mission, goals, and objectives. Management's consistent application of the production unit is just as important as its choice of unit in effective cost finding.

Patient financial services managers are responsible for selecting and/or recommending production units that most equitably measure services rendered by the patient financial services department and in turn maximize the healthcare facility's reimbursement for those services. Since cost allocation is an integral part of the rate-setting process, it is imperative that managers test the production units thoroughly to ensure that they accurately represent the department's total costs. Equally important is that the production unit managers select for cost allocation does not have to be the same as the production unit they use to evaluate employee performance. Indeed, in all probability the units will not be the same.

Developing Production Standards

Managers have numerous systems at their disposal to develop production standards. These systems fall into two major groups:

1. predetermined

2. involvement

The predetermined production standard approach uses motion time measurement (MTM) studies that usually require trained industrial or management engineering personnel to perform detailed studies. Since this approach is highly detailed, it is very sensitive to any change in work procedure and must be adjusted accordingly. This approach does have the advantage of being a proven scientific method. However, at times, its highly impersonal, scientific procedures can be extremely costly and relatively difficult to implement. Many employees feel that the production standards resulting from this method are not relevant to their work because they were not involved in establishing the standards.

The involvement approach to developing production standards requires the active participation of the employees who will be evaluated. Historical information, self-logging, and time studies of relevant functions are some of the techniques managers use in this approach.

Employees accept production standards established with their involvement more readily because

- the standards are derived from actual department performance;

- the department personnel actually participate with their manager in developing the standards; and

- the time standards and the system as a whole are relatively easy to understand.

Also, according to Berman, Weeks, and Kukla, the more challenging an objective, be it a production standard or another area, the higher is employee performance, so long as employees joined management in setting and agreeing to this objective. If an objective is too easy, employees are not as motivated to achieve. Similarly, if it is too difficult, employees will ignore it. Only if they accept the difficult objective and make it their level of aspiration does it tend to lift performance, these authors conclude.[20]

How to Develop Production Standards

Step 1. Develop the normal task time per production unit for each employee position. The normal time is the average time a qualified employee takes under normal circumstances to perform a task or group of tasks, not including normal personal, fatigue, and delay (P, F,&D) time.

a. Classify all tasks into productive work for each production unit and respective P,F,&D factor (see table 5–3). Complete this activity before beginning the employees on the daily task self-logging process (see exhibit 5–2).

b. Calculate the normal time for each task by purging the non-representative logged time from the raw data (see the Daily Employee Self-logging Worksheet shown in exhibit 5–2) and computing the average of all the logged task times (see tables 5–4 and 5–5). The average, which is calculated by dividing the total of all the individual task times by the number of occurrences, represents the normal time it should take an average experienced employee to perform the task. It should not require any adjustment unless there is a change in department methods, procedures, or equipment.

c. Develop task frequency mix factors to indicate the number of times a task is performed per production unit by paid employees on a normal shift (see tables 5–4 and 5–5). (A task that constitutes part of a production unit need not be performed every time the unit occurs.) This percentage figure reflects the number of times the task is performed.

d. Multiply normal task times by frequency/mix factors to compute the average normal task time per production unit. For example, if an admitting clerk admits 50 percent of all patients admitted on a normal shift and the normal task time is ten minutes, the normal task time average per production unit—that is, number of admissions—is 50 percent of ten minutes, or five minutes.

TABLE 5–3
Departmental Task List

Memorial Medical Center
Anytown, U.S.A.

DEPARTMENTAL TASK LIST
Department: Admitting   **Section:** Inpatient Admitting

Task No.	Task Description	Production Unit
10	file admissions, pull preadmissions, and maintain files	patient admitted
11	log inpatient admission	patient admitted
12	type and distribute reports	patient admitted
13	order and store supplies	week
15	perform secretarial and clerical duties	week
16	perform receptionist duties	week
17	perform messenger duties	week
20	clean up area and assist others	week
21	answer telephone and complete telephone reports	week

EXHIBIT 5–2
Daily Employee Self-logging Worksheet

Memorial Medical Center
Anytown, U.S.A.

DAILY EMPLOYEE SELF-LOGGING WORKSHEET

Employee Name _____ Section _____
Position _____ Date _____ 19 ____
Department _____

Task No.	Task Description and Equipment	Units	Start	Stop	Minutes

Time

Total

TABLE 5–4

Standard Time Development Worksheet for Logging Inpatient Admissions

Memorial Medical Center
Anytown, U.S.A.

STANDARD TIME DEVELOPMENT WORKSHEET FOR LOGGING INPATIENT ADMISSIONS

Department: Admitting   **Section:** Inpatient Admitting
Production Unit: Patients Admitted   **Employee Position:** Admitting Clerk

Date: _____ 19____

No.	TASK Description	Normal Minutes per Task	Frequency per Production Unit	Refer to Matrix	Normal Minutes per Production Unit
11	log inpatient admissions	.528	1.00	2A	.528
12	type and distribute reports	3.451	1.00	3A	3.451
10	file admissions, pull pre-admissions, and maintain files	4.579	1.00	4A	4.579

Total Normal Minutes per Production Unit	8.558

Standard Hours per Production Unit (Including 6.4% P,F,&D Factor)	.152

Step 2. Using the standard time development sheets (tables 5–4 and 5–5), calculate standard production unit time for each employee classification. Standard production unit time is the total of all normal task time per production unit plus an allowance for personal, fatigue, and delay (P,F,&D) time. To calculate standard production unit time, follow these steps:

a. Total the normal task times for all the tasks that make up the production unit.

b. Develop a P,F,&D factor to convert normal time to standard time. The P,F,&D factor calculation is based on actual time recorded during a self-logging period, supervisor's estimates, and hospital policy guidelines. The formula is as follows:

$$\text{P,F,\&D Factor} = \frac{\text{Personal Time}}{\text{Reported Productive Time} + \text{Delay Time}}$$

TABLE 5–5

Standard Time Development Worksheet

Memorial Medical Center
Anytown, U.S.A.

STANDARD TIME DEVELOPMENT WORKSHEET

Department: *Admitting*   Section: *Inpatient Admitting*
Production Unit: *Week*   Employee Position: *Admitting Clerk*
                                            Date: _____ 19____

No.	TASK Description	Normal Minutes per Task	Frequency per Production Unit	Refer to Matrix	Normal Minutes per Production Unit
13	order and store supplies				
15	perform secretarial and clerical duties	5.323	1.00		5.323
16	perform receptionist duties				
17	perform messenger duties	.572	1.00		.572
20	clean up area and assist others	.288	1.00		.288
21	answer telephone and complete telephone reports	.761	1.00		.761

Total Normal Minutes per Production Unit	6.944

Standard Hours per Production Unit (Including 6.4% P,F,&D Factor)	.123

c. To compute the standard production unit time, multiply the total normal task time by the P,F,&D factor:

$$\begin{array}{ccc} \text{Standard Production} & \text{Normal} & \text{P,F,\&D} \\ \text{Unit Time} \quad = & \text{Production Time} \quad \times & \text{Factor} \end{array}$$

Step 3. Since standard minutes may be too cumbersome for developing staffing requirements, convert the standard minutes to standard hours as follows:

$$\begin{array}{c} \text{Standard} \\ \text{Production Unit Hour} \ = \end{array} \ \dfrac{\text{Total Standard Production Unit Minutes}}{60}$$

Step 4. Since employees cannot always perform their tasks in the normal time, nor be engaged in productive tasks 100 percent of the working day, a performance factor is calculated to make allowances for

- unavoidable delays, such as waiting for a patient, doctor, elevator, etc.;

- normal fluctuations in the work flow; and

- abnormal occurrences encountered during the performance of productive work.

The formula for calculating the performance factor is

$$\text{Performance Factor} = \frac{\text{Normal Productive Time}}{\text{Total Reported Productive Time} + \text{Delay Time}}$$

Provided there have been no significant changes in departmental procedures or methods, the performance factor's unique feature is that it allows patient financial services managers to adjust expectancy levels of performance to the production standards. For example, management could initially establish expectancy levels at 60 percent of production standards. Next time period the expectancy levels could be adjusted to 70 percent, or any other percentage that the manager and the employees believe to be the most accurate and fair expectancy level of performance.

Step 5. Next, compute the adjusted standard hours required (ASHR). The ASHR represents the total paid work hours that a department or section should require to perform a given volume of work over a specified period of time during the regularly scheduled shift (excluding on-call and non-normal hours worked). (See table 5–6.) The formula to compute the ASHR is

$$\text{ASHR} = \frac{\text{Total Standard Hours Required}}{\text{Performance Factor}}$$

Step 6. Identify and total all unmeasurable time, such as on-call hours, and all other time that employees must spend or use even if the work load is negligible.

Step 7. Determine the target production level (TPL) for each employee classification in each department or section. The TPL is the result of the calculations of Steps 5 and 6. The formula is

TABLE 5–6
Performance Factor Calculation Worksheet

Memorial Medical Center
Anytown, U.S.A.

PERFORMANCE FACTOR CALCULATION WORKSHEET

Department: Admitting   **Section**: Inpatient Admitting

Date: _____ 19____

Number of Personnel Measured: Full-time _____

Part-time _____

Unmeasured: Administrative _____

Physician _____

		Hours
1.	Total Paid Hours for All Measured Personnel	16,622
2.	Less: Hours Paid for but Not Measured	
	Vacation	
	Holiday	
	Illness, Absence	
	Others*	
	On-Call—Not Worked	
	On-Call—Worked	
	Total #2	1,511
3.	Total Hours Applied to Measured Work	
	(#1 Less #2) Total #3	15,111
4.	Standard Hours Produced—All Employee Classifications:	

Reporting Unit (Specify)	Standard Hours per Reporting Units (a)	Number of Reporting Units (b)	Standard Hours Produced (a × b)
Inpatient Admissions	.152	46,800	7,114
Weeks	123.1	52	6,401

	Hours
Total Hours Produced #4	13,515
Variance Hours (#3 Less #4)	1,596
5. Performance factor $\left(\dfrac{\text{Total \#4}}{\text{Total \#3}}\right)$	89.4

*Example: Special assignment hours, such as attending conference outside
healthcare facility by a "measured" employee.

$$\begin{array}{ccc} \text{Adjusted Standard} \\ \text{Hours Produced} \end{array} + \begin{array}{ccc} \text{Other Scheduled} \\ \text{Staff Hours} \end{array} + \begin{array}{ccc} \text{On-Call Scheduled} \\ \text{Hours} \end{array}$$

$$= \text{TPL for All Reporting Units}$$

Please note that management should not use the self-logging, employee involvement method of production standard development and productivity improvement as a tool for external evaluation and comparison of performance. Rather, it is an internal management tool that enables patient financial services managers to measure and evaluate employee and departmental performance. Again, graphs are an excellent medium for recording and monitoring production standards and performance. Figure 5–5 shows how a graph conveys this information.

In summary, the scientific exactness of a production standard is not as important as its acceptance and consistent use by both supervisor and subordinate. The key point is that even loosely defined production standards that are mutually accepted, used, and refined are preferable to nonexistent standards or employee-rejected, albeit scientifically accurate, standards. Production standards are merely a means of measuring actual performance against what the patient financial services manager desires and expects from a given work effort or dollar expenditure. Productivity is the first test of management's competence, as well as labor's competence.

The Need for Productivity Improvement

Since 1980 factory productivity has improved by 44 percent as U.S. manufacturers responded to foreign competition by slashing costs and restructuring their operations. During the same period in the nonmanufacturing or service sector, productivity rose only 1.4 percent. However, the rate of productivity in the healthcare industry generally has been negative.[21]

To combat this problem, the healthcare industry's primary challenge for the next decade needs to be productivity improvement. It is unlikely that major increases in federal and state funding for health care will take place soon, at least not in a way that greatly aids the private payer, who often bears the brunt of cost increases in the health sector. Further, U.S. firms contend that out-of-control healthcare costs hamper their ability to compete in international markets.[22]

Healthcare managers, then, must control, if not reduce, these spiraling costs; if they don't act, the government will. Because it decreases operating costs and consequently the cost to the consumer, improved productivity is one solution to the rising cost of health care, if not the only solution. And the organization that works earnestly on its output will soon have the means to reward its staff.[23]

FIGURE 5–5
Production Trend Chart

For the Period from ⎯⎯⎯⎯⎯⎯ 19⎯⎯ to ⎯⎯⎯⎯⎯⎯ 19⎯⎯

Department: Admitting   **Section:** Inpatient Admitting
Production Unit: Inpatient Admissions   **Employee Position:** Admitting Clerk

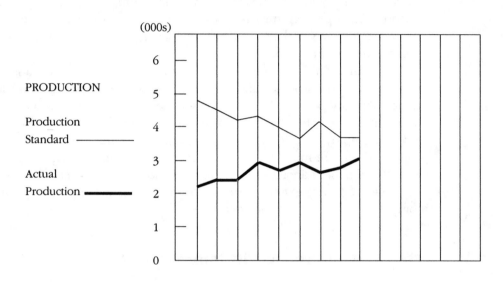

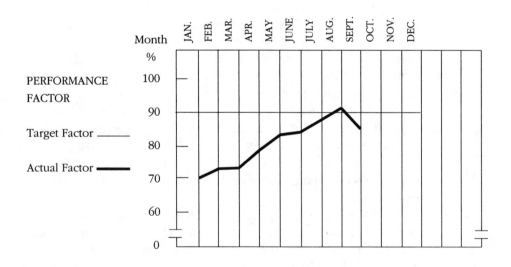

NOTES

1. Peter F. Drucker, *The Frontiers of Management: Where Tomorrow's Decisions Are Being Shaped Today* (New York: Dutton Signet, a division of Penguin Books USA, Inc., 1986), 120.

2. Drucker, *Frontiers of Management*, 130.

3. Drucker, *Frontiers of Management*, 131.

4. Allen G. Herkimer Jr., *Understanding Hospital Financial Management*, 2nd ed. (Rockville, Md.: Aspen Publishers, Inc., 1986), 91.

5. Herkimer, *Understanding Hospital Financial Management*, 90.

6. Herkimer, *Understanding Hospital Financial Management*, 90.

7. Herkimer, *Understanding Hospital Financial Management*, 90.

8. Drucker, *Frontiers of Management*, 220.

9. Allen G. Herkimer Jr., *Understanding Health Care Budgeting* (Rockville, Md.: Aspen Publishers, Inc., 1988), 47.

10. Herkimer, *Understanding Health Care Budgeting*, 49.

11. Herkimer, *Understanding Health Care Budgeting*, 49.

12. Herkimer, *Understanding Health Care Budgeting*, 49.

13. Herkimer, *Understanding Health Care Budgeting*, 49.

14. Herkimer, *Understanding Health Care Budgeting*, 49–50.

15. Herkimer, *Understanding Health Care Budgeting*, 50.

16. Herkimer, *Understanding Hospital Financial Management*, 96.

17. *"Definition of and Payment for Uncompensated Services"* and *"Special Problems of Disproportionate Share,"* a monograph series ed. (Westchester, Ill.: Healthcare Financial Management Association, 1987), 12.

18. Chris Argyris, *Integrating the Individual and the Organization*, 2nd ed. (New Brunswick, N.J.: Transaction Publishers, 1990), 249, 250.

19. Allen G. Herkimer Jr., *Understanding Health Care Accounting* (Rockville, Md.: Aspen Publishers, Inc., 1989), 197.

20. Howard J. Berman, Lewis E. Weeks, and Steven F. Kukla, *The Financial Management of Hospitals,* 7th ed. (Ann Arbor, Mich.: Health Administration Press Division of the Foundation of the American College of Healthcare Executives, 1990), 513.

21. William O. Cleverley, "Productivity Improvement Is a Must," *Healthcare Bottom Line* 8, no. 4 (May 1991), 1.

22. Cleverley, "Productivity Improvement Is a Must," 1.

23. Drucker, *Frontiers of Management*, 269.

CHAPTER 6

The Budgetary
Control System

An effective budgetary control system keeps the overall healthcare organization and its departments on their planned courses of action: achieving departmental and organizational missions, goals, objectives, and performance standards. To establish a system this far-reaching, management must plan carefully for its effective implementation. This chapter will identify and describe tactics patient financial services managers can employ in developing their department's and healthcare organization's budgetary control systems, from promoting employee participation to selecting the appropriate budgetary type and approach.

The Budgetary Control System: An Overview

The *budgetary control system* is a process that guides and assists all levels of healthcare management in achieving its established financial and statistical mission, goals, objectives, and performance standards. An effectively installed budgetary control system helps to assure management that it is on its planned course of action and that it is realizing planned results from operations.[1] The *budget,* the foundation of the budgetary control system, is a formal plan for future operations expressed quantitatively and serving as a basis of measurement for the subsequent control of these operations.[2]

To obtain the correct perspective on the budgetary control system, it is necessary to examine several key words and phrases:

- process

- assist

- achieve

- financial and statistical

- performance standards

- planned course

- results

- formal plan

- future operations

The word *process* implies that budgetary control is an ongoing, day-to-day series of functions and tasks that management must continually perform, evaluate, and/or monitor to identify weaknesses and strengths within the budgetary control system. The system itself, a management tool, has evolved into a management style that keeps all managers mindful of their respective department's mission, goals, objectives, and other desired results in light of their facility's overall mission, goals, and objectives.

The Importance of Staff Involvement

For the budgetary control system to be completely effective, all levels of the department's managers must participate actively in the budgetary control process. An effective program not only assists in management development and aids in stabilizing the department's financial and productivity positions; it also promotes cooperation, mutual understanding, and sharing of the decision-making process. Coordinating management's involvement in the budgetary control process with employee participation will enable the department to meet the demand for improved patient care through dynamic, imaginative, and concerned management.[3] The budgetary control system assists managers in obtaining the results they have planned for; however, it cannot achieve these results without the involvement of people.

Many budgetary program shortcomings stem from poor human relations and improper attitudes on the part of management. In the case of weak management, executives often use management tools such as budgets as a means of unilaterally imposing performance expectations on employees. A technique in and of itself, however, can do nothing; the individuals using it determine its effective or poor administration. Managers must base their budgetary control system upon such motivational essentials as recognition of accomplishments, consideration for the rights of individuals, fairness, and mutual trust.

The human element of budgeting, or "humantology," is the tempered and responsive management application of a structured, individual assignment of functional responsibilities within a relevant authority range based on the principles of

- mutual trust and faith among and between managers and staff members, and

- knowledgeable and active participation of these individuals in the endeavor to achieve the organization's established mission, goals, and objectives.[4]

The real values of participation in the budgetary control process at all management and employee levels, aside from effective and productive planning and budgeting, are the resulting psychological benefits—a high degree of employee participation is conducive to higher morale, increased initiative and incentive, and a more creative work environment.

Managers must be ever-vigilant against insufficient employee participation in the budgetary control process. When this condition exists, the primary elements of humantology, faith and trust, are jeopardized. If employees suspect that managers are placating or ignoring them, then management's credibility is at stake.

As Seawell points out, despite the healthcare industry's increasing use of sophisticated statistical and mathematical techniques in conjunction with computers in financial management and accounting, managers must keep in mind that a budget is merely a device to control costs through people. He warns that the most advanced budgetary program will actually tend to decrease efficiency unless management ranks the human element equally with the program's technical aspects. In other words, no plan, no matter how scientific, will work unless people are willing to *make* it work.[5]

Identifying and Quantifying Desired Results

Achievement is the hallmark of successful planning, but patient financial services managers will never know what their department has accomplished unless they identify and quantify specific goals and objectives. Once they detail these goals and objectives in this manner, they can properly evaluate departmental and employee performance for a given time period in terms of whether desired results were achieved. Although the budgetary control system is not exclusively financial—it has many other components, such as goals and objectives—it is the quantitative statistics, such as patient days and patient admissions, that never change. The net result of the budgetary control system, then, is a documented financial plan based on sound logic and firm, quantifiable statistical bases.

Performance or production standards, which managers establish before employees actually perform a specific task, are another way to describe managers' desired results for the department and each staff member. They also form the basis on which management evaluates actual performance. To organize and staff effectively, patient financial services managers must start with proper delegation and then establish the quality level at which they expect individuals to perform. These expectancy levels of performance or production standards are discussed in detail in chapter 5.

Multilateral vs. Unilateral Approaches to Budgeting

The budgetary control system charts a planned course of action with a set of planned results, two things that top management justifiably expects from each department head. Patient financial services managers should plot this course of action for their department as well. To plan effectively, patient financial services managers must take the multilateral approach to budgeting by seeking input from the supervisors reporting to them and indirectly from their subordinates. It is foolhardy for patient financial services managers to plan their department's course of action unilaterally, identifying desired results without full consultation with, and agreement of, their supervisory staff. The budgetary control system requires teamwork, which calls for a multilateral approach.

Managing for Economic Results

Managing for economic results begins by analyzing result areas—in other words, defining the output or services that the department generates. For example, in the patient financial services department, output units might include the following:

- patients admitted

- bills processed

- interviews conducted

According to Drucker, concentration is the key to economic results; managers need to focus their efforts on the smallest number of products or services that will produce the largest amount of revenue. He also observes that managers must minimize the amount of attention they devote to services that are not cost-effective because their volume is too small or too splintered.[6] The word *concentration* is key in the management-for-results concept. Before they can begin the concentration process, however, managers must identify desired results. This step is a prerequisite for the entire budgetary control system.

The Budget

In most healthcare organizations, an approved budget is a formal financial plan and course of action that the facility's board of trustees (directors) and chief executive officer refer to department managers, including the patient financial services manager, for implementation. Ideally, patient financial services managers have been actively involved in identifying their department's mission, goals, objectives, volume, and financial and performance standards for incorporation into the comprehensive budget.

The last key word in understanding the budgetary control system is the word *future* used in our definition of *budget*. Predicting the future entails a considerable amount of risk for the forecaster—in this case, the patient financial services manager. This is especially true when the healthcare system depends on the forecast to know what its cash inflow will be for the next twelve months, the next three years, and so forth. The patient financial services managers' role in this process is critical for two reasons. First, their forecast has a short-term impact on the financial plan of the patient financial services department. Second, and more important, is the forecast's impact on the more sensitive task of projecting the healthcare organization's total cash inflow. Certainly, any major miscalculation will adversely affect the entire organization and its service area and patients. The organization's ultimate survival may very well depend on accurate cash flow forecasting.

To summarize, the budgetary control system is a management process that uses the optimum skills of the healthcare system's entire management team in a well-documented, forward-thinking plan designed to carry out the organization's mission and to achieve its goals and objectives. An essential part of the systemwide strategic plan is the synchronization of each departmental strategic plan with the overall plan.

The Patient Financial Services Managers' Role

All department managers and supervisors must be actively involved in the development of their department's financial plan—the budget. Patient financial services managers should also play a leading role in cash forecasting and management for their entire healthcare organization, a responsibility that is discussed more fully in chapter 10.

The patient financial services manager's position is crucial in the process of setting goals and objectives for the department because it links the plans of the organization's board and administration with the work of the department staff. If the patient financial services manager fails to understand the plan, it will never filter down to each employee correctly. Perhaps the worst situation would occur when the manager understands the plan but fails to communicate appropriate information to the department staff. Effective two-way communication is essential. Without complete and active cooperation, as well as total commitment to the plan on the part of the patient financial services manager and the staff, the budgetary control system cannot succeed. There must be no credibility gap between management and employees.

Patient financial services managers have come to recognize their role as leaders of people, not just as skilled technicians. In this leadership role, managers should be able to distinguish between the goal-oriented employee and the task-oriented employee. The goal-oriented employee does not like close supervision while working but is interested in finding out results. This individual is also eager to accept challenges, wants definite goals, and feels a need to reach objectives. Task-oriented employees, on the other hand, just want to do their particular job and aren't very interested in overall results. By recognizing these differences, patient financial services managers are better equipped to set realistic goals for individual employees and for the department.

Approaches to the Budgetary Control System

Functional Accounting and Budgeting

Broadly speaking, there are two major approaches to the budgetary control system. One approach, functional accounting and budgeting, assigns costs and revenues to a specific function, such as admitting, billing, and collection, without regard to who is responsible for managing the function. Theoretically, the primary purpose of functional accounting and budgeting is to enable the analyst to compare the functional costs of one healthcare organization with the same functional costs in another institution. In theory, the approach seems reasonable; in practice, the approach has proven to be relatively difficult to apply. The functional methodology is usually used by external agencies such as cost commissions to survey and compare a facility's departmental costs with those of similar departments in other healthcare facilities.

Responsibility Accounting and Budgeting

The second approach, responsibility accounting and budgeting, is the most universally accepted budgetary control method in the healthcare industry because its primary purpose is to control and manage costs and revenues. This system allocates costs and revenues in line with the facility's organizational structure and delegation of responsibility and authority. It is based on the premise that each manager should be held accountable for a specific responsibility center and its related controllable costs and revenues.

To illustrate how these two budgeting systems work, assume that the following inpatient and outpatient functions have been identified for the patient financial services department (see figure 6–1):

- preadmission
- admitting
- discharging
- counseling
- billing
- collection

Further assume that a patient service representative (PSR) system organizational structure (see figure 6–2) has replaced the traditional patient financial services department structure (see figure 6–3). In this system, one PSR unit performs all the functions previously handled by separate units such as billing, admitting, and so forth. If management were to use a functional accounting and budgeting system, it would have to reallocate time and related expenses from the PSR responsibility center to an individual functional area. On the other hand, under the responsibility accounting and budgeting

FIGURE 6–1

Functions of the Patient Financial Services Department

Memorial Medical Center
Anytown, U.S.A.

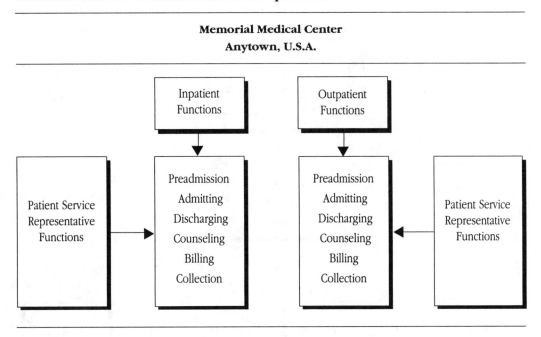

FIGURE 6–2

PSR-Patient Financial Services Department Organizational Structure

Memorial Medical Center
Anytown, U.S.A.

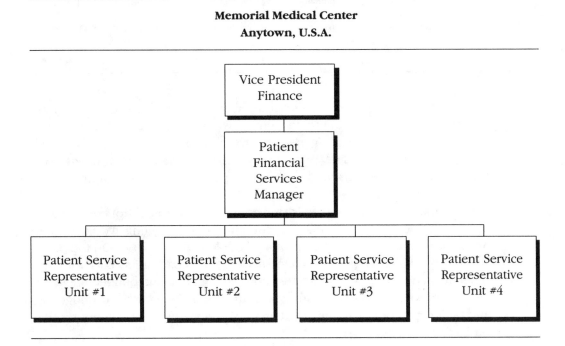

FIGURE 6–3

Traditional Patient Financial Services Department Organizational Structure

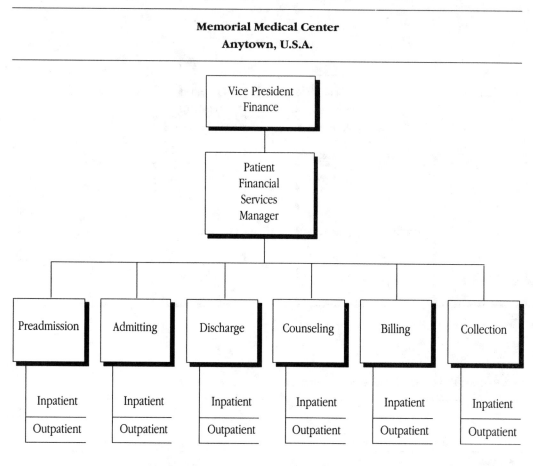

Memorial Medical Center
Anytown, U.S.A.

system, each PSR unit becomes a responsibility center regardless of the facility's organizational structure, and management would hold one person accountable for costs and revenues generated by that center. However, it is totally unacceptable in the budgetary control system for a department manager or supervisor to be responsible for costs incurred or caused by another individual or department.

Assuming that management's primary purpose is to control costs and to operate efficiently, responsibility accounting and budgeting would be the most appropriate budgetary control methodology for it to use. On the other hand, if management is more concerned with comparing its costs with another institution's costs, perhaps functional accounting and budgeting would be the appropriate system. Throughout this book, references to budgeting and budgetary control systems pertain only to responsibility accounting and budgeting.

Budget Types

There are two primary systems of budgeting used in the healthcare setting:

1. fixed or target

2. variable or flexible

The fixed or target budget system does not necessarily distinguish between cost behaviors—that is, fixed, variable, or step-variable—of a department's cost items (see chapter 4). Rather, it considers all costs to be fixed for the budget's projected fixed volume of activity.

The variable or flexible system of budgeting, on the other hand, requires each cost item to be identified as one of three types: fixed, variable, or step-variable. Typically, only fixed and variable costs are identified by this system.

The primary purpose of variable budgeting is to allow the analyst or manager to adjust the variable expense items according to the actual volume of activity. The fixed approach does not allow for this adjustment; consequently, any budget variance resulting from volume changes must be rationalized by the user rather than mathematically adjusted. The application of variable budgeting to the patient financial services department is discussed in chapter 7.

Another way of classifying budgeting systems is based on time. Budgets may be either of two types:

1. fixed-period

2. rolling or moving

The fixed-period approach to budgeting identifies a period of time—for example, one month, one year, or two years—and develops a budget to cover that period of time. A rolling or moving budget deletes the projection for the most recent month, quarter, or year and extends the budget by the corresponding time period. The rolling-budget methodology is especially effective in a department or organization that experiences dynamic growth because management can make adjustments easily and routinely.

Other types of budgets include the following:

- appropriation

- program or project

- zero-base

The appropriation budget is used primarily by government agencies and municipalities. In this approach, the user establishes fixed expenditures for each department or cost center. Expense overruns or underruns cannot be transferred to another department without formal approval. This approach to budgeting is relatively archaic due to its cumbersome methodology and lack of incentive to control costs. Critics of the appropriation budget refer to it as a systematic way to go into debt because the principal thesis behind the system is to spend this year, or lose it next year; witness the federal and state governments. As a result, the appropriation approach to budgetary control does not encourage cost savings, nor does it reward those managers who do or could save costs.

The program budget, also called a project budget, outlines costs and revenues for one specific program; for example, in-house collection of accounts. This approach to budgeting is especially effective when management wants to monitor the costs and revenues of a new program or project. Users of the program budget usually develop it apart from the traditional budgetary process, so it is simply a supplement to the overall budget. The program budget approach is a very effective management tool for determining the cost/benefit of a specific new program or project, but it should never replace the responsibility budgetary control system.[7]

Zero-base budgeting adopts the premise that a department or program will continue only as long as it can justify its existence. The approach has two basic steps:

1. development of decision packages, and

2. ranking of decision packages.

Each decision package identifies the project, department, or unit and includes its mission, goals, objectives, revenues, expenses, and its benefits to the entire organization.[8]

Once management develops decision packages and ranks them in order of priority, it can allocate resources accordingly, funding the most important decision packages whether they are new or existing. It produces the final budget by sorting decision packages approved for funding into appropriate budget units and totaling the revenues and costs of individual packages to produce the budget for each unit or department.[9]

Zero-base budgeting can be a time-consuming process, but it can also be valuable for any floundering healthcare organization that is trying to recover its overall profitability.[10] On the other hand, as Wildavsky points out, this approach builds the budget entirely from the bottom up, thereby divorcing the justification for expenditures from their connections to other activities and purposes. Another flaw of zero-base budgeting is that it ranks objectives without considering whether available resources would limit those goals.[11]

In summary, the Budgeting Classification Tree (figure 6–4) illustrates the various types and approaches that managers can use in the budgetary control process.

FIGURE 6–4
Budgeting Classification Tree

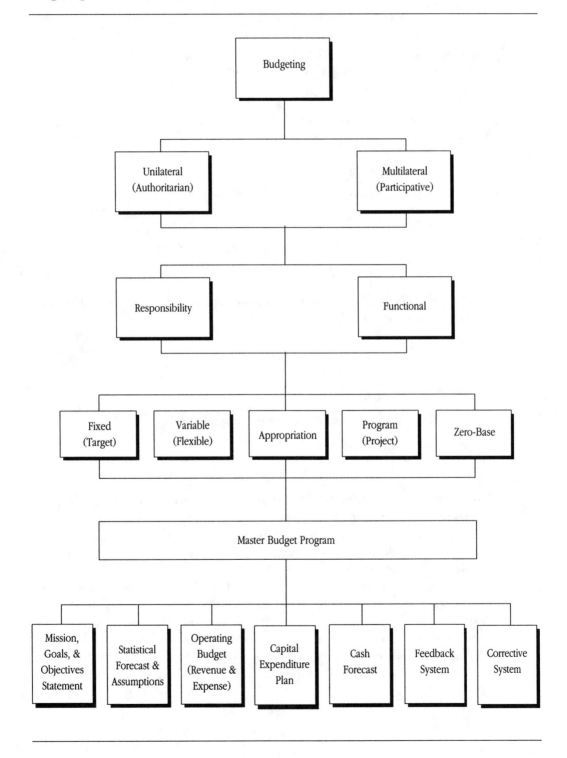

The Budgetary Control System's Typical Elements

As long as hospitals and other healthcare organizations exist, there will be variations in the approaches and techniques of budgetary control. However, there are eight basic components, as shown in figure 6–5, that are likely to remain constant in most budgetary control systems:

1. statement of purpose

2. statistical forecast

3. operating budget

4. capital expenditure plan

5. cash flow forecast

6. operations

7. performance evaluation and corrective measures

8. budget review and adjustment

The *statement of purpose* is a narrative report that identifies and quantifies the department's

- mission;

- goals and objectives;

- assumptions;

- strategy to be used to obtain these goals and objectives;

- required resources; and

- standards of acceptable or expected performance.

This report requires information and involvement from top and middle management. When both management levels accept the statement and performance standards, the data are documented and subsequently serve as the foundation for all the budgets and evaluating mechanisms in the total budgetary control system.

The *statistical forecast* forms the basis for all financial projections. Volume or statistical forecasting is so vital to the success of any healthcare institution's budget that it is frequently referred to as the budget's keystone; it projects revenue and expenses—especially variable expenses—and literally ties the revenue and expense plans together.[12] The statistical forecast includes such inpatient and outpatient statistics as the following:

- admissions

- discharges

FIGURE 6–5
The Budgetary Control System

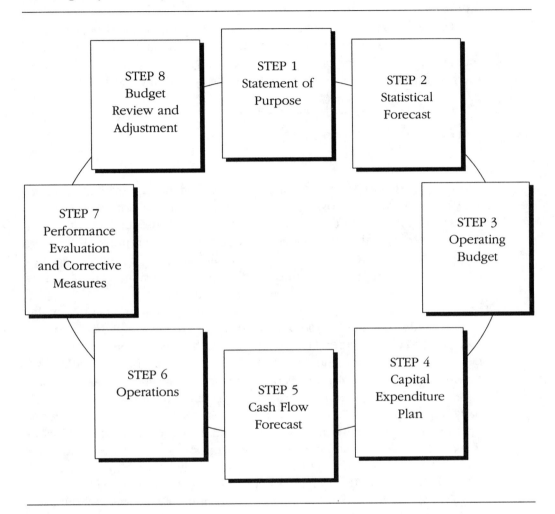

- preadmissions
- initial billings
- follow-up billings
- accounts in file
- patient consultations
- telephone calls
- letters typed

Management uses these and other assumptions, as well as many other statistics and established performance standards, to determine staffing requirements. The number and variety of statistics and/or production units patient financial services managers use are limited only by their imagination and needs.

The *operating budget* is the statement of purpose and statistical forecast expressed in financial terms. Because the patient financial services department is a cash-collecting department rather than a revenue-producing center, the primary components of the department's operating budget are

- salary and fringe benefit expenses,

- nonsalary and supply expenses, and

- provision for depreciation.

The first two expense categories, salary and nonsalary expenses, represent eventual cash outflows, whereas depreciation is a noncash item that represents only an accounting provision to amortize the purchase of capital assets. It is essential that management separates cash and noncash items to facilitate cash flow forecasting. Essentially, the operating budget is a tool to assist management in short-term or tactical planning and the control of current operating needs. It usually spans a minimum of one year.

The *capital expenditure plan* represents management's perception of the capital needs for a long period of time—usually a minimum of three years. A well-devised capital expenditure plan ensures that the equipment and facilities needed to support the overall healthcare organization and individual department programs will be available at the proper time. According to Berman, Weeks, and Kukla, developing a capital expenditure decision package essentially requires two decisions: the capital investment decision focuses on the investment opportunity's intrinsic merits, and the capital budgeting decision focuses on which of the better investment opportunities can be funded by the capital budget. These two decisions frequently become intertwined because the capital budget preparation process addresses both matters.[13]

The *cash flow forecast* is a plan for projecting cash inflows and outflows and the resulting cash balances. The forecast serves as the mechanism or instrument that expresses the operating budget and capital expenditure plan in cash terms. Chief among the forecast's objectives is determining whether sufficient cash resources will be available at the appropriate time to meet all the planned operating and capital cash requirements. A secondary purpose of cash flow forecasting is to determine when the healthcare organization will have an excess of operating cash on hand so that management can make capital and/or temporary investments. Before the cash flow forecast can begin, however, management must complete the operating budget and capital expenditure plan.

All the time and resources management spends in developing the aforementioned planning instruments would be futile if it fails to include feedback and performance evaluation in the comprehensive budgetary control system.

A well-designed budgetary control system should be a self-regulating arrangement with built-in provisions for reporting to the responsible individual actual performance as compared with the plan. The system should also require individual employees to report to the supervisor reasons for unfavorable variances and the corrective measures to be taken. When management evaluates performance and takes corrective measures, its next step is to review the original plan for the system and make any necessary adjustments to it.

As illustrated in figure 6–5, the budgetary control system is a continual cycle. A responsive budgetary control system (see figure 6–6) is a constantly revolving sequence of the following tasks:

- plan
- perform

FIGURE 6–6
Budgetary Control Cycle

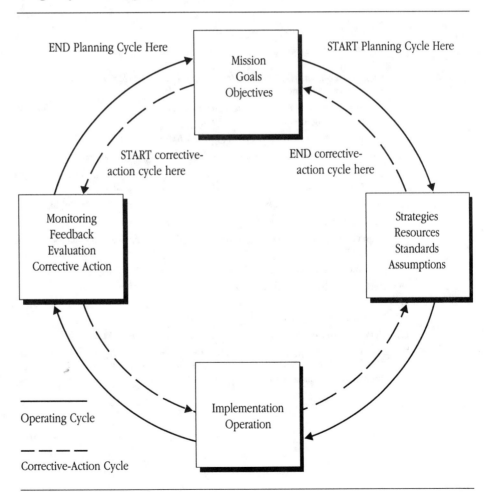

- two-way feedback

- performance evaluation

- corrective action

In an effective budgetary control system, the completion of one cycle begins another.

In summary, an effective budgetary control system helps create a management style that involves all levels of the management hierarchy. It also uses the hands-on experience of employees at every level to help formulate a cohesive plan that will improve the quality as well as the quantity of work performed. However, one word of caution: the budgetary control system is not a panacea, nor does it work by itself. It not only requires management's constant nurturing and evaluation, but it also requires the total cooperation of all levels of people—the skilled and the nonskilled, the managers and the managed. Simply speaking, it requires dedication, commitment, and involvement.

NOTES

1. Allen G. Herkimer Jr., *Understanding Hospital Financial Management,* 2nd ed. (Rockville, Md.: Aspen Publishers, Inc., 1986), 143.

2. L. Vann Seawell, *Introduction to Hospital Accounting,* 3rd ed. (Westchester, Ill.: Healthcare Financial Management Association, 1992), 473.

3. Herkimer, *Understanding Hospital Financial Management,* 146.

4. Herkimer, *Understanding Hospital Financial Management,* 64–65.

5. L. Vann Seawell, *Hospital Financial Accounting: Theory and Practice,* 2nd ed. (Westchester, Ill.: Healthcare Financial Management Association, 1987), 161.

6. Peter F. Drucker, *Managing for Results* (New York: Harper & Row, Publishers, Inc., 1986), 11.

7. Herkimer, *Understanding Hospital Financial Management,* 155–56.

8. Allen G. Herkimer Jr., *Understanding Health Care Budgeting* (Rockville, Md.: Aspen Publishers, Inc., 1988), 17.

9. Herkimer, *Understanding Health Care Budgeting,* 17.

10. Herkimer, *Understanding Health Care Budgeting,* 17.

11. Aaron Wildavsky, *Budgeting: A Comparative Theory of Budgetary Processes,* rev. ed. (New Brunswick, N.J.: Transaction Publishers, 1986), 322, 323.

12. Herkimer, *Understanding Hospital Financial Management,* 117.

13. Howard J. Berman, Lewis E. Weeks, and Steven F. Kukla, *The Financial Management of Hospitals,* 7th ed. (Ann Arbor, Mich.: Health Administration Press Division of the Foundation of the American College of Healthcare Executives, 1990), 565.

CHAPTER 7

Application of Variable Budgeting

To maximize their department's cost-effectiveness, patient financial services managers need to establish a variable budgeting system. This chapter explains the concept and purpose of variable budgeting and the relationship of standard costs to this system. Next, it explains how to develop standard rates and costs as part of the groundwork for the variable budget itself. The rest of the chapter covers developing the variable control budget, analyzing salary budget and nonsalary expense variances, and analyzing step-variable staffing and expense variances.

The Variable Budgeting Concept

Variable budgeting, occasionally known as flexible budgeting, eliminates any variance between actual and budgeted volumes of activity. It is also based on the principle of cost variability: certain costs arising from work volume or output are influenced by time and volume. Under this principle, costs related to activity are classified as fixed, variable, or step-variable (see chapter 4). To sort costs into these three categories, the healthcare organization's management must use its organizational chart of accounts to clearly define each natural cost classification. Classification of costs for the patient financial services department are discussed later in this chapter.

In applying the variable budgeting concept to the patient financial services department, managers need to remember that the degree of accuracy that they require determines how sound the eventual budgetary analysis and decision making will be. They should also keep in mind that although data for managerial use must be accurate, that requirement does not preclude the use of nonquantifiable information, such as conversations and newspaper articles,[1] in making judgments. Sound judgment is the basis of any effective budgetary control system.

The Purpose of Variable Budgeting

The primary purposes of variable budgeting are to

- assist management in controlling expenses and

- eliminate budget variances due to volume changes.

Variable budgets provide expense information that makes it possible to compensate for differences between actual and budgeted volumes and rates. Essentially, the variable budget develops a methodology for classifying every expense in any department. In turn, that methodology establishes the relationship of these expense categories to the production units that a given department generated.

In addition, the variable budget shows the planned behavior of costs at various volume levels. Management uses budgeted costs at one volume level in this budget as part of its healthcare organization's master or comprehensive budget; that volume level becomes the volume at which the organization plans to operate during the budget period.[2] In this manner, the variable budget is a planning tool, helping managers identify the volume level that will serve as the organization's target level of activity for the coming period. This budget is also a control device in that it helps managers analyze actual performance results,[3] a process that is covered later in this chapter.

Relationship of Standard Costs to Variable Budgeting

Standard costs are the building blocks of a variable budgeting control system. Based on standards that management established to indicate the resources—labor, supplies, equipment—that employees need to perform specific tasks or groups of tasks, standard costs express in financial terms what specific tasks should cost per production unit. Standard costs can be segmented into three types:

1. basic

2. ideal

3. attainable

Basic cost standards are static, thereby providing a basis for comparing actual costs. Since this type of standard is inflexible, basic cost standards are seldom used because they cannot reflect market fluctuations or changes in costs and methods.

Ideal cost standards represent the absolute minimum cost possible under the best conceivable operating conditions.[4] Use of this standard in the healthcare industry is relatively limited; however, managers can use it to motivate employees to achieve greater productivity. The danger is that ideal cost standards may, instead, discourage employees from improving productivity.

The third and most commonly used standard cost is the attainable cost. This standard tends to be less restrictive than the ideal cost standard because it allows for downtime and lost time. However, the attainable standard is strict enough to encourage improved productivity and to give employees a sense of achievement when they reach the standard. The major benefits of using attainable standard costs are that managers can use them to

- develop production unit costs,

- develop departmental and total organizational costs, and

- motivate employees.

Regardless of the type of standard managers select, it serves as the bridge that allows the budget analyst to adjust a target budget to a variable budget; that is, the analyst can adjust a *fixed*-volume departmental or production-unit cost to the *actual*-volume departmental or unit cost. This capacity of cost standards is essential for effective and prudent management, especially during times in which the healthcare industry is experiencing dynamic changes in consumers' use of healthcare services coupled with ravaging inflation.

The variable budgeting system offers management a unique tool for expense control and evaluation. The basic objectives of any cost control program are to

- control the production unit cost and

- maintain or increase production per employee.

Variable budgeting enables managers to meet these objectives.

Developing Standard Rates and Costs

Standard rates and costs can be developed for the healthcare institution as a whole, for each department, or for individual services or items. Managers can establish institutional and/or departmental standards for use in determining the volume of service that their healthcare organization and/or a department requires to break even, as illustrated below.

Computation of Break-Even Daily Census	*Amount*	*Percent*
1. Average net charge per patient day	$600	100%
2. Average variable cost per patient day	200	$33^1/_3$
3. Contribution	$400	
4. Contribution margin		$66^2/_3$
5. Fixed expenses per calendar day	$40,000	
6. Desired profit per calendar day	20,000	
7. Total fixed expenses and desired profit per calendar day	$60,000	

Computation of Break-Even Daily Census (Cont'd)   Amount

8. Break-even census per calendar
    day (line 7 ÷ line 3 = line 8)   150 patient days

9. Break-even net charges per calendar
    day (line 7 ÷ line 4 = line 9,
    or line 8 × line 1 = line 9) $90,000

For standard rates and costs to be most effective, management should develop them for each revenue service, expense item, and salaried position. This step enables the budget analyst to localize any major variance between actual performance and the standard. Developing individual standards will be discussed in more detail in the case study at the end of this chapter.

The basic formulas for developing standards are as follows:

A. *Standard Rate Formula*

$$\frac{\text{Total Annual Revenue}}{\text{Total Annual Relevant Production Units}} = \text{Standard Rate}$$

For example:

$$\frac{\$3,285,000}{36,500} = \$90.00 \text{ Standard Rate (price)}$$

B. *Standard Cost Formula*

$$\frac{\text{Total Annual Variable Expense}}{\text{Total Annual Relevant Production Units}} = \text{Standard Cost}$$

For example:

$$\frac{\$2,865,250}{36,500} = \$78.50 \text{ Standard Cost}$$

As illustrated, standards can be developed for revenue and expenses. Generally, the term *standard rate* refers either to an average or actual charge for an individual service generated by a revenue-producing department, the average rate an employee is paid per hour, or the average cost per production unit. The term *standard cost* refers to the amount of any specific expense-variable item per production unit.

Developing the Variable Budget

Although the fixed budget methodology cannot satisfy the objectives of the variable budgeting concept, it serves effectively as the target or forecast budget from which management establishes standard rates and costs for the variable budgetary control system. The following is a step-by-step approach to developing a variable budget for the patient financial services department of Memorial Medical Center of Anytown, U.S.A.

Step 1. Identify the fixed salary and nonsalary expense items in the department's chart of accounts. These fixed expenses will not change within a relevant range of activity or volume, yet they are incurred no matter how many production units the department produces. (Please note that costs identified as fixed in one department or healthcare facility will not necessarily be fixed costs in another setting.) Next, the budget analyst must relate cost behavior to the specific environment and the manner in which management chooses to control the cost item. Using the chart of accounts shown in table 7–1, the patient financial services manager classified the following expense items as fixed (see table 7–2):

Fixed Expenses: Patient Financial Services Department Salaries and Wages

.01 Management and Supervision

.02 Executive Secretary

.10 Employee Benefits—Management

Nonsalary Expenses

.21 Dues and Subscriptions

.22 Equipment Rentals and Leases

.24 Travel

.29 Training Programs

.30 Depreciation

Step 2. Using this methodology, assume that all remaining items are variable costs, even though some expense categories, such as salaries for the admitting, billing, and collection clerks, actually may be step-variable expenses. (This matter will be discussed more fully later in this chapter.) The department's cost classification chart of accounts is illustrated in table 7–2.

TABLE 7–1

Chart of Accounts

Memorial Medical Center
Anytown, U.S.A.

Patient Financial Services Department
CHART OF ACCOUNTS

Dept. Code No.	Natural Code No.	Description

Salaries and Wages

Dept. Code No.	Natural Code No.	Description
8244	.01	Management and Supervision
8244	.02	Executive Secretary
8244	.03	Admitting Clerks
8244	.04	Billing Clerks
8244	.05	Collection Clerks
8244	.10	Employee Benefits—Management
8244	.11	Employee Benefits—Staff

Nonsalary Expenses

Dept. Code No.	Natural Code No.	Description
8244	.21	Dues and Subscriptions
8244	.22	Equipment Rentals and Leases
8244	.23	Telephone
8244	.24	Travel
8244	.25	Postage
8244	.26	Collection Fees
8244	.27	Printed Forms
8244	.28	Other Office Supplies
8244	.29	Training Programs
8244	.30	Depreciation

Step 3. Select a production unit that represents with reasonable accuracy the work performed in the department. For illustration purposes, note that Memorial Medical Center's patient financial services department uses the number of inpatient and outpatient admissions as its macro or gross departmental production unit. Selecting this unit does not preclude using other production units to measure individual position or expense categories. In this case,

TABLE 7–2

Cost Classification—Chart of Accounts

Memorial Medical Center
Anytown, U.S.A.

Patient Financial Services Department
DEPARTMENT EXPENSES

Department Production Unit:
Number of Admissions (Inpatient and Outpatient)

Dept. Code No.	Natural Code No.	Description	Cost Behavior	
			Variable Method	*Step-Variable Method*
Salaries and Wages				
8244	.01	Management and Supervision	Fixed	Fixed
8244	.02	Executive Secretary	Fixed	Fixed
8244	.03	Admitting Clerks	Variable	Step-Variable
8244	.04	Billing Clerks	Variable	Step-Variable
8244	.05	Collection Clerks	Variable	Step-Variable
8244	.10	Employee Benefits—Management	Fixed	Fixed
8244	.11	Employee Benefits—Staff	Variable	Step-Variable
Nonsalary Expenses				
8244	.21	Dues and Subscriptions	Fixed	Fixed
8244	.22	Equipment Rentals and Leases	Fixed	Fixed
8244	.23	Telephone	Variable	Variable
8244	.24	Travel	Fixed	Fixed
8244	.25	Postage	Variable	Variable
8244	.26	Collection Fees	Variable	Variable
8244	.27	Printed Forms	Variable	Variable
8244	.28	Other Office Supplies	Variable	Variable
8244	.29	Training Programs	Fixed	Fixed
8244	.30	Depreciation	Fixed	Fixed

the number of admissions will be the basis for establishing departmental production and cost standards.

Step 4. Using the target or fixed budget (see table 7–3), record these expense classifications and amounts in columns 4, 5, and 6 of the variable budget worksheet shown in table 7–4.

TABLE 7–3

Target or Fixed Budget

Memorial Medical Center
Anytown, U.S.A.

Patient Financial Services Department
TARGET OR FIXED BUDGET
For the Fiscal Year Ending September 30, 19x1

	Total	
	Amount	*Hours*
Volume		
Number of Admissions:		
Inpatient	6,738	
Outpatient	31,025	
Total Admissions	37,763	
Salaries and Wages		
Management and Supervision	$ 55,000	4,160
Executive Secretary	18,000	2,080
Admitting Clerks	85,000	17,680
Billing Clerks	60,000	12,480
Collection Clerks	48,000	8,320
Employee Benefits—Management	18,250	n/a
Employee Benefits—Staff	48,250	n/a
Total Salaries and Wages	$332,500	44,720
Nonsalary Expenses		
Dues and Subscriptions	$ 1,000	
Equipment Rentals and Leases	21,600	
Telephone	10,800	
Travel	6,000	
Postage	32,000	
Collection Fees	180,000	
Printed Forms	75,500	
Other Office Supplies	38,000	
Training Programs	6,000	
Depreciation	12,000	
Total Nonsalary Expenses	$382,900	
Total Expenses	$715,400	

Step 5.   Record the target budget hours in columns 1 and 2 of table 7–4.

Step 6.   Using the total volume of production units (column 5, lines 6 and 7 in table 7–4), compute the variable expense standard for each variable item and record in column 7. For example:

$$\frac{\text{Total Admitting Clerk Expense (column 6, line 1(c))}}{\text{Total Relevant Number of Admissions (column 5, line 7)}} = \text{Standard Costs per Admission}$$

or

$$\frac{\$85,000}{37,763} = \$2.25$$

Step 7.   Using the total volume of production units (column 5, line 7), compute the variable production standard for each variable salary and wage expense position as follows:

$$\frac{\text{Total Number of Admissions (column 5, line 7)}}{\text{Total Relevant Admitting Clerk Hours (column 2, line 1(c))}} = \text{Variable Production Standard}$$

or

$$\frac{37,763}{17,680} = 2.14 \text{ Admissions per Hour}$$

Record in column 3, line 1(c).

Completing Step 7 results in variable production standards for each position and for the department:

Salaries and Wages	*Variable Production Unit Standard*	
Admitting clerks	2.14	admissions per hour
Billing clerks	3.03	admissions per hour
Collection clerks	4.54	admissions per hour
Total variable positions*	0.98	admissions per hour

* $\dfrac{37,763 \text{ Admissions}}{38,480 \text{ Var. Hours}} = 0.98$

TABLE 7–4

Variable Budget Worksheet

Memorial Medical Center
Anytown, U.S.A.

VARIABLE BUDGET WORKSHEET
For the Fiscal Year Ending September 30, 19x1

Department: Patient Financial Services
Production Unit: Number of Admissions (Inpatient and Outpatient)

HOURS				EXPENSES		
TARGET BUDGET				TARGET BUDGET		
Fixed (1)	Variable (2)	Variable Production Standard (3)	ACCOUNT DESCRIPTION (4)	Fixed (5)	Variable (6)	Variable Expense Standard (7)
			Salaries and Wages			
4,160		n/a	1. (a) Management and Supervision	$ 55,000		$ n/a
2,080		n/a	(b) Executive Secretary	18,000		n/a
	17,680	2.14	(c) Admitting Clerks		$ 85,000	2.25
	12,480	3.03	(d) Billing Clerks		60,000	1.59
	8,320	4.54	(e) Collection Clerks		48,000	1.27
			(f) Employee Benefits— Management	18,250		n/a
			(g) Employee Benefits—Staff		48,250	1.28
6,240	38,480	0.98	2. Total Salaries and Wages	$ 91,250	$241,250	$6.39
Computation of Variable Standard Hourly Rates			*Nonsalary Expenses*			

Computation of Variable Standard Hourly Rates

Position	Standard Hourly Rate
Admitting Clerks	$4.81
Billing Clerks	4.81
Collection Clerks	5.77
Employee Benefits— Staff	1.25
Total	6.27

Formula:

$$\frac{\text{Total Salary Expense (from col. 6)}}{\text{Total Hours (from col. 2)}} = \frac{\text{Variable Standard Hourly Rate}}{}$$

For Example: Admitting Clerks

$$\frac{\$85,000}{17,680} = \$4.81$$

Account Description	Fixed (5)	Variable (6)	Variable Expense Standard (7)
3. (a) Dues and Subscriptions	$ 1,000		n/a
(b) Equipment Rentals and Leases	21,600		n/a
(c) Telephone		$ 10,600	.28
(d) Travel	6,000		n/a
(e) Postage		32,000	.85
(f) Collection Fees		180,000	4.77
(g) Printed Forms			2.00
(h) Other Office Supplies		38,000	1.01
(i) Training Programs	6,000		n/a
(j) Depreciation	12,000		n/a
4. Total Nonsalary Expenses	$ 46,600	$336,100	$ 8.91
5. Grand Total Expenses	$137,850	$577,350	
Number of Admissions (Volume)			
6. (a) Inpatient	6,738		
(b) Outpatient	31,025		
7. Total Admissions	37,763		

Variable expense (cost) standards for each expense category and for the department are as follows:

Salaries and Wages	*Variable Standard Cost*	
Admitting clerks	$2.25	per admission
Billing clerks	1.59	per admission
Collection clerks	1.27	per admission
Employee benefits—staff	1.28	per admission
Total salaries and wages	$6.39	per admission

Nonsalary Expenses	*Variable Standard Cost*	
Telephone	$0.28	per admission
Postage	0.85	per admission
Collection fees	4.77	per admission
Printed forms	2.00	per admission
Other office supplies	1.01	per admission
Total nonsalary expenses	$8.91	per admission

These standards will remain relatively consistent throughout Memorial Medical Center's budget year, barring any major changes in systems or costs, and will lay the groundwork for its variable control budgets. *Control budgets* are budgets that show targeted fixed-expense levels with variable-expense categories adjusted according to the actual work volume. The variable-expense categories are adjusted by multiplying standard rates by the actual volume of work performed. By adjusting the target budget to the actual volume of activity, the variable budget eliminates performance variances due to volume changes. Developing and using control budgets will be discussed in more detail later in this chapter.

For further illustration of the application of the variable budget, assume that during the course of the year, the patient financial services department at Memorial Medical Center experienced a decrease of 2,873 in the amount of budgeted admissions, from 37,763 to 34,890. Assume further that the patient financial services manager retained the variable staff level budgeted on the basis of a higher volume of work. Table 7–5 is a comparative analysis of the original target (fixed-volume) budget and the actual performance. The patient financial services manager initially reviewing this analysis (see summary below) would be very pleased with department performance because there is a favorable variance of $17,500 for nonsalary expense, and salary and wage expense is exactly as budgeted, as illustrated in the comparative summary below:

TABLE 7–5

Comparative Analysis of Fixed Target Budget to Actual Performance

Memorial Medical Center
Anytown, U.S.A.

Patient Financial Services Department
COMPARATIVE ANALYSIS OF FIXED TARGET BUDGET
TO ACTUAL PERFORMANCE
For the Fiscal Year Ending September 30, 19x1

	Amount		*Variance:* *Favorable/(Unfavorable)*	
	Actual	*Budgeted*	*Amount*	*Percent*
Salaries and Wages				
Management and Supervision	$ 56,000	$ 55,000	$(1,000)	(1.82)
Executive Secretary	18,000	18,000	–0–	–0–
Admitting Clerks	83,000	85,000	2,000	2.35
Billing Clerks	62,000	60,000	(2,000)	(3.33)
Collection Clerks	47,000	48,000	1,000	2.08
Employee Benefits—Management	19,250	18,250	(1,000)	(5.48)
Employee Benefits—Staff	47,250	48,250	1,000	2.07
Total Salaries and Wages	$332,500	$332,500	–0–	–0–
Nonsalary Expenses				
Dues and Subscriptions	$ 900	$ 1,000	$ 100	10.00
Equipment Rental and Leases	21,600	21,600	–0–	–0–
Telephone	9,400	10,600	1,400	12.96
Travel	5,000	6,000	1,000	16.67
Postage	30,000	32,000	2,000	6.25
Collection Fees	170,000	180,000	10,000	5.56
Printed Forms	74,000	75,500	1,500	1.99
Other Office Supplies	36,500	38,000	1,500	3.95
Training Programs	6,000	6,000	–0–	–0–
Depreciation	12,000	12,000	–0–	–0–
Total Nonsalary Expenses	$365,400	$382,700	$17,500	4.57
Total Expenses	$697,900	$715,200	$17,500	2.45

	Actual	Budgeted	Variance
Total salaries and wages	$332,500	$332,500	$ -0-
Total nonsalary expenses	365,400	382,700	17,300 (Favorable)
Total expenses	$697,900	$715,200	$17,300 (Favorable)

However, extending the analysis to include evaluating the work volume and paid hours is essential; table 7–6 analyzes and compares these data. The first indication of any problem is the unfavorable variance of 2,873 in the number of admissions. This figure represents a 7.6-percent decrease in work volume. The second indication of a possible problem is the relatively small favorable decrease of 350 variable hours. This decrease, less than 1.0 percent, is small compared with the 7.6-percent decrease in work volume. At this point, developing a control budget would allow for these volume variances and would adjust variable expenses to match the actual volume of work.

TABLE 7–6

Comparative Analysis of Volume to Variable Paid Hours

Memorial Medical Center
Anytown, U.S.A.

Patient Financial Services Department
COMPARATIVE ANALYSIS OF VOLUME TO VARIABLE PAID HOURS
For the Fiscal Year Ending September 30, 19x1

	Amount		Variance: Favorable/(Unfavorable)	
	Actual	Budgeted	Amount	Percent
Volume				
Number of Admissions:				
Inpatient	6,280	6,738	(458)	(6.80)
Outpatient	28,610	31,025	(2,415)	(7.78)
Total Admissions	34,890	37,763	(2,873)	(7.61)
Variable Paid Hours				
Admitting Clerks	17,500	17,680	180	1.02
Billing Clerks	12,480	12,480	-0-	-0-
Collection Clerks	8,150	8,320	170	2.04
Total Variable Paid Hours	38,130	38,480	350	0.91

Developing the Variable Control Budget

A step-by-step approach to developing a variable control budget is presented below. This control budget uses the variable standard costs developed for the target budget and adjusts the department's total variable expenses according to the actual volume of work.

Step 1.   Record actual performance, that is, 34,890 admissions, in the control budget as the volume of work (see table 7–7, columns 3 and 4).

Step 2.   Separate fixed expenses into two categories: (1) salaries and wages, and (2) nonsalary expenses. Record the exact amount of each expense as it was projected in the target budget (see column 3).

Step 3.   Record the standard costs developed in the variable budget worksheet (table 7–4, column 7) for each variable-expense item in the appropriate column (table 7–7, column 2). Multiply these costs by the actual volume of work (34,890 admissions) to obtain the control budget variable cost for these expense items. For example:

Standard rate for admitting clerks = $2.25 per admission

Volume × Rate = Total Control Budget Variable Cost

or

34,890 × $2.25 = $78,503

Step 4.   Record the actual fixed and variable performance in column 4; adjust the subtotals and totals.

Table 7–8 provides a comparative summary of data from the target and variable control budgets and the actual performance. Comparing the total target budget of $715,200 with the total actual performance of $697,900 indicates a favorable variance of $17,300. However, this comparison does not take into consideration the unfavorable variance of 2,873 from the target budget's volume forecast of 37,763 to the actual volume of 34,890. The variable budget makes provision for this volume variance and thus identifies an unfavorable variance of $26,582 from the control budget's total of $671,318 to the actual performance total of $697,900.

TABLE 7–7

Comparative Analysis of Variable Control Budget to Actual Performance

Memorial Medical Center
Anytown, U.S.A.

Patient Financial Services Department
COMPARATIVE ANALYSIS OF VARIABLE CONTROL BUDGET
TO ACTUAL PERFORMANCE

(1)	Standard Cost per Admission (2)	Control Budget (3)	Actual (4)	Variance: Favorable/ (Unfavorable) Amount (5)	Percent (6)
Volume					
Number of Admissions		34,89	34,890	–0–	–0–
Fixed Expenses					
Salaries and Wages					
Management and Supervision		$ 55,000	$ 56,000	$ (1,000)	(1.82)
Executive Secretary		18,000	18,000	–0–	–0–
Employee Benefits—Management		18,250	19,250	(1,000)	(5.48)
Total Fixed Salaries and Wages		$ 91,250	$ 93,250	$ (2,000)	(2.19)
Nonsalary Expenses					
Dues and Subscriptions		$ 1,000	$ 900	$ 100	10.0
Equipment Rental and Leases		21,600	21,600	–0–	–0–
Travel		6,000	5,000	1,000	16.67
Training Programs		6,000	6,000	–0–	–0–
Depreciation		12,000	12,000	–0–	–0–
Total Fixed Nonsalary Expenses		$ 46,600	$ 45,500	$ (1,100)	2.36
Total Fixed Expenses		$137,850	$138,750	$ (900)	(0.65)
Variable Expenses					
Salaries and Wages					
Admitting Clerks	$ 2.25	$ 78,503	$ 83,000	$ (4,497)	(5.73)
Billing Clerks	1.59	55,475	62,000	(6,525)	(11.76)
Collection Clerks	1.27	44,310	47,000	(2,690)	(6.07)
Employee Benefits—Staff	1.28	44,659	47,250	(2,591)	(5.80)
Total Variable Salaries and Wages	$ 6.39	$222,947	$239,250	$(16,303)	(7.31)
Nonsalary Expenses					
Telephone	$ .28	$ 9,769	$ 9,400	$ 369	3.78
Postage	.85	29,657	30,000	(343)	(1.16)
Collection Fees	4.77	166,425	170,000	(3,575)	(2.15)
Printed Forms	2.00	69,780	74,000	(4,220)	(6.05)
Other Office Supplies	1.01	35,239	36,500	(1,261)	(3.58)
Total Variable Nonsalary Expenses	$ 8.91	$310,870	$319,900	$ (9,030)	(2.90)
Total Variable Expenses	$15.30	$533,817	$559,150	$(25,333)	(4.74)
Total Fixed and Variable Expenses		$671,667	$697,900	$(26,233)	(3.90)

TABLE 7–8

Comparative Summary Analysis

Memorial Medical Center
Anytown, U.S.A.

Patient Financial Services Department
COMPARATIVE SUMMARY ANALYSIS OF TARGET
AND VARIABLE CONTROL BUDGET TO ACTUAL PERFORMANCE
For the Fiscal Year Ending September 30, 19x1

	Target (1)	Control (2)	Actual (3)	*Actual Performance Variance: Favorable/(Unfavorable)* To Target (4)	To Control (5)
Volume					
Number of Admissions	37,763	34,890	34,890	(2,873)	–0–
Fixed Expenses					
Salaries and Wages	$ 91,250	$ 91,250	$ 93,250	$(2,000)	$ (2,000)
Nonsalary Expenses	46,600	46,600	45,500	1,100	1,100
Total Fixed Expenses	$137,850	$137,850	$138,750	$ (900)	$ (900)
Variable Expenses					
Salaries and Wages	$241,250	$222,947	$239,250	$ 2,000	$(16,303)
Nonsalary Expenses	336,100	310,521	319,900	16,400	(9,379)
Total Variable Expenses	$577,350	$533,468	$559,150	$18,200	$(25,682)
Total Fixed and Variable Expenses	$715,200	$671,318	$697,900	$17,300	$(26,582)

Analyzing Salary Budget Variances

The next series of steps will indicate how to analyze specific favorable and unfavorable variances between actual performance and the control budget. Analyzing specific budget variances in the fixed-cost category is relatively simple; see column 5 of table 7–7. Here is a summary of these variances:

	Budget Variances	
Account Description	Favorable	Unfavorable
Fixed Salaries and Wages		
Management and Supervision		$1,000
Employee Benefits—Management		1,000
Fixed Nonsalary Expenses		
Dues and Subscriptions	$ 100	
Travel	1,000	
Total Fixed Variances	$1,100	$2,000
Net Unfavorable Variance		$ 900

Patient financial services managers should be prepared to explain not only the unfavorable variances but also the favorable variances in their department budget.

Variable budget variances generally fall under one of two categories: efficiency variances or rate variances. The *efficiency variance* attaches a dollar amount to the difference between the number of hours budgeted for a given task and the number of hours actually used to perform it, multiplied by the position's standard hourly rate. The formula for calculating the efficiency variance is as follows:

$$\text{Efficiency Variance} = (\text{Budgeted Hours} - \text{Actual Hours}) \times \text{Standard Hourly Rate}$$

or

$$\text{Hourly Variance} \times \text{Standard Hourly Rate}$$

For example: *Admitting clerks*

Target budget	17,680 hours
Actual performance	17,500 hours
Hourly variance	180 hours (Favorable)
Standard hourly rate	= $4.81

Efficiency variance	=	(17,680 − 17,500) × $4.81
	=	180 × $4.81
	=	$866.00 (Favorable)

The *rate variance* is the difference between the standard hourly rate and the actual rate paid times the actual volume. The formula for calculating the rate variance is as follows:

$$\text{Rate Variance} = (\text{Standard Rate} - \text{Actual Rate}) \times \text{Actual Hours}$$

For example: *Admitting clerks*

	Target	*Actual*
Volume	37,763	34,890
Total expenses	$85,000	$83,000
Total hours	17,680	17,500
Average hourly rate	$4.81	$4.74

Rate variance	=	($4.81 − $4.74) × 17,500
	=	$0.07 × 17,500
	=	$1,225 (Favorable)

Table 7–9 shows the computation and analysis of efficiency and rate variances for each of the variable positions in Memorial Medical Center's patient financial services department. Here is a summary of the variances:

	Variance: Favorable/(Unfavorable)		
Position	Efficiency (Line IV. 14)	Rate (Line V. 19)	Total (Line VI. 20)
Admitting Clerks	$ 866	$1,225	$2,091
Billing Clerks	None	(1,997)	(1,997)
Collection Clerks	981	None	981
Employee Benefits—Staff	588	381	969
Total	$2,435	$ (391)	$2,044

By exceeding their original targeted performance, the admitting and collection clerks experienced a total favorable variance of $2,435. The billing clerks, on the other hand, performed just as efficiently as they had been targeted to do. However, because the billing clerks were paid an average of $0.16 per hour more than had originally been budgeted, there was an unfavorable variance of $1,997 in their wages. Conversely, the admitting clerks' average hourly wage was $0.07 less than the target budget amount, resulting in a favorable variance of $1,225.

This exercise calls for analyzing each variable position in the patient financial services department and computing corresponding efficiency and rate variances. Memorial Medical Center's patient financial services manager could use the department's total variable salary and wage expense figures (see table 7–8) to compute these variances in the following manner:

I. Efficiency Variance
    1. Standard hours   38,480
    2. Actual hours   38,130
    3. Hourly variance   350 (Favorable)
        (line 1 − line 2 = line 3)
    4. Standard hourly rate $6.27
        ($241,250 ÷ 38,480)
    5. Efficiency variance $2,195 (Favorable)
        (line 3 × line 4 = line 5)

II. *Rate Variance*
    6. Actual hours   38,130
    7. Actual hourly rate $6.27
        ($239,250 ÷ 38,130)
    8. Standard hourly rate $6.27
    9. Hourly rate variance   None
        (line 7 − line 8 = line 9)
    10. Rate variance   None
        (line 6 × line 9 = line 10)
    11. Net total variance $2,195 (Favorable)
        (line 5 + line 10 = line 11)

TABLE 7–9

Computation and Analysis of Variances of Variable Salary and Wage Expenses

Memorial Medical Center
Anytown, U.S.A.

Patient Financial Services Department
COMPUTATION AND ANALYSIS OF VARIANCES OF VARIABLE SALARY AND WAGE EXPENSES
For the Fiscal Year Ending September 30, 19x1

Description (1)	*Admitting Clerks* (2)	*Billing Clerks* (3)	*Collection Clerks* (4)	*Employee Benefits —Staff* (5)	*Total* (6)
I. *Target Standard*					
1. Standard Hourly Rate	$ 4.81	$ 4.81	$ 5.77	$ 1.25	
2. Standard Hours	17,680	12,480	8,320	38,480	
3. Target Budget (line 1 × line 2 = line 3)	$85,000	$60,000	$48,000	$48,250	
II. *Control Standard*					
4. Standard Hourly Rate (line 1)	$ 4.81	$ 4.81	$ 5.77	$ 1.25	
5. Actual Hours	17,500	12,480	8,150	38,130	
6. Control Standard (line 4 × line 5 = line 6)	$84,175	$60,029	$47,026	$47,663	
III. *Actual Performance*					
7. Actual Hourly Rate	$ 4.74	$ 4.97	$ 5.77	$ 1.24	
8. Actual Hours (line 5)	17,500	12,480	8,150	38,130	
9. Actual Performance (line 7 × line 8 = line 9)	$83,000	$62,000	$47,000	$47,250	
IV. *Efficiency Variance*					
10. Standard Hours (line 2)	17,680	12,480	8,320	38,480	
11. Actual Hours (line 5)	17,500	12,480	8,150	38,130	
12. Hour Variance (line 10 − line 11 = line 12)	180 Favorable	None	170 Favorable	350 Favorable	
13. Standard Hourly Rate (line 1)	$ 4.81	$ 4.81	$ 5.77	$ 1.25	
14. Efficiency Variance (line 12 × 13 = line 14)	$ 866 Favorable	None	$ 981 Favorable	$ 438 Favorable	$2,285 Favorable
V. *Rate Variance*					
15. Actual Hours (line 5)	17,500	12,480	8,150	38,130	
16. Actual Hourly Rate (line 7)	$ 4.74	$ 4.97	$ 5.77	$ 1.24	
17. Standard Hourly Rate (line 1)	$ 4.81	$ 4.81	$ 5.77	$ 1.25	
18. Hourly Rate Variance (line 16 − line 17 = line 18)	$ .07 Favorable	$ .16 Unfavorable	None	$ .01 Favorable	
19. Rate Variance (line 15 × line 18 = line 19)	$ 1,225 Favorable	$ 1,997 Unfavorable	None	$ 381 Favorable	$ 391 Unfavorable
VI. 20. *Net Total Variances* (line 14 + line 19 = line 20)	$ 2,091 Favorable	$ 1,997 Unfavorable	$ 981 Favorable	$ 819 Favorable	$1,894 Favorable
VII. *Proof*					
21. Target Budget (line 3)	$85,000	$60,000	$48,000	$48,250	
22. Actual Performance (line 9)	$83,000	$62,000	$47,000	$47,250	
23. Variance—Target to Actual (line 21 − line 22 = line 23)	$ 2,000 Favorable	$ 2,000 Unfavorable	$ 1,000 Favorable	$ 1,000 Favorable	$2,000 Favorable

NOTE: Differences between net total variance (line 20) and variance between target and actual (line 23) are due to rounding off all rates and totals to the nearest dollar or hundredths of a dollar; there is no substantial difference.

We may compare these two methods of analyzing variances as follows:

	Position by Position	*Every Position*
Efficiency variance	$2,285	$2,195
Rate variance	(391)	None
Net total variance	$1,894	$2,195

Differences in these variances, representing less than 1 percent of the department's total variable salary and wage expense, are probably due to rounding off totals and rates to the nearest dollar or hundredths of a dollar.

Analyzing Nonsalary Expense Variances

Usage variances and rate variances are two common methods of analyzing the differences between budgeted and actual performance for nonsalary expenses. The usage variance is computed by multiplying the standard rate by the difference between the actual volume and the target volume. The formula follows; refer to tables 7–4 and 7–6 for the volume and rate figures.

Usage Variance = (Target Volume − Actual Volume) × Standard Rate

For example: *Telephone* = (37,763 − 34,890) × $0.29
Usage Variance = 2,873 × $0.29
= $833 (Favorable)

This amount represents the savings experienced due to a lower volume of service.

The rate variance represents the favorable or unfavorable variance costs experienced when the actual rate differs from the rate in the target budget. The formula for the variance is as follows:

Rate Variance = (Standard Unit Cost − Actual Unit Cost) × Actual Volume

For example: *Telephone*
Rate Variance = ($0.29 − $0.27) × 34,890
= $0.02 × 34,890
= $698 (Favorable)

As is the case with salary and wage expense, we can analyze nonsalary expense variances either by individual item, as in table 7–10, or as a composite of all variable expenses:

I. *Usage Variance*
    1. Target volume   37,763
    2. Actual volume   34,890
    3. Volume variance   3,873
       (line 1 − line 2 = line 3)
    4. Standard unit cost $8.90
    5. Usage variance $25,570 (Favorable)
       (line 3 × line 4 = line 5)

II. *Rate Variance*
    6. Standard unit cost $8.90
    7. Actual unit cost $9.17
    8. Unit cost variance $0.27
       (line 6 − line 7 = line 8)
    9. Actual volume   34,890
    10. Rate variance $9,420 (Unfavorable)
       (line 8 × line 9 = line 10)

III. *Net Total Variance*
     (line 5 + line 10 = line 11) $16,150 (Favorable)

Analyzing wage and salary expenses using these two methods results in minimal differences, which are due to the rounding off of the numbers used. The important point is that the analyst can find out why variances occurred. These examples illustrate the variable application of the variable budget concept: all variable expenses are adjusted in direct proportion to the volume of work. Some may argue that variable salary and wage expense cannot be adjusted in direct proportion to the volume of work. Patient financial services managers would not hire an additional admitting clerk just because admissions increase by 20, nor would they release one clerk just because admissions drop by 20. As noted earlier in this book, any staff exhibits a certain amount of elasticity over a relevant period of time. This elasticity tends to create certain plateaus in the staffing of the patient financial services department. These plateaus, in turn, result in a step-variable condition that serves as a lag factor, helping the department to adjust to volume changes.

Analyzing Step-Variable Staffing and Expense Variances

Step-variable expenses are costs that may change abruptly at intervals according to relevant ranges of activity that are measurable in discrete segments. In practice, most clerks often experience uneven work loads. The staff elasticity factor means that the clerks can maintain an intensive or leisurely work pace for long periods of time or for a relevant range of activity, as illustrated in figure 7–1. On the other hand, expenses such as office supplies and forms tend to vary in direct proportion to the actual volume of work, as illustrated in figure 7–2. Table 7–11

TABLE 7–10

Computation and Analysis of Variances of Variable Nonsalary Expenses

Memorial Medical Center
Anytown, U.S.A.

Patient Financial Services Department
COMPUTATION AND ANALYSIS OF VARIANCES OF VARIABLE
NONSALARY EXPENSES
For the Fiscal Year Ending September 30, 19x1

Description	Telephone	Postage	Collection Fees	Printed Forms	Other Office Supplies	Total
I. *Target Standard*						
1. Target Volume	37,763	37,763	37,763	37,763	37,763	
2. Standard Unit Cost	$ .29	$ .85	$ 4.76	$ 2.00	$ 1.01	
3. Target Budget	$10,800	$32,000	$180,000	$75,500	$38,000	
(line 1 × line 2 = line 3)						
II. *Control Standard*						
4. Actual Volume	34,890	34,890	34,890	34,890	34,890	
5. Standard Unit Cost	$ .29	$ .85	$ 4.76	$ 2.00	$ 1.01	
6. Control Cost	$10,118	$29,657	$166,076	$34,890	$34,890	
(line 4 × line 5 = line 6)						
III. *Actual Performance*						
7. Actual Volume	34,890	34,890	34,890	34,890	34,890	
8. Actual Unit Cost	$ .27	$ .86	$ 4.87	$ 2.12	$ 1.05	
9. Actual Total Cost	$ 9,400	$30,000	$170,000	$74,000	$36,500	
(line 7 × line 8 = line 9)						
IV. *Usage Variance*						
10. Target Volume	37,763	37,763	37,763	37,763	37,763	
11. Actual Volume	34,890	34,890	34,890	34,890	34,890	
12. Volume Variance	2,873	2,873	2,873	2,873	2,873	
(line 10 − line 11 = line 12)	Favorable	Favorable	Favorable	Favorable	Favorable	
13. Standard Unit Cost	$ .29	$ .85	$ 4.76	$ 2.00	$ 1.01	
14. Usage Variance	$ 833	$ 2,442	$ 13,675	$ 5,746	$ 2,873	$25,569
(line 12 × line 13 = line 14)	Favorable	Favorable	Favorable	Favorable	Favorable	Favorable
V. *Rate Variance*						
15. Standard Unit Cost	$ .29	$ .85	$ 4.76	$ 2.00	$ 1.01	
16. Actual Unit Cost	$ .27	$ .86	$ 4.87	$ 2.12	$ 1.05	
17. Unit Cost Variance	$ .02	$ .01	$ .11	$ .12	$ .05	
(line 15 − line 16 = line 17)	Favorable	Unfavorable	Unfavorable	Unfavorable	Unfavorable	
18. Actual Volume	34,890	34,890	34,890	34,890	34,890	
19. Rate Variance	$ 698	$ 349	$ 3,838	$ 4,187	$ 1,745	$ 9,421
(line 17 × line 18 = line 19)	Favorable	Unfavorable	Unfavorable	Unfavorable	Unfavorable	Unfavorable
VI. 20. *Net Total Variance*	$ 1,531	$ 2,093	$ 9,832	$ 1,559	$ 1,128	$16,148
(line 14 + line 19 = line 20)	Favorable	Favorable	Favorable	Favorable	Favorable	Favorable
VII. *Proof*						
21. Target Budget	$10,800	$32,000	$180,000	$75,000	$38,000	
22. Actual Total Cost	$ 9,400	$30,000	$170,000	$74,000	$36,500	
23. Variance—Target to Actual	$ 1,400	$ 2,000	$ 10,000	$ 1,000	$ 1,500	$15,900
(line 21 − line 22 = line 23)	Favorable	Favorable	Favorable	Favorable	Favorable	Favorable

NOTE: Differences between net total variances (line 20) and variance between target and actual (line 23) are due to rounding off all rates and totals to the nearest dollar or hundredth of a dollar; there is no substantial difference.

FIGURE 7–1
Step-Variable Cost Behavior

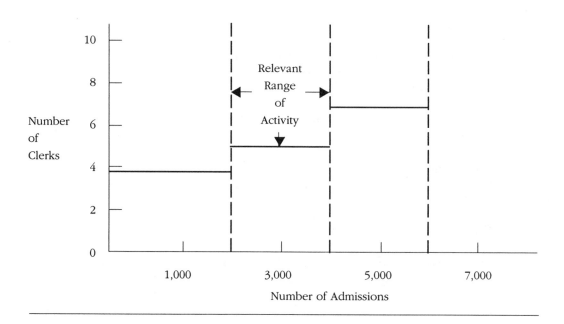

FIGURE 7–2
Variable Cost Behavior

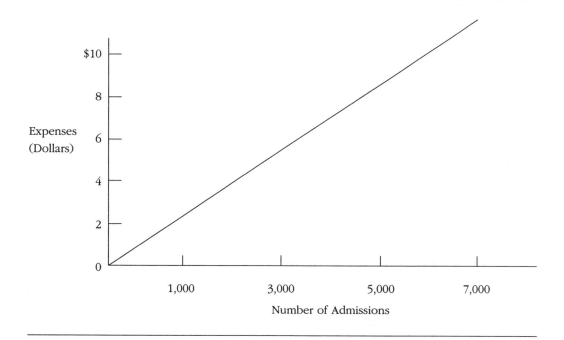

TABLE 7–11

Computation of Step-Variable Adjustment to Actual Volume of Work

Memorial Medical Center
Anytown, U.S.A.

Patient Financial Services Department
**COMPUTATION OF STEP-VARIABLE ADJUSTMENT TO ACTUAL
VOLUME OF WORK**
For the Fiscal Year Ending September 30, 19x1

Description (1)	Admitting Clerks (2)	Billing Clerks (3)	Collection Clerks (4)	Employee Benefits—Staff (5)	Total (6)
1. Target Budget Volume	37,763	37,763	37,763	37,763	37,763
2. Budget Hours (Paid)	17,680	12,480	8,320	38,480	38,480
3. Units per Paid (line 1 ÷ line 2 = line 3)	2.14	3.03	4.54	0.98	0.98
4. Average Hours per Week	40	40	40	40	40
5. Average Weeks per Year	52	52	52	52	52
6. Average Hours per Year (line 4 × line 5 = line 6)	2,080	2,080	2,080	2,080	2,080
7. Average Annual Production (line 3 × line 6 = line 7)	4,451	6,302	9,443	2,038	2,038
8. Budget Volume (line 1)	37,763	37,763	37,763	37,763	37,763
9. Actual Volume	34,890	34,890	34,890	34,890	34,890
10. Volume Variance (line 8 – line 9 = line 10)	2,873	2,873	2,873	2,873	2,873
11. Average Annual Production (line 7 – Length of Step-Variable)	4,451	6,302	9,443	2,038	2,038
12. Average Number of Steps (line 10 ÷ line 11 = line 12)	0.65	0.46	0.30	1.41	1.41
13. Standard Hourly Wage	$ 4.81	$ 4.81	$ 5.77	$ 1.25	$ 6.27
14. Average Cost per Step (line 6 × line 13 = line 14)	$10,005	$10,005	$12,002	$2,600	$13,042
15. Step-Variable Adjustment (line 12 × line 14 = line 15)	None	None	None	$2,600	$13,042
				Unfavorable	Unfavorable

NOTE: Use only whole numbers on line 12.

exemplifies the use of step-variable expense analysis to examine budget variances. The step-variable adjustment for each variable position, as computed by individual position in table 7–11, line 15, is as follows:

Position	Step-Variable Adjustment
Admitting Clerks	None
Billing Clerks	None
Collection Clerks	None
Employee Benefits—Staff	$2,600
Total Step-Variable Adjustment	$2,600 Unfavorable

TABLE 7–12

Comparative Analysis of Step-Variable Budget to Actual Performance

Memorial Medical Center
Anytown, U.S.A.

Patient Financial Services Department
COMPARATIVE ANALYSIS OF STEP-VARIABLE BUDGET
TO ACTUAL PERFORMANCE
For the Fiscal Year Ending September 30, 19x1

Description (1)	Control Budget (2)	Actual (3)	Variance: Favorable/ (Unfavorable) Amount (4)	Percent (5)
Volume				
Number of Admissions	34,890	34,890	–0–	–0–
Fixed Expenses				
Salaries and Wages	$ 91,250	$ 93,250	$ (2,000)	(2.19)
Nonsalary Expenses	46,600	45,500	1,100	2.36
Total Fixed Expenses	$137,850	$138,750	$ (900)	(0.65)
Variable Expenses				
Salaries and Wages	$228,208	$238,250	$(11,042)	(4.84)
Nonsalary Expenses	310,521	319,900	(9,379)	(3.02)
Total Variable Expenses	$538,729	$559,150	$(20,421)	(3.79)
Total Fixed and Variable Expenses	$676,579	$697,900	$(21,321)	(3.15)

When the step-variable adjustment is computed in the aggregate, there is a total unfavorable adjustment of $13,042.

The step-variable adjustment becomes part of the step-variable control budget and is compared with actual departmental performance (see table 7–12). In this example, Memorial Medical Center's patient financial services manager uses the total unfavorable step-variable variance of $13,042 to arrive at the summary adjusted step-variable salary and wage control total, as follows:

Original target budget salary and wage expense	
Variable expense (table 7–8, column 1)	$241,250
Less: unfavorable step-variable	13,042
Adjusted step-variable salary and wage expense	$228,208

The summary analysis in table 7–13 compares actual performance, the target budget, the variable control budget, and the step-variable control budget. In all cases, fixed budget expenses are the same in all budgets, while management has adjusted budgeted variable expenses according to the actual volume. Nonsalary expenses have been adjusted to $310,521 in each of the variable control budgets. The major differences are in the variable salary and wage expenses, as summarized below:

Description	Actual	Budget	Variance
Target budget	$239,250	$241,250	$ 2,000
Variable budget	$239,250	$222,947	$(16,303)
Step-variable budget	$239,250	$228,208	$(11,042)

In summary, there is no precise or perfect method for establishing a variable budgeting system. Instead, patient financial services managers need to design a system that best fits the needs of their individual department or healthcare organization. These managers, their supervisors, and their subordinates should agree on which departmental costs are fixed, variable, or step-variable. Once management classifies costs in this manner, it can develop

TABLE 7–13

Comparative Summary Analysis

Memorial Medical Center
Anytown, U.S.A.

Patient Financial Services Department
COMPARATIVE SUMMARY ANALYSIS OF ACTUAL PERFORMANCE TO TARGET, VARIABLE, AND STEP-VARIABLE CONTROL BUDGETS
For the Fiscal Year Ending September 30, 19x1

Description (1)	Actual Performance (2)	Target Budget (3)	Variable Control Budget (4)	Step-Variable Control Budget (5)
Volume				
Number of Admissions	34,890	37,763	34,890	34,890
Fixed Expenses				
Salaries and Wages	$ 93,250	$ 91,250	$ 91,250	$ 91,250
Nonsalary Expenses	45,500	46,600	46,600	46,600
Total Fixed Expenses	$138,750	$137,850	$137,850	$137,850
Variable Expenses				
Salaries and Wages	$239,250	$241,250	$222,947	$228,208
Nonsalary Expenses	319,900	336,300	310,521	310,521
Total Variable Expenses	$559,150	$577,550	$533,468	$538,729
Total Fixed and Variable Expenses	$697,900	$715,400	$671,318	$676,579

management reports that will produce the desired results: a variable budgetary control system that provides a more realistic report of cost variances, leading to greater cost-effectiveness.

NOTES

1. Robert N. Anthony, Glenn A. Welsch, and James S. Reece, *Fundamentals of Management Accounting*, 4th ed. (Homewood, Ill.: Richard D. Irwin, Inc., 1985), 10.

2. Anthony, Welsch, and Reece, *Fundamentals of Management Accounting*, 632.

3. Charles T. Horngren and Walter T. Harrison Jr., *Accounting* (Englewood Cliffs, N.J.: Prentice Hall Inc. Division of Simon & Schuster, 1989), 938.

4. Ralph S. Polimeni, Frank J. Fabozzi, and Arthur H. Adelberg, *Cost Accounting: Concepts and Applications for Managerial Decision Making* (New York: McGraw-Hill Book Company, 1986), 378.

CHAPTER 8

The Cost-finding Process

Cost finding is an integral part of the healthcare organization's budgetary control system because it is the process by which management allocates the costs of nonrevenue-producing departments to each other and to revenue-producing departments. Moreover, it is the only process that reasonably assures that managers have distributed all direct and indirect costs to the appropriate revenue centers. As such, cost finding forms the basis for *rate setting,* the process a healthcare organization uses to establish the price for each service it provides (see chapter 9). This chapter will discuss the importance of cost finding in addition to its applications in the healthcare industry. Next, chapter 8 covers cost-finding objectives and methods, concluding with keys to valid results and a cost-finding case study.

Why Cost Finding?

Patient financial services managers may be questioning why they should concern themselves with cost finding and its function in the budgetary control system. One of the primary reasons they need to become involved in this process is because the results generated from cost finding help to determine the rate (price), gross or net, that the healthcare facility is going to charge the purchaser of its services. Ultimately, this process relates directly to the amount of cash patient financial services managers should collect for healthcare services on behalf of their organization. Armed with the knowledge of how cost finding helps establish rates for services, these managers are better equipped to negotiate the final settlement of a patient's bill and/or a managed-care contract.

Traditionally, the healthcare industry has considered cost finding to be merely a means of establishing the amount to be reconciled at the end of the year between the healthcare organization and third-party payers such as Blue Cross and Medicare. Cost finding, however, is much more than that. Only in recent years have healthcare financial managers effectively used the cost-finding process as a basic management tool that can help ensure their healthcare organization's financial viability—if it is properly used.[1]

Cost-finding Applications

A unique feature of cost finding is that managers can apply it to both budgeted and actual costs incurred by the organization. It is applied to budgeted costs for *prospective rate setting,* which is the establishment of rates before the organization renders service. The most common use of prospective rate setting is to establish a published charge list. The past ten to fifteen years have seen increased use of prospective rate setting by state hospital commissions and Blue Cross plans. In most of these instances, the established rate is final with no retrospective settlement. If the healthcare organization's costs exceed the prospective rate, the healthcare facility must assume the loss. On the other hand, if the healthcare organization's costs are less than the prospective rate, the care provider can keep the surplus.

Financial managers apply cost finding to actual costs in healthcare organizations primarily to determine the cost of providing services that are reimbursed under third-party contracts. For example, the costing and pricing of many managed-care contracts require prospective rate setting, as does assessing the payment level of each of the diagnosis-related groups (DRGs). DRGs are used in the Medicare program to establish reimbursement rates in its prospective payment system (PPS).

The managers use the information resulting from cost finding to determine the third party's financial obligation to the care provider at the time of the final settlement for the fiscal year. In some cases, the results of the cost-finding process lead to retrospective negotiations or settlements with a third party. For example, a third party may agree to reimburse a healthcare provider for its costs or charges, whichever is less. If the provider billed the third party for $3 million, received interim payments totaling $2.5 million, and subsequently determined that its actual cost of providing the services was $2.75 million, the retrospective settlement would amount to $250,000:

1.	Total patient charges	$3,000,000
2.	Third-party interim payments to provider	2,500,000
3.	Provider's third-party cost	2,750,000
4.	Due from third party	250,000

To illustrate further the retrospective settlement process, assume the following:

1.	Total patient charges	$2,650,000
2.	Third-party interim payments	2,500,000
3.	Provider's third-party cost	2,750,000
4.	Due from third party	150,000

In the first example, the provider's charges were greater than its costs; therefore, it received its costs ($2,750,000). The retrospective settlement of $250,000 represents the difference between the provider's costs and the third party's interim payments. In the second example, the facility's charges of $2,650,000 were less than its costs, so it was entitled to receive only its charges. The retrospective settlement of $150,000 is the difference between the provider's charges and the third party's interim payments.

These examples highlight the need for healthcare facilities to keep established charges sufficiently higher than costs to not only generate the profit necessary to protect their assets but also to preclude being required to accept less than their costs from third-party payers. The Medicare program's PPS, as administered by the Health Care Financing Administration (HCFA) for the federal Department of Health and Human Services, allows healthcare facilities to reduce their costs below the PPS payment rate, thereby generating the profits necessary for the facility's future growth. To earn profits under this system, however, Seawell advises that healthcare organizations be managed on cost-efficiency principles similar to those employed by other industries; it is also essential that management deal successfully with competitive pressures.[2]

To guard further against the penalty of less-than-cost reimbursement, the provider must monitor costs and charges at least on a monthly basis. Financial managers can accomplish this task by applying the cost-finding process to the facility's actual costs and comparing the results with the facility's third-party charges and interim payments. This procedure should be done every month.

With the advent of DRGs, managed-care contracts, and other prospective payment systems, retrospective payments are not as prevalent in the healthcare industry as they once were. However, even Medicare's PPS allows for certain payments to be settled retrospectively by any program fiscal intermediary (FI) because final data were not available when the FI made interim payments. These reimbursements include payments to hospitals serving a disproportionate share of low-income patients; payments for the indirect costs of medical education programs; and "pass-through" cost items (costs excluded from the prospective rate and still paid by the FI based on what Medicare considers to be a reasonable cost), including

- ancillary medical education programs (e.g., nursing, clinical pastoral care, paramedical education)

- bad debts arising from patient default on coinsurance and deductible amount related to inpatient services

- costs of Certified Nurse Anesthetists in certain rural facilities containing fewer than fifty beds

- capital-related costs of "old capital" for healthcare facilities paid under the "hold harmless" methodology of capital PPS (please refer to the *Federal Register* of August 30, 1991, for specific details)

- certain organ procurement costs for qualifying facilities

Furthermore, certain Medicare providers, such as rural hospitals containing less than 100 beds and healthcare facilities having a disproportionate-share percentage of at least 5.1percent, still qualify for interim payments from the FI in biweekly lump sums (periodic interim payments, or PIP). These payments may differ from the actual claim submitted by the provider. Therefore, the FI needs to make a retrospective settlement adjustment.

Ultimately, then, through either Medicare's compliance audit or its payment appeal process, all payments to providers are subject to some sort of retrospective settlement.

Cost-finding Objectives

Some of the objectives of cost finding in a healthcare facility or department are to provide information for

- determining the total cost of a revenue-producing department or facility;

- determining a department or facility's profitability by matching total operating expenses to its total net revenue;

- determining the price of a production unit of a revenue-producing department or facility;

- conducting price-sensitivity testing to establish optimal profits and/ or competitive position;

- conducting break-even analyses to assist management in risk-based contract negotiating;[3] and

- satisfying the reporting requirements of external organizations, such as health associations, commissions, and other regulatory agencies.[4]

For the cost-finding process to fulfill these objectives and operate efficiently, Berman, Weeks, and Kukla recommend that the system meet the following prerequisites.

- The system should employ an organization chart and a related chart of accounts.

- Management has identified all cost centers as either general-service cost centers or as final cost centers to which managers ultimately assign all costs.

- The system should feature an accurate accounting system capable of accumulating financial data by cost center.

- The cost-finding process should include a comprehensive information system capable of collecting nonfinancial data by cost center and by the total healthcare facility, providing (1) the basis for distributing costs from general service centers to final cost centers; and (2) the basis for calculating unit cost by final cost center.

- Management should select a cost-finding method that is the most practicable for its facility's situation.[5]

Cost-finding Methods

While this chapter will concentrate on the results of cost finding, it is important for patient financial services managers to be familiar with the mechanics of cost finding, too, so that they can respond knowledgeably to any criticism about "ridiculously high" charges for patient services.

There are four basic cost-finding methods commonly used in the healthcare industry:

1. direct allocation

2. stepdown

3. double apportionment

4. algebraic

These methods differ primarily in the manner in which they allocate costs between and from nonrevenue-producing (support) centers. The above list places each method in order from the simplest to the most complex, and the order also proceeds from the least correct to the most accurate cost representation.[6] The first three methods were orginally developed and approved by the American Hospital Association.

Direct Allocation

The direct-allocation method allocates the costs of the nonrevenue-producing centers only to the revenue-producing centers. Certainly, most nonrevenue-producing centers render services to each other as well as to revenue-producing centers, but this system ignores that fact. The direct-allocation method does not allocate any of the costs of the nonrevenue-producing centers to the other nonrevenue-producing centers, and it does not compensate for the different demand levels for nonrevenue-producing departments' services to revenue-producing departments. As a result, the direct-allocation system is the least accurate cost-finding method.[7] The Health Care Financing Administration does not permit healthcare facilities' use of direct allocation for Medicare cost-reporting purposes, but it permits the remaining three categories.[8]

Stepdown

This system, also called the single-apportionment method, recognizes the important fact that services rendered by certain nonrevenue-producing centers are used by other nonrevenue-producing centers, as well as by revenue-producing centers or departments. Therefore, the stepdown method allocates the accumulated costs in a nonrevenue-producing center to those nonrevenue-producing centers and revenue-producing centers that use its services. The significant feature of this method is that once the costs of a nonrevenue-producing center have been allocated to other centers, the center is considered "closed." This means that no portion of the costs of other nonrevenue-producing centers whose costs have yet to be allocated will be applied to it.[9]

Exhibit 8–1 is a spreadsheet illustrating the stepdown approach to cost finding. It is separated into two major segments. The upper segment lists all of the healthcare facility's nonrevenue-producing departments, such as administration, housekeeping, laundry, and medical records. The cost centers are generally ranked so that the cost center providing the greatest amount of services to other cost centers but receiving the least amount of services heads the list. This spreadsheet segment concludes with the cost center providing the least amount of services to the other cost centers.

The lower segment of the cost study lists all of the healthcare organization's revenue-generating departments. The ancillary or special-services cost centers are usually grouped together and separated from the routine nursing services and ambulatory services.

Once management segments the organization's cost centers, it systematically distributes the nonrevenue-producing department expenses to the revenue-producing cost centers using a statistical analysis that serves as the basis to determine the amount of work or services provided to other cost centers. For example, laundry expenses are distributed to nursing services in proportion to the amount of the pounds of laundry used by nursing; the laundry's remaining expenses are allocated in a similar manner. The cost study is concluded when management has distributed all of the nonrevenue-producing expenses to the revenue-producing departments. When these allocated indirect (overhead) costs of the nonrevenue-producing departments are combined with the revenue-producing department's direct expenses, the resulting costs serve as the basis to establish the selling price for the department's services.

Double Apportionment

This cost-finding approach, the most complex of the three original American Hospital Association methods, is also called the double-distribution method. It gives more recognition to the fact that nonrevenue-producing centers render services to other nonrevenue-producing centers as well as to revenue-producing centers. Under this method, nonrevenue-producing centers are not considered permanently closed after management has allocated their

EXHIBIT 8–1

Cost-finding Spreadsheet

Memorial Medical Center
Anytown, U.S.A.

COST-FINDING SPREADSHEET
For the Budget Year 19x1

| Department | Direct Costs | Allocated Costs | | | | | | | | | | Total Costs |
		II	AG	HK	LL	OP	RM	NA	IR	MR	SS	
Nonrevenue-producing												
Departments												
Insurance and Interest	xxxxx	xx										
Administrative and General	xxxxx	xx	xx									
Housekeeping	xxxxx	xx	xx	xx								
Laundry and Linen	xxxxx	xx	xx	xx	xx							
Operation of Plant	xxxxx	xx	xx	xx	xx	xx						
Repairs and Maintenance	xxxxx	xx	xx	xx	xx	xx	xx					
Nursing Administration	xxxxx	xx	xx	xx	xx	xx	xx	xx				
Interns and Residents	xxxxx	xx	xx	xx	xx	xx	xx	xx	xx			
Medical Records and Quality												
Assurance	xxxxx	xx	xx	xx	xx	xx	xx	xx	xx	xx		
Social Service	xxxxx	xx	xx	xx	xx	xx	xx	xx	xx	xx	xx	
Subtotal												
Revenue-producing												
Departments												
Medical and Surgical Nursing	xxxxx	xx	xx	xx	xx	xx	xx	xx	xx	xx	xx	xxxxxx
ICU/CCU Nursing	xxxxx	xx	xx	xx	xx	xx	xx	xx	xx	xx	xx	xxxxxx
Operating Rooms	xxxxx	xx	xx	xx	xx	xx	xx	xx	xx	xx	xx	xxxxxx
Postoperative Room	xxxxx	xx	xx	xx	xx	xx	xx	xx	xx	xx	xx	xxxxxx
Anesthesiology	xxxxx	xx	xx	xx	xx	xx	xx	xx	xx	xx	xx	xxxxxx
Radiology	xxxxx	xx	xx	xx	xx	xx	xx	xx	xx	xx	xx	xxxxxx
Pathology	xxxxx	xx	xx	xx	xx	xx	xx	xx	xx	xx	xx	xxxxxx
Physical Therapy	xxxxx	xx	xx	xx	xx	xx	xx	xx	xx	xx	xx	xxxxxx
Respiratory Therapy	xxxxx	xx	xx	xx	xx	xx	xx	xx	xx	xx	xx	xxxxxx
Pharmacy	xxxxx	xx	xx	xx	xx	xx	xx	xx	xx	xx	xx	xxxxxx
Emergency Services	xxxxx	xx	xx	xx	xx	xx	xx	xx	xx	xx	xx	xxxxxx
Ambulatory Clinic	xxxxx	xx	xx	xx	xx	xx	xx	xx	xx	xx	xx	xxxxxx
Total	xxxxxxx	xx	xx	xx	xx	xx	xx	xx	xx	xx	xx	xxxxxxx

SOURCE: Allen G. Herkimer Jr., *Understanding Health Care Budgeting* (Rockville, Md: Aspen Publishers, Inc., 1988), 142.

costs. Instead, they are re-opened in the second part of the apportionment process to receive allocated costs from other nonrevenue-producing centers from which they have received services. After management has allocated the costs of each nonrevenue-producing center once, some costs will remain in some departments, representing services received from other departments. Management then needs to make a second apportionment to close out every nonrevenue-producing center's total direct and accumulated costs.[10]

Algebraic

Other methods of cost finding are based on the use of algebraic formulas and the computer. These formulas are designed to identify costs in departments that serve each other by recognizing the relationship that exists between those departments. Through the use of simultaneous equations, the cost allocation process for the nonrevenue-producing departments continues to accumulate cost and allocate it to other nonrevenue-producing centers as well as to revenue-producing centers until there is virtually no more cost left to allocate. The simultaneous-equation method is by far the most sophisticated method of cost finding.

A much simpler method of cost finding is the "short-formula 1" algebraic approach, which uses the healthcare organization's most recent comprehensive cost finding report. Initially, this abbreviated cost-finding method assumes that there has been no major change in revenue-producing departments' use of the nonrevenue-producing departments' services. Once the analyst confirms this condition, the percentage distribution of each revenue-producing departments' share of the indirect expenses (see table 8–5, column 5) is calculated and used to distribute any current actual or budgeted expenses, thereby establishing the total expenses of each revenue-producing department.

The short-formula 1 method, which the analyst may implement either manually or by computer, is fairly accurate and requires much less time than completing a comprehensive cost-finding study. In addition, this method usually can serve as a basis for evaluating a healthcare facility's departmental profitability, as illustrated in table 8–6. However, if there has been a major change in statistical or expense distribution since the comprehensive cost was completed (for example, increased square footage in a department), the analyst must adjust the overhead cost percentage to reflect the change.

Keys to the Cost-finding Process

One of the keys to valid results in any cost-finding or rate-setting process is understandable, meaningful cost-allocation techniques. For optimal managerial decision making, those persons responsible for cost allocation in their organization need to standardize this process to the extent possible. Although external agencies such as Medicare and Medicaid require the use of specific allocation techniques in allocating indirect costs to their patients, internal managers still require that allocation information be presented in a format meaningful to their decision making.[11]

Another key to the validity of the cost-finding or rate-setting process is the quality of the statistics used to distribute the nonrevenue-producing departments' cost to the revenue-producing departments. In selecting statistical bases, management needs to employ the statistics that are most appropriate for its particular healthcare organization. Furthermore, the statistical bases managers choose for each department or cost center should be the ones that are most appropriate for that department or cost center. Each statistical base should be the one that most accurately represents the proportionate amount of service a given nonrevenue-producing center renders to other nonrevenue-producing centers and to revenue-producing centers. It is also important that the chosen statistic be easy to identify, gather and count, and audit, subject to minimal probability of error.

The third key to valid cost finding and rate setting lies in the selection of the proper production unit for each revenue-producing department. Although the production unit is a minor part of the cost-finding process, it plays a major role in the rate-setting process. (Chapter 5 discusses the distinction between macro and micro production units.) In the cost-finding and rate-setting process, micro production units, that is, relative value units such as person-minutes, usually serve as the basis for rate setting. In the cost-finding process, managers identify direct and allocated or indirect costs for each revenue center. For example:

Laboratory

Direct costs	$716,509
Allocated or indirect costs	195,955
Total costs	$912,464

Assuming that a volume of 8,850,000 relative value units has been projected for this laboratory for the budget year, we can use the above data to develop the average cost per production unit:

$$\frac{\text{Total Departmental Costs}}{\text{Total Relevant Departmental Production Units}} = \text{Average Cost per Production Unit}$$

or

$$\frac{\$912,464}{8,850,000} = \$0.103$$

After computing average cost per micro production unit, it is relatively simple to continue the process and establish an average charge or selling price for the production unit. This procedure is discussed in more detail in chapter 9.

A Cost-finding Case Study

The case study that follows uses the double-apportionment method, which, along with the stepdown method, is arguably the most practical in terms of time and cost for the typical healthcare organization to use.[12] As with any other cost-finding system, the process illustrated in the case study starts with the gathering of the healthcare organization's direct departmental costs, as illustrated in table 8–1. The total net expenses are $6,041,776 (see column 6, line 64); this amount will serve as a "proof total" at each cost allocation checkpoint in table 8–3, column 12, line 64 and in table 8–4, column 15, line 64.

An interesting feature of the case study is its distribution of depreciation (see table 8–2). Note that major or movable and fixed equipment expenses are allocated directly to the using department; however, depreciation expense for buildings is allocated on the basis of square feet. The total depreciation expense of $224,138 is distributed to individual centers as shown in table 8–1, column 3, lines 1 through 64.

Memorial Medical Center managers used the following statistical bases to allocate the remaining cost centers:

Cost Center	Statistical Base
Administration	Average number of employees (full-time equivalents)
Housekeeping	Hours of service
Laundry and Linen	Pounds of clean laundry processed
Operation of Plant	Square feet
Repairs and Maintenance	Square feet
Dietary	Number of meals served
Loss on Pay Cafeteria	Number of meals served
Maintenance of Personnel	Number of personnel living in
Nursing Service Administration	Hours of service
Nursing Education	Weighted student hours
Interns and Residents	Hours of service
Pharmacy	Requisitioned costs
Central Sterile Supply	Requisitioned costs
Medical Records and Library	Weighted discharges
Social Service	Weighted visits
Administration (second allocation)	Accumulated costs

TABLE 8–1

General Fund Expense Summary

Memorial Medical Center
Anytown, U.S.A.

(OMIT CENTS)

GENERAL FUND EXPENSE SUMMARY (12 MONTHS ENDED SEPT. 30, 19__)	1 SALARY & FEE EXPENSE	2 NON-SALARY EXPENSE	3 DEPRECIATION EXPENSE (FORM 5)	4 DEBIT & (CREDIT) ADJUSTMENTS (FORM 8)	5 CREDITS TO EXPENSE (FORM 8)	6 NET EXPENSE
GENERAL SERVICE DEPARTMENTS						
1 *ADMINISTRATION & GENERAL	518,015	580,551	28,391	20,982	2,811	1,145,128
2 DIETARY	213,980	221,310	9,944		141	445,093
3 HOUSEKEEPING	150,733	29,466	1,905			182,104
4 LAUNDRY	80,957	8,984	6,571			96,512
4A LINEN SERVICE	9,258	12,956	1,634		4,770	19,078
5 MAINTENANCE OF PERSONNEL	9,312	723	12,188		3,046	19,177
6 OPERATION OF PLANT	37,601	64,084	13,929			115,614
7 REPAIRS & MAINTENANCE	158,411	79,509	4,391		13,456	228,875
PROFESSIONAL SERVICE DEPARTMENTS						
8 NURSING SERVICE ADMINISTRATION	101,111	5,023	2,093			108,227
9 NURSING EDUCATION						
10 INTERNS, RESIDENTS & PHYSICIANS	63,016	20,266	1,396	(11,274)		73,404
11 MEDICAL RECORDS & LIBRARY	91,018	16,460	4,810		8,449	103,839
12 SOCIAL SERVICE	16,307	132	405			16,844
SPECIAL SERVICE DEPARTMENTS						
13 OPERATING ROOMS	142,392	85,266	10,007			237,665
14 POST OPERATIVE ROOM	62,269	598	1,511			64,378
15 ANESTHESIOLOGY	146,430	19,872	957			167,259
16 DELIVERY ROOMS	64,418	13,339	4,394		368	81,783
17 RADIOLOGY	262,152	121,038	15,364	(16,310)	2,323	379,921
18 LABORATORY	463,361	123,035	16,988	(8,979)		504,405
19 ELECTROENCEPHALOGRAPHY	11,959	513	889			13,361
20 ELECTROCARDIOLOGY	67,244	6,013	1,392	645		75,294
21 PHYSICAL THERAPY	26,352	572	2,413	(52)		29,285
22 MEDICAL & SURGICAL SUPPLIES		35,009				35,009
23 CENTRAL STERILE SUPPLY	42,839	903	3,191			46,933
24 INHALATION THERAPY	31,576	16,561	2,908	1,311		52,356
25 INTRAVENOUS THERAPY	59,214	63,488	139			122,841
26 PHARMACY	38,335	145,642	1,561	(127)	173	185,238
27 EMERGENCY SERVICE	59,818	19,415	4,432	(6)		83,659
28 ISOTOPE THERAPY	39,599	46,806	3,881			90,286
29 COST OF DRUGS SOLD						
30 ROUTINE SPECIAL SERVICES						
31 M.HEALTH	46,492	562	1,022		55,000	(6,924)
32 R. THERAPY	5,496	3,987	108			9,591
33						
34						
35 RADIUM THERAPY						
36 SHOCK THERAPY						
37 OCCUPATIONAL THERAPY						
38 NON-CHC SPECIAL SERVICES						
39						
40						
41						
42						
43						
ROUTINE SERVICE						
44 NON-MATERNITY	964,138	82,202	51,289	(1,966)		1,095,663
45						
46						
47						
48						
TOTAL (Lines 44-48)						
49 MATERNITY	61,523	8,762	4,375			74,660
50 NEWBORN INFANTS	55,819	9,625	1,589			67,032
51 OUTPATIENT CLINICS	12,013	2,771	1,871			16,655
52 PRIVATE REFERRED OUTPATIENTS						
OTHER EXPENSE						
53 REAL ESTATE & PROPERTY TAXES						
54 RESEARCH						
55 FUND RAISING EXPENSE			638			638
56 AMBULANCE SERVICE						
57 SPECIAL NURSES & GUEST MEALS						
58 PAY CAFETERIA	33,499	1,761	4,188	15,776	85,706	(30,482)
59 COFFEE & GIFT SHOPS			1,375			1,375
60 BLOOD & BLOOD DERIVATIVES						
61						
62						
63 MISCELLANEOUS						
64 TOTAL	4,146,677	1,847,204	224,138	-0-	176,243	6,041,776

*INTEREST EXPENSE IN THE AMOUNT OF $ 39,441 INCLUDED.

POST TO FORM 9 COL 1

TABLE 8–2

Schedule of Depreciation

Memorial Medical Center
Anytown, U.S.A.

(OMIT CENTS)

SCHEDULE OF DEPRECIATION 12 MONTHS ENDED SEPT. 30, 198___	1 MOVABLE EQUIPMENT	2 FIXED EQUIPMENT	3 *BUILDINGS	4 TOTAL
GENERAL SERVICE DEPARTMENTS				
1 ADMINISTRATION & GENERAL	7,900	813	19,678	28,391
2 DIETARY	4,612	420	4,912	9,944
3 HOUSEKEEPING	1,075	5	825	1,905
4 LAUNDRY	4,429	140	2,002	6,571
4A LINEN SERVICE			1,634	1,634
5 MAINTENANCE OF PERSONNEL	689	5	11,494	12,188
6 OPERATION OF PLANT	285	9,664	3,980	13,929
7 REPAIRS & MAINTENANCE	1,125	217	3,049	4,391
PROFESSIONAL SERVICE DEPARTMENTS				
8 NURSING SERVICE ADMINISTRATION	468		1,625	2,093
9 NURSING EDUCATION				
10 INTERNS, RESIDENTS & PHYSICIANS	131		1,265	1,396
11 MEDICAL RECORDS & LIBRARY	1,506	75	3,229	4,810
12 SOCIAL SERVICE	12		393	405
SPECIAL SERVICE DEPARTMENTS				
13 OPERATING ROOMS	3,908	2,265	3,834	10,007
14 POST OPERATIVE ROOM	357	194	960	1,511
15 ANESTHESIOLOGY	648		309	957
16 DELIVERY ROOMS	1,204	512	2,678	4,394
17 RADIOLOGY	10,069	1,142	4,153	15,364
18 LABORATORY	8,345	1,969	6,674	16,988
19 ELECTROENCEPHALOGRAPHY	565		324	889
20 ELECTROCARDIOLOGY	1,068		324	1,392
21 PHYSICAL THERAPY	553	194	1,666	2,413
22 MEDICAL & SURGICAL SUPPLIES				
23 CENTRAL STERILE SUPPLY	977	285	1,929	3,191
24 INHALATION THERAPY	2,237		671	2,908
25 INTRAVENOUS THERAPY			139	139
26 PHARMACY	258	242	1,061	1,561
27 EMERGENCY SERVICE	722	1,554	2,156	4,432
28 ISOTOPE THERAPY	3,326		555	3,881
29 COST OF DRUGS SOLD				
30 ROUTINE SPECIAL SERVICES				
31 MENTAL HEALTH	69	141	812	1,022
32 RAD. THERAPY			108	108
33				
34				
35 RADIUM THERAPY				
36 SHOCK THERAPY				
37 OCCUPATIONAL THERAPY				
38 NON-CBC SPECIAL SERVICES				
39				
40				
41				
42				
43				
ROUTINE SERVICE				
44 NON-MATERNITY	9,647	4,978	36,664	51,289
45				
46				
47				
48				
TOTAL (Lines 44-48)				
49 MATERNITY	901	229	3,245	4,375
50 NEWBORN INFANTS	299	106	1,183	1,588
51 OUTPATIENT CLINICS	168	7	1,696	1,871
52 PRIVATE REFERRED OUTPATIENTS				
OTHER EXPENSE				
53 REAL ESTATE & PROPERTY TAXES				
54 RESEARCH				
55 FUND RAISING EXPENSE	46		592	638
56 AMBULANCE SERVICE				
57 SPECIAL NURSES & GUEST MEALS				
58 PAY CAFETERIA	1,378		2,810	4,188
59 COFFEE & GIFT SHOPS	832		543	1,375
60 BLOOD & BLOOD DERIVATIVES				
61				
62				
63 MISCELLANEOUS				
64 TOTAL	69,809	25,157	129,172	224,138

Depreciation of Fixed Equipment and Buildings should be on the basis of Floor Area as defined on Page 13 of the Cost Analysis Manual. The depreciation on buildings occupied solely by one department should be charged in full to that department.

*Includes Depreciation on Land Improvements in the amount of $ 26,834

POST TO FORM 3 COL 3

Since most healthcare organizations are not organized or operated the same way, many costs may not be equitably or appropriately distributed in a specific facility if typical statistical bases are used. If this is the case, alternate statistical bases may permit more equitable allocation of costs. Where third-party reimbursement is concerned, changing the bases for allocating costs requires intermediary approval before the beginning of the reporting period to which the change applies. However, management should examine ongoing studies to refine and improve its organization's cost-finding process. These studies should be adequately documented and should support the provider's decision to change the basis of allocation. Because the decision to change the statistical basis for allocating a cost or the order in which costs are allocated must be made before the beginning of the reporting period to which the change applies, it is absolutely necessary to carefully analyze the full effect of the change before requesting it. A sensitivity computer program can be used for this analysis as well as for determining the impact of reclassification entries.

There is no single generally accepted cost-finding procedure in the healthcare industry. The Medicare program's stepdown approach to cost finding is probably the most commonly used method; unfortunately, as is the case with other third-party reimbursement cost-finding methods, it tends to minimize reimbursement to the healthcare facility rather than develop the true cost of a revenue-producing department. For this reason, the Medicare cost-finding system should *not* be used for rate setting. After gaining the permission of its Medicare fiscal intermediary, the healthcare organization may use a more sophisticated cost-finding method to allocate allowable overhead costs to user departments (cost centers). The organization's request to change methods must be in writing and must be made no later than the end of the fourth month of the cost-reporting period to which the change is to apply.

To continue with the case study, examine table 8–3, which illustrates Memorial Medical Center's first apportionment of costs. Note that the nonrevenue-producing cost centers are *not* closed out after the first distribution as in the stepdown method. Instead, they are kept open for a second or double apportionment, as shown in table 8–4. In the double-apportionment method, the nonrevenue-producing departments pick up the costs of other nonrevenue-producing departments as well as those of revenue-producing departments. For example, table 8–3 (column 1, line 3) indicates that housekeeping has total direct expenses of $182,104 and accumulates the following indirect expenses:

Administration	$69,933
Laundry and Linen	466
Operation of Plant	794
Repairs and Maintenance	1,560
Loss on Pay Cafeteria	9,089
Total	$81,842

TABLE 8–3
Preliminary Direct Expense Apportionment

Memorial Medical Center
Anytown, U.S.A.

PRELIMINARY APPORTIONMENT 12 MONTHS ENDED SEPT. 30, 198__	1 NET EXPENSE	2 ADMINIS- TRATION	3 HOUSE- KEEPING	4 LAUNDRY & LINEN SERVICE	5 OPERATION OF PLANT	6 REPAIRS & MAINTENANCE SERVICE
		WORK SHEET 1	WORK SHEET 2	WORK SHEET 3	WORK SHEET 4	WORK SHEET 5
GENERAL SERVICE DEPARTMENTS						
1 ADMINISTRATION & GENERAL	1,145,128		29,057		18,931	37,190
2 DIETARY	445,093	96,825	7,253	522	4,726	9,283
3 HOUSEKEEPING	182,104	69,933		466	794	1,560
4 LAUNDRY & LINEN SERVICE	115,590	38,303	5,369		3,498	6,871
5 MAINTENANCE OF PERSONNEL	19,177	4,481	9,554	1,138	6,225	12,228
6 OPERATION OF PLANT	115,614	10,696	5,877	129		7,522
7 REPAIRS & MAINTENANCE	228,875	44,223	4,502	142	2,933	
PROFESSIONAL SERVICE DEPARTMENTS						
8 NURSING SERVICE ADMINISTRATION	108,227	27,331	2,399	49	1,563	3,071
9 NURSING EDUCATION						
10 INTERNS, RESIDENTS & PHYSICIANS	73,404	16,906	1,868	288	1,217	2,391
11 MEDICAL RECORDS & LIBRARY	103,839	39,094	4,768		3,107	6,103
12 SOCIAL SERVICE	16,844	5,241	581	46	379	744
SPECIAL SERVICE DEPARTMENTS						
13 OPERATING ROOMS	237,665					
14 POST OPERATIVE ROOM	64,378	12,753	1,418	741	924	1,815
15 ANESTHESIOLOGY	167,259	18,571	456	236	297	583
16 DELIVERY ROOMS	81,783	18,551	3,955	4,919	2,577	5,052
17 RADIOLOGY	379,921	52,243	6,132	1,641	3,955	7,848
18 LABORATORY	594,405	117,816	9,856	329	6,421	12,615
19 ELECTROENCEPHALOGRAPHY	13,361	3,981	478	175	312	612
20 ELECTROCARDIOLOGY	75,294	13,774	478	171	312	612
21 PHYSICAL THERAPY	29,285	9,448	2,461	526	1,603	3,149
22 MEDICAL & SURGICAL SUPPLIES	35,009					
23 CENTRAL STERILE SUPPLY	46,933	18,592	2,849	296	1,856	3,646
24 INHALATION THERAPY	52,356	11,930	991	184	646	1,268
25 INTRAVENOUS THERAPY	122,841	16,907	205		134	262
26 PHARMACY	185,238	12,139	1,566	56	1,021	2,005
27 EMERGENCY SERVICE	83,659	19,290	3,184	2,754	2,074	4,075
28 ISOTOPE THERAPY	90,286	8,501	820		534	1,050
29 COST OF DRUGS SOLD						
30 ROUTINE SPECIAL SERVICES						
31 Mental Health	(6,924)	8,150	1,199		782	1,535
32 Radiation Therapy	9,591	1,955	159		104	204
33						
34						
35 RADIUM THERAPY						
36 SHOCK THERAPY						
37 OCCUPATIONAL THERAPY						
38 NON-CRC SPECIAL SERVICES						
39						
40						
41						
42						
43						
ROUTINE SERVICE						
44 NON-MATERNITY	1,095,663	335,106	54,138	71,984	35,273	69,292
45						
46						
47						
48						
TOTAL (Lines 44–48)						
49 MATERNITY	74,660	19,299	4,792	3,274	3,122	6,134
50 NEWBORN INFANTS	67,032	18,825	1,747	2,248	1,139	2,237
51 OUTPATIENT CLINICS	16,655	3,899	2,505	391	1,631	3,206
52 PRIVATE REFERRED OUTPATIENTS						
OTHER EXPENSE						
53 REAL ESTATE & PROPERTY TAXES						
54 RESEARCH						
55 FUND RAISING EXPENSE	638		875		570	1,120
56 AMBULANCE SERVICE						
57 SPECIAL NURSES & GUEST MEALS						
58 PAY CAFETERIA	(30,482)	17,542	4,149	105	2,703	5,310
59 COFFEE & GIFT SHOPS	1,375		802	101	522	1,026
60 BLOOD & BLOOD DERIVATIVES						
61						
62						
63 MISCELLANEOUS						
64 TOTAL	6,041,776	1,145,128	182,104	115,590	115,614	228,875
	NET EXPENSE FROM FORM 3, COL. 6	TOTAL EQUALS COL. 1, LINE 1	TOTAL EQUALS COL. 1, LINE 3	TOTAL EQUALS COL. 1, LINE 4	TOTAL EQUALS COL. 1, LINE 6	TOTAL EQUALS COL. 1, LINE 7

(OMIT CENTS)

7 TOTAL COLUMNS 2-6 (WORK SHEET 6)	8 DIETARY (WORK SHEET 7)	9 LOSS ON PAY CAFETERIA (WORK SHEET 7)	10 MAINTENANCE OF PERSONNEL (WORK SHEET 8)	11 COLUMN 1 LINES 8 TO 64	12 TOTAL COLUMNS 7 TO 11		
						GENERAL SERVICE DEPARTMENTS	
85,178					108,431	ADMINISTRATION & GENERAL	1
118,609						DIETARY	2
72,753		9,089			81,842	HOUSEKEEPING	3
54,041		4,934			58,975	LAUNDRY & LINEN SERVICE	4
33,626		584				MAINTENANCE OF PERSONNEL	5
24,224		1,307			25,531	OPERATION OF PLANT	6
51,800		5,384			57,184	REPAIRS & MAINTENANCE	7
						PROFESSIONAL SERVICE DEPARTMENTS	
34,413		3,309		108,227	145,949	NURSING SERVICE ADMINISTRATION	8
						NURSING EDUCATION	9
22,670	19,810	2,149	15,951	73,404	133,984	INTERNS, RESIDENTS & PHYSICIANS	10
53,072		5,042		103,839	161,953	MEDICAL RECORDS & LIBRARY	11
6,991		652		16,844	24,487	SOCIAL SERVICE	12
						SPECIAL SERVICE DEPARTMENTS	
92,098				237,665	342,650	OPERATING ROOMS	13
17,651		1,457		64,378	83,486	POST OPERATIVE ROOM	14
20,143	1,534	2,273	5,860	167,259	197,069	ANESTHESIOLOGY	15
35,064		2,271		81,783	119,118	DELIVERY ROOMS	16
71,859	5,920	6,527	3,906	379,921	468,133	RADIOLOGY	17
147,037	1,991	14,857	11,719	594,405	770,009	LABORATORY	18
5,558		498		13,361	19,417	ELECTROENCEPHALOGRAPHY	19
15,347		1,603	1,953	75,294	94,197	ELECTROCARDIOLOGY	20
17,187		1,194	1,953	29,285	49,619	PHYSICAL THERAPY	21
				35,009	35,009	MEDICAL & SURGICAL SUPPLIES	22
27,239		2,401		46,933	76,573	CENTRAL STERILE SUPPLY	23
15,019		1,517	1,953	52,356	70,845	INHALATION THERAPY	24
17,508		2,056		122,841	142,415	INTRAVENOUS THERAPY	25
16,787		1,508		185,238	203,533	PHARMACY	26
31,377		2,402	1,953	83,654	119,391	EMERGENCY SERVICE	27
10,905		982		90,286	102,173	ISOTOPE THERAPY	28
						COST OF DRUGS SOLD	29
						ROUTINE SPECIAL SERVICES	30
11,666		1,001		(6,924)	5,743		31
2,422		247		9,591	12,260		32
							33
							34
						RADIUM THERAPY	35
						SHOCK THERAPY	36
						OCCUPATIONAL THERAPY	37
						NON-CBC SPECIAL SERVICES	38
							39
							40
							41
							42
							43
						ROUTINE SERVICE	
565,793	355,317	42,162		1,095,663	2,058,935	NON-MATERNITY	44
							45
							46
							47
							48
						TOTAL (Lines 44-48)	
36,621	25,848	2,394	1,953	74,660	141,476	MATERNITY	49
26,196		2,359		67,032	95,587	NEWBORN INFANTS	50
11,632		486		16,655	28,773	OUTPATIENT, CLINICS	51
						PRIVATE REFERRED OUTPATIENTS	52
						OTHER EXPENSE	
						REAL ESTATE & PROPERTY TAXES	53
						RESEARCH	54
2,565				638	3,203	FUND RAISING EXPENSE	55
						AMBULANCE SERVICE	56
						SPECIAL NURSES & GUEST MEALS	57
29,809	153,282					PAY CAFETERIA	58
2,451				1,375	3,826	COFFEE & GIFT SHOPS	59
						BLOOD & BLOOD DERIVATIVES	60
							61
							62
						MISCELLANEOUS	63
6,787,311	563,702	152,609	53,387	3,820,677	6,041,776	TOTAL	64
TOTAL EQUALS COLS. 2-6 LINE 64	TOTAL EQUALS COLS. 167 LINE 2	TOTAL EQUALS COLS. 1,7, & 8 LINE 58	TOTAL EQUALS COLS. 1,7,8,&9 LINE 5		TOTAL EQUALS COL.1, LINE 64		

TABLE 8–4
Secondary Direct Expense Apportionment

Memorial Medical Center
Anytown, U.S.A.

Line	1 FORM 9 LINES 13-64 IN COL. 12	2 HOUSE-KEEPING	3 LAUNDRY & LINEN SERVICE	4 OPERATION OF PLANT	5 REPAIRS & MAINTENANCE SERVICE	6 NURSING SERVICE ADMINISTRATION	7 NURSING EDUCATION	8 INTERNS RESIDENTS & PHYSICIANS
		WORK SHEET 9	WORK SHEET 10	WORK SHEET 11	WORK SHEET 12	WORK SHEET 13	WORK SHEET 14	WORK SHEET 15
13	342,650							
14	83,486	1,088	387	339	760			
15	197,059	349	123	109	244			
16	119,118	3,033	2,574	946	2,119	5,477		6,959
17	468,133	4,702	859	1,467	3,285			
18	770,009	7,558	172	2,359	5,282			43,133
19	19,417	367	91	114	256			
20	94,197	367	89	114	256			15,191
21	49,619	1,887	275	589	1,318			
22	35,009							
23	76,573	2,185	155	682	1,526	5,759		
24	70,845	760	97	237	531			
25	142,415	157		49	110	4,957		10,135
26	203,533	1,201	29	375	839			
27	119,391	2,441	1,442	762	1,705			2,347
28	102,173	629		196	439			1,269
29								
30								
31	5,743	920		287	643			
32	12,260	122		38	85			
33								
34								
35								
36								
37								
38								
39								
40								
41								
42								
43								
44	2,058,935	41,514	37,668	12,951	29,006	101,143		17,530
45								
46								
47								
48								
49	141,476	3,675	1,713	1,146	2,568	5,742		2,603
50	95,587	1,340	1,176	417	936	5,659		3,446
51	28,773	1,920	204	599	1,342	1,166		11,138
52								
53								
54								
55	3,203	671		209	469			
56								
57								
58								
59	3,826	615	53	192	430			
60								
61								
62								
63								
64	5,243,440	81,842	58,975	25,531	57,184	145,949	None	133,984
		TOTAL EQUALS FORM 9 COLUMN 12 LINE 3	TOTAL EQUALS FORM 9 COLUMN 12 LINE 4	TOTAL EQUALS FORM 9 COLUMN 12 LINE 6	TOTAL EQUALS FORM 9 COLUMN 12 LINE 7	TOTAL EQUALS FORM 9 COLUMN 12 LINE 8	TOTAL EQUALS FORM 9 COLUMN 12 LINE 9	TOTAL EQUALS FORM 9 COLUMN 12 LINE 10

NOTE A: Add Line 26, Columns 1-8 and post as a credit on Line 26, Column 9.
Redistribute on Worksheet 15.

NOTE B: Add Line 23, Columns 1-9 and post as a credit on Line 23, Column 10.
Redistribute on Worksheet 17.

(OMIT CENTS)

SECONDARY APPORTIONMENT 12 MONTHS ENDED SEPT. 30, 1968	9 PHARMACY	10 CENTRAL STERILE SUPPLY	11 MEDICAL RECORDS & LIBRARY	12 SOCIAL SERVICE	13 TOTAL COLUMNS 1 TO 12	14 ADMINISTRATION	15 TOTAL COLUMNS 13 AND 14	
	WORK SHEET 16	WORK SHEET 17	WORK SHEET 18	WORK SHEET 19		WORK SHEET 20		
SPECIAL SERVICE DEPARTMENTS								
OPERATING ROOMS					435,163		443,116	13
POST OPERATIVE ROOM	97	873			87,030	1,590	88,620	14
ANESTHESIOLOGY	3,444				201,338	3,679	205,017	15
DELIVERY ROOMS	2,037	10,043			152,288	2,783	155,071	16
RADIOLOGY	386	13,100			491,932	8,990	500,922	17
LABORATORY	738	873			830,124	15,170	845,294	18
ELECTROENCEPHALOGRAPHY	26				20,271	370	20,641	19
ELECTROCARDIOLOGY	2	437	1,739		112,392	2,054	114,446	20
PHYSICAL THERAPY	24				53,712	982	54,694	21
MEDICAL & SURGICAL SUPPLIES		23,580			58,589	1,071	59,660	22
CENTRAL STERILE SUPPLY	453	(87,333)						23
INHALATION THERAPY	447				72,917	1,333	74,250	24
INTRAVENOUS THERAPY	141				157,964	2,887	160,851	25
PHARMACY	(205,977)							26
EMERGENCY SERVICE	9,887	2,620	3,432		144,028	2,632	146,660	27
ISOTOPE THERAPY	6				104,712	1,914	105,626	28
COST OF DRUGS SOLD	172,034				172,034	3,144	175,178	29
ROUTINE SPECIAL SERVICES								30
Mental Health					7,593	139	7,732	31
Radiation Therapy					12,505	229	12,734	32
								33
								34
RADIUM THERAPY								35
SHOCK THERAPY								36
OCCUPATIONAL THERAPY								37
NON-CRC SPECIAL SERVICES								38
								39
								40
								41
								42
								43
ROUTINE SERVICE								
NON-MATERNITY	8,084		142,327	20,066	2,469,224	45,125	2,514,349	44
								45
								46
								47
								48
TOTAL (Lines 44-48)								
MATERNITY	2,410		4,938	1,391	167,662	3,064	170,726	49
NEWBORN INFANTS	936	3,493	4,140	35	117,165	2,140	119,305	50
OUTPATIENT CLINICS	647	673	1,716	2,995	51,373	939	52,312	51
PRIVATE REFERRED OUTPATIENTS			3,661		3,661	67	3,728	52
OTHER EXPENSE								
REAL ESTATE & PROPERTY TAXES								53
RESEARCH								54
FUND RAISING EXPENSE					4,552	83	4,635	55
AMBULANCE SERVICE								56
SPECIAL NURSES & GUEST MEALS								57
PAY CAFETERIA								58
COFFEE & GIFT SHOPS					5,116	93	5,209	59
BLOOD & BLOOD DERIVATIVES								60
								61
								62
MISCELLANEOUS								63
TOTAL	-0-	-0-	161,953	24,487	5,933,345	108,431	6,041,776	64
	TOTAL EQUALS ZERO (NOTE A)	TOTAL EQUALS ZERO (NOTE B)	TOTAL EQUALS FORM 9 COLUMN 12 LINE 11	TOTAL EQUALS FORM 9 COLUMN 12 LINE 12		TOTAL EQUALS FORM 9 COLUMN 12 LINE 1	TOTAL EQUALS FORM 3 COLUMN 6 LINE 64	

Housekeeping's total accumulated indirect or allocated expenses of $81,842 are transferred to table 8–4 (column 2, line 64) for the second allocation to departments that use housekeeping's services. The first and second distribution of nonrevenue-producing costs to using departments is concluded in table 8–4 (column 10, lines 13 and 14). Table 8–5 summarizes the medical center's revenue-producing departments' direct and indirect expenses. Note that one of the checkpoints or "proof totals" mentioned earlier is the $6,041,776, which appears at the end of table 8–5.

Regardless of which system the healthcare organization selects for cost finding, it is important to keep in mind the purposes the cost-finding method is intended to achieve. If cost finding is to be used for rate setting, the system design should enable the costs of nonrevenue-producing departments to be allocated in such a manner that they are accurately reflected in the healthcare organization's published charges.

If, on the other hand, the organization's cost-finding process is the basis for third-party reimbursement, the provider will find that it must use designated forms and conform to regulatory reporting requirements. However, this does not preclude the use of imaginative or creative cost finding that maximizes reimbursement. The provider should document any deviations from prescribed reporting requirements and be prepared to support its position all the way through an appeal to the Provider Reimbursement Review Board (PRRB), the body which adjudicates Medicare reimbursement disputes.

In summary, the cost-finding process is a management tool that can be used to the healthcare organization's advantage or disadvantage. It all depends on who designs the cost-finding methodology and what the designer intends to accomplish with it. Cost finding will become increasingly important when negotiating managed-care contracts.

NOTES

1. Allen G. Herkimer Jr., *Understanding Hospital Financial Management,* 2nd ed. (Rockville, Md.: Aspen Publishers, Inc., 1986), 173.

2. L. Vann Seawell, *Hospital Financial Accounting: Theory and Practice,* 2nd ed. (Westchester, Ill.: Healthcare Financial Management Association, 1987), 167.

3. Allen G. Herkimer Jr., *Understanding Health Care Budgeting* (Rockville, Md.: Aspen Publishers, Inc., 1988), 140.

4. Allen G. Herkimer Jr., *Understanding Health Care Accounting* (Rockville, Md.: Aspen Publishers, Inc., 1989), 198.

5. Howard J. Berman, Lewis E. Weeks, and Steven F. Kukla, *The Financial Management of Hospitals,* 7th ed. (Ann Arbor, Mich.: Health Administration Press Division of the Foundation of the American College of Healthcare Executives, 1990), 111.

6. James D. Suver, Bruce R. Neumann, and Keith E. Boles, *Management Accounting for Healthcare Organizations,* 3rd ed. (Westchester, Ill.: Healthcare Financial Management Association; Chicago: Pluribus Press, Inc. Division of Teach'em, Inc., 1992), 287.

TABLE 8–5

Summary of Revenue-Producing Departments' Direct and Indirect Expenses

Memorial Medical Center
Anytown, U.S.A.

SUMMARY OF REVENUE-PRODUCING DEPARTMENTS' DIRECT
AND INDIRECT EXPENSES
For the Year Ending September 30, 19x1

Department	Direct Expense	Indirect Expense	Total Expense	Percentage of Indirect Expense
(1)	(2)	(3)	(4)	(5)
Operating Room	$ 237,665	$ 205,451	$ 443,116	8.0
Postoperative Room	64,378	24,242	88,620	.9
Anesthesiology	167,259	37,758	205,017	1.4
Delivery Room	81,783	73,288	155,071	2.8
Radiology	379,921	121,001	500,922	4.6
Laboratory	504,405	340,889	845,294	13.0
EEG	13,361	7,280	20,641	.3
EKG	75,294	39,152	114,446	1.5
Physical Therapy	29,285	25,409	54,694	.9
Central Sterile Supply	81,942	(22,282)	59,660	(.8)
Inhalation Therapy	52,356	21,894	74,250	.8
Intravenous Therapy	122,841	38,010	160,851	1.5
Pharmacy	185,238	(10,060)	175,178	(.4)
Emergency Room	83,659	63,001	146,660	2.4
Isotope Therapy	90,286	16,340	106,626	.6
Mental Health	(6,924)	14,656	7,732	.6
Radiation Therapy	9,591	3,143	12,734	.1
Nonmaternity Nursery	1,095,663	1,418,686	2,514,349	54.4
Maternity Nursery	74,660	96,066	170,726	3.8
Newborn Nursery	67,032	52,273	119,305	2.0
Outpatient Clinic	16,655	39,385	56,040	1.6
Total	$3,426,350	$2,605,582	$6,031,932	100.0
Plus:				
Other Expenses				
Fund Raising			4,635	
Coffee and Gift Shop			5,209	
Total Expenses			$6,041,776	

TABLE 8–6

Application of Short-Formula 1 Method of Cost Finding to the Revenue-producing Departmental Operations

Memorial Medical Center
Anytown, U.S.A.

APPLICATION OF SHORT-FORMULA 1 METHOD OF COST FINDING TO THE REVENUE-PRODUCING DEPARTMENTAL OPERATIONS
For the Year Ending September 30, 19x1

Department	Percentage of Gross Charges (A)	Overhead Ratio	Gross Charges to Patients	Less: Deductions & Allowances (B)	Net Charges to Patients	Direct Expense	Indirect Expense (C)	Total Expense	Net Gain or Loss
Operating Room	7.4	8.0	$ 509,583	$ 48,444	$ 461,139	$ 261,143	$ 174,385	$ 435,528	$ 25,611
Postoperative Room	1.5	0.9	101,913	9,820	92,093	70,815	19,618	90,433	1,660
Anesthesiology	3.4	1.4	235,770	22,258	213,512	183,985	30,517	214,502	(990)
Delivery Room	1.9	2.8	132,332	12,438	119,894	89,960	61,035	150,995	(31,101)
Radiology	8.4	4.6	576,060	54,990	521,070	417,913	100,271	518,184	2,886
Laboratory	14.2	13.0	972,088	92,960	879,128	554,845	283,375	838,220	40,908
EEG	0.3	.3	23,737	1,964	21,773	14,697	6,539	21,236	537
EKG	1.9	1.5	131,613	12,438	119,175	82,823	32,697	115,520	3,655
Physical Therapy	0.9	.9	62,898	5,892	57,006	32,213	19,618	51,831	5,175
Central Sterile Supply	1.0	(.8)	68,909	6,546	62,363	90,136	(17,438)	72,698	(10,335)
Inhalation Therapy	1.2	.8	85,388	7,856	77,532	57,592	17,438	75,030	2,502
IV Therapy	2.7	1.5	184,979	17,675	167,304	135,125	32,697	167,822	(518)
Pharmacy	2.9	(.4)	201,455	18,985	182,470	203,760	(8,719)	195,041	(12,571)
Emergency Room	2.4	2.4	168,659	15,711	152,948	92,025	52,315	144,340	8,608
Isotope Therapy	1.8	.6	122,620	11,784	110,836	99,315	13,079	112,394	(1,558)
Mental Health	0.1	.6	8,892	655	8,237	7,616	13,079	20,695	(12,458)
Radiation Therapy	0.2	.1	14,644	1,309	13,335	10,550	2,180	12,730	605
Nonmaternity Nursery	42.0	54.4	2,891,501	274,952	2,616,549	1,205,229	1,185,817	2,391,046	225,503
Maternity Nursery	2.8	3.8	196,335	18,330	178,005	82,126	82,833	164,959	13,046
Newborn Nursery	2.1	2.0	137,200	13,748	123,453	73,735	43,596	117,331	6,122
Outpatient Clinic	0.9	1.6	64,446	5,892	58,554	18,320	34,877	53,197	5,357
Total	100.0	100.0	$6,891,022	$654,647	$6,236,375	$3,783,923	$2,179,809	$5,963,732	$272,643

(A) Source: Percent of departmental charges to total gross charges to patients.
For example: Operating Room $\frac{\$\ 509,583}{\$6,891,022} = 0.74$ or 7.4%

(B) Source: Departmental percent of total gross charges to patients multiplied by total deductions and allowances.
For example: Operating Room .074 x $654,647 = $48,444.

(C) Source: Total indirect expense represents the balance of expenses after direct expenses have been deducted.
For example: $5,963,732 less $3,783,923 = $2,179,809.
Departmental indirect expenses are computed by multiplying overhead ratio by total indirect expenses.
For example: Operating Room .08 x $2,179,809 = $174,385.

Source: Allen G. Herkimer Jr., *Understanding Hospital Financial Management,* 2nd ed. (Rockville, Md.: Aspen Publishers, Inc., 1986), 187.

7. Berman, Weeks, and Kukla, *The Financial Management of Hospitals,* 113.

8. Suver, Neumann, and Boles, *Management Accounting for Healthcare Organizations,* 288.

9. Herkimer, *Understanding Hospital Financial Management,* 177–78.

10. Herkimer, *Understanding Hospital Financial Management,* 180.

11. Suver, Neumann, and Boles, *Management Accounting for Healthcare Organizations,* 281, 278.

12. Berman, Weeks, and Kukla, *The Financial Management of Hospitals,* 131.

Financial Requirements and Rate Setting

One of the fundamental purposes of any business is to provide a product or service that meets a consumer need. Ideally, the customer and the business negotiate a fair exchange that satisfies them both.

Consequently, the business executive focuses on developing and maintaining the organization's financial viability and growth. Key to accomplishing these duties is the business' rate-setting or pricing structure—that is, if the business' long-range financial plan identifies and incorporates financial requirements and operating costs into that structure.

This chapter will address effective rate-setting objectives and techniques, including a discussion of the impact of Medicare and other third-party payers on published rates. Chapter 9 also contains a description of sensitivity testing, a process that can guide patient financial services managers and other healthcare executives in making optimal pricing decisions.

The Healthcare Organization as a Business

Crass as this may sound, a healthcare oganization is a business! Management must conduct it as such if the organization is to survive and serve its patients, employees, and community responsibly. To remain viable, the healthcare provider must receive full compensation for its financial or economic requirements as well as its accounting or operating costs. *Full financial requirements* of any healthcare organization are those resources necessary for

- meeting current operating needs;

- permitting the physical plant's replacement when appropriate; and

- allowing for changing community health and patient needs, education and research, and all other factors necessary to the institutional provision of healthcare services.[1]

Operating costs, on the other hand, are the actual expenses a healthcare facility incurs during the normal course of carrying out its day-to-day responsibilities and functions.

Accounting and economic costs differ from each other in that analysts determine accounting costs in accordance with generally accepted accounting principles, whereas the more-inclusive economic costs include a return to all suppliers of capital to the organization and focus on cash flows; in other words, economic costs consider the organization's total financial requirements.[2] The one thing that accounting and economic requirements have in common is their recognition of normal, day-to-day, out-of-pocket costs such as

- salaries and wages,

- nonsalary supplies and expenses,

- purchased services, and

- depreciation (amortized at cost).

Although these costs are generally accepted accounting costs in the healthcare industry, the Medicare and Medicaid payment systems have not always recognized all of these costs. Moreover, most third-party purchasers of health care do not accept completely the healthcare provider's economic costs. The purchasers' definitions of "reasonable" and "reimburseable" costs have frequently been at odds with the healthcare industry's view ever since third-party contracts began.[3]

Arguably, third-party payers, by virtue of their reduced business risk, create a slightly lower expense for healthcare services to their patients than do the self-paying patients. Berman, Weeks, and Kukla, however, stress the necessity of third-party payers paying their appropriate share of full costs so that the healthcare organization maintains a sound financial position. This approach to charging or billing for services remains consistent with the common business practice of offering price discounts to reliable purchasers. Unfortunately, third parties want to exclude several real operational cost elements from the items included in determining their share of cost, so they pay for services based on adjusted cost that falls short of full cost.[4]

Financial Requirements

At one time, the healthcare industry followed the philosophy that the rates the healthcare organization charged for each service should cover the service's operating expenses, along with an amount earmarked for the patient's share of the organization's other financial needs. As Berman, Weeks, and Kukla point out, while this is a reasonable, financially realistic philosophical guideline for rate setting, it does not indicate the specific cost elements the charges must include to properly reflect operating expenses and other financial needs.[5] These authors also observe that (1) third-party, cost-based payment systems would have to be modified substantially to cover all the economic costs of a healthcare facility's operation so that payment would equal full economic cost; and (2) healthcare executives should base their facility's rates on economic cost, not financial expediency.[6]

Any discussion of a healthcare organization's economic costs must include a crucial cost element: profit. In the past, healthcare executives operated and managed hospitals so that the facilities broke even or even operated in the red. From a public relations standpoint, the industry viewed the provision of health care at a profit as detrimental, at best. Today, as healthcare facilities have become big businesses no longer receiving vast amounts of philanthropic donations, the industry generally recognizes that adopting businesslike methods and financial policies would relieve much of its financial distress. As Seawell stresses, any organization will fail if its revenues are insufficient to finance its current operating activities and maintain its long-run productive capacity. Earning reasonable amounts of profit is essential, he concludes, because in an extended period of price inflation, technological advancements, and other fiscal pressures, the healthcare organization must obtain revenues in excess of the costs of providing its services.[7]

Profitability measures how well the healthcare organization conducts its operations to serve the community and the patient. Drucker declares that there is no virtue in being nonprofit—any activity that could produce a profit yet does not is antisocial. A business' first responsibility, he continues, is to produce an adequate surplus. Otherwise, the organization would be stealing from the commonwealth, depriving society and the economy of the capital needed to provide tomorrow's jobs. A business cannot speak of a profit, he concludes, unless it has earned the true cost of capital—and, in most cases, the cost of capital is much higher than what businesses tend to consider as "record profits."[8]

The plain fact is that any healthcare organization—or any other business, for that matter—requires payment not only for its operating costs but also for its economic costs if it is to grow, especially in an inflationary economy. Furthermore, healthcare executives must base their organization's economic costs on its current budget, not past experience.

Third-Party Impact on Published Rates

A *third-party payer* is one who pays for a service or product on behalf of another individual or subscriber. The Medicare program, for example, pays a healthcare facility for services rendered to the program's subscribers. Many of the major third-party healthcare service purchasers—Medicare, Medicaid, and some Blue Cross plans—purchase these services under a contract in which the party agrees to pay the provider only those costs it deems to be allowable. This amount frequently falls short of the facility's published rates. The difference between published rate and allowable cost is called contractual allowance, and the healthcare provider has no recourse to the beneficiary; in other words, the healthcare facility cannot collect from the patient.[9]

Someone has to make up the cost of nonallowable expenses and enable the healthcare facility to meet its full financial requirements. The only persons able (or left) to do so are the self-paying and commercial insurance patients. These patients, in effect, make up the difference between the facility's total financial requirements and the amount paid by the third-party contractor,[10] as in the following example:

	Third-Party Payment System	Full-Charge Payment System
Total Gross Charges to Patient	$5,000	$5,000
Less: Deductible and Coinsurance from Patient	500	500
Net Balance Due	$4,500	$4,500
Less: Amount Due from Third-Party Contract	4,050	
Contractual Allowance	$ 450	$ –0–
Cash Inflow Analysis		
Due from Patient	$ 500	$ 500
Due from Patient's Insurance	4,050	4,500
Total Cash Inflow	$4,550	$5,000

This payment procedure is unique in that:

- The third party is the major purchaser of healthcare services. In fact, third-party contractors pay more than 90 percent of patients' bills.[11]

- The third party determines what costs are reasonable, appropriate, and allowable.

- Any difference between the third party's cash payment and the healthcare provider's published charge (the contractual allowance) is lost income.

- The healthcare provider has no recourse to the patient or any other party; its only course of action is to recover the contractual allowance somehow from the full-charge patient.

What is really happening? The self-paying patient and the patient with commercial insurance coverage are actually subsidizing the third-party patients and their guarantors. The following case study illustrates this situation.

Case Study of Payment Procedures

Assume that Memorial Medical Center of Anytown, U.S.A., has computed its actual accounting costs for one thousand patient days as follows:

Total Operating Costs for One Thousand Patient Days

Salaries and Wages	$210,000
Nonsalary Expenses	80,000
Depreciation	10,000
Total Operating Costs	$300,000

Assume further that the medical center has been experiencing a loss of 10 percent of total operating costs due to bad debts and charity allowances. In addition, the organization's board of trustees has decided that the medical center requires a minimum of 10 percent of total operating costs as profit to provide for growth and development. Here is a summary of the organization's total financial requirements:

Total Financial Requirements for One Thousand Patient Days

	Total Amount	Average Cost per Patient Day	Percent
Operating Costs			
Salaries and Wages	$210,000	$210	58.34%
Nonsalary Expenses	80,000	80	22.22
Depreciation	10,000	10	2.78
Total Operating Costs	$300,000	$300	83.34%
Plus:			
(a) Provision for Bad Debts and Charity Allowances	30,000	30	8.33
(b) Growth and Development	30,000	30	8.33
Total Financial Requirements	$360,000	$360	100.00%

Figure 9–1 illustrates these amounts. This illustration assumes that all patients are charged the same average rate of $360 per patient day—a two-party, or full-charge, payment system.

FIGURE 9–1

Memorial Medical Center's Financial Requirements per Patient Day for One Thousand Patients—Two-Party Payment System

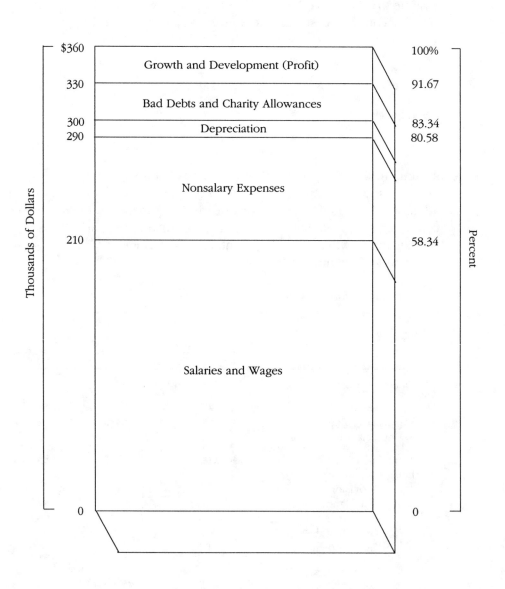

To continue with the case study, assume that half of Memorial Medical Center's patients are covered by a third-party payment system. These payment systems reimburse the medical center only for its accounting costs of $300 per patient day, even though the facility must provide for bad debts and charity care along with its profit or growth and development—costs that management distributes over the entire patient population. The following computation shows the redistribution of the medical center's financial requirements:

Description	Full-Charge Patient	Cost-based Patient	Total
Number of Patients	500	500	1,000
Direct Costs			
Salaries and Wages	$105,000	$105,000	$210,000
Nonsalary Expenses	40,000	40,000	80,000
Depreciation	5,000	5,000	10,000
Total Direct Costs	$150,000	$150,000	$300,000
Plus:			
(a) Provision for Bad Debts and Charity Allowances	30,000	-0-	30,000
(b) Profit (Growth and Development)	30,000	-0-	30,000
Total Financial Requirements	$210,000	$150,000	$360,000
Average Charge Per Patient Day	$ 420	$ 300	$ 360

Figure 9–2 depicts the cost redistribution. Looking at this case study, it is easy to see how management has no recourse but to shift the financial burden from the patient with cost-based coverage, who pays $300 per patient day, to the full-charge patient, who pays $420 per patient day.

In the next step, assume that the patient mix at Memorial Medical Center is as follows:

Patient Description	Number	Percent
Full-Charge (Private)	250	25%
Cost-based (Medicare)	500	50
80% of Cost (Medicaid)	250	25
Total Patients	1,000	100%

FIGURE 9–2

Comparison of Memorial Medical Center's Average Charge per Patient Day with Its Cost-based Patients

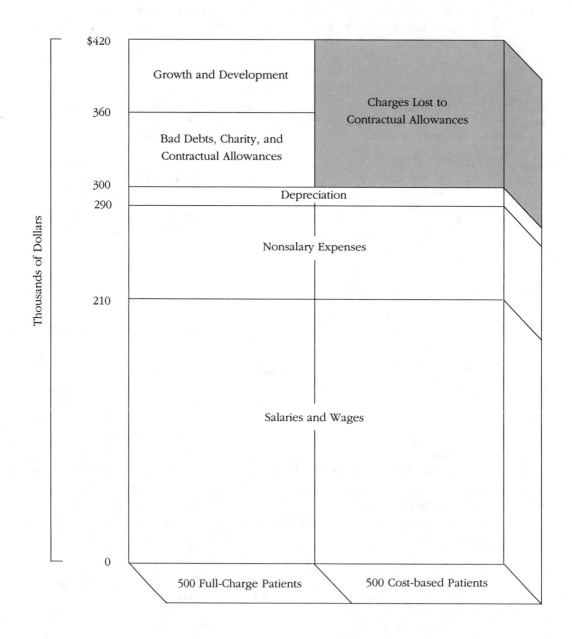

Although the medical center's total financial requirements remain the same, management would distribute the costs as follows:

Description	Full-Charge Patient	Cost-based Patient	80%-of-Cost Patient	Total
Number of Patients	250	500	250	1,000
Direct Costs				
Salaries and Wages	$ 52,500	$105,000	$52,500	$210,000
Nonsalary Expenses	20,000	40,000	20,000	80,000
Depreciation	2,500	5,000	2,500	10,000
Total Direct Costs	$ 75,000	$150,000	$75,000	$300,000
Less:				
(a) Provision for Bad Debts and Charity Allowances	$ 30,000	-0-	-0-	$ 30,000
(b) Growth and Development	30,000	-0-	-0-	30,000
(c) Loss on 80%-of-Cost Patients	15,000	-0-	(15,000)	-0-
Total Financial Requirements	$150,000	$150,000	$60,000	$360,000
Average Charge per Patient Day	$ 600	$ 300	$ 240	$ 360

As figure 9–3 shows, Memorial Medical Center's financial officers had to shift the burden of meeting the facility's financial requirements for revenue losses and growth more markedly to the full-charge patient. Memorial Medical Center charges this patient an average cost of $600 per patient day, while the cost-based patient pays $300 per day and the 80-percent-of-cost patient pays $240 per day.

Although Memorial Medical Center charges an average daily rate of $600 to *all* patients for its services, only the self-paying patients and/or their private (commercial) insurance companies pay this amount. The other patients and their third-party healthcare service purchasers pay either $300 or $240 per day, with the medical center writing off as contractual allowances the differences between these payments and the $600 gross charge (price). In other words, the facility's operating costs of doing business have not increased, but management needed to inflate the published (gross) charges to compensate for losses due to contractual arrangements.

This case study illustrates payment conditions that go far beyond the original congressional intent of the Medicare program. Congress designed the program to pay

- all costs of program beneficiaries and none of the nonparticipants' costs, and

FIGURE 9–3

Comparison of Memorial Medical Center's Average Charge per Patient Day (25 Percent) with Cost-Based Patients (50 Percent) and 80%-of-Cost Patients (25 Percent)

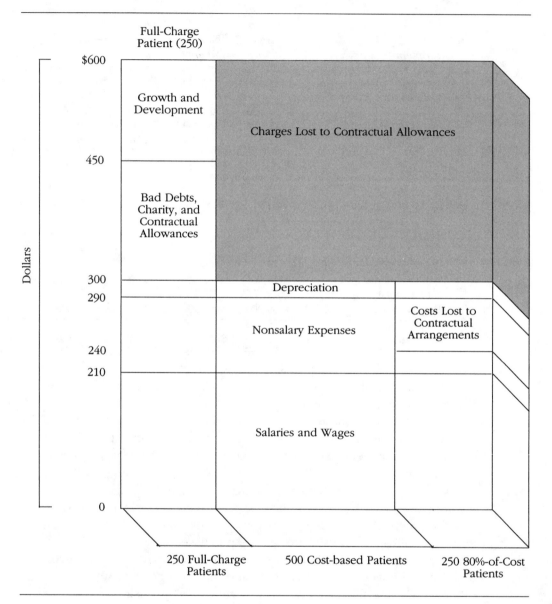

- actual costs, however widely they may vary from one institution to another, unless such costs (in the aggregate) are substantially in excess of those costs incurred by similarly situated providers in the same area.[12]

It is doubtful, then, that Congress intended to impose additional social costs upon full-charge patients.

Reasonable-Cost Reimbursement

As a general policy, the Medicare program does not pay for providers' costs that exceed reasonable and prudent expenses of similarly situated providers. Currently, fiscal intermediaries, or FIs—typically Blue Cross or commercial insurance companies serving as Medicare claims agents and payers on behalf of the Department of Health and Human Services—do not tend to view providers' total expenses in the aggregate except for certain small providers such as home health agencies and comprehensive outpatient rehabilitation facilities.

Apparently, FIs' applying this "reasonable cost" rule to other providers' aggregate costs would be easily refuted by these organizations based on detailed analyses of patient needs, market prices, and other relevant factors. Indeed, the *Code of Federal Regulations* (42 CFR § 413.5) notes that costs may vary from provider to provider, and that the objective of reasonable-cost reimbursement is to pay actual costs, no matter how widely they do vary.

Nonetheless, reasonable costs form the basis of reimbursement under the Medicare program for only a few healthcare services:

- hospital outpatient services (except for clinical diagnostic lab); some fee schedule blending is used for radiology and other diagnostic procedures;

- skilled nursing facility services, subject to a per-diem cap on routine inpatient costs;

- home health agency services, subject to limits applied to each visit discipline (skilled nursing, physical therapy, occupational therapy, speech pathology, home health aide); and

- comprehensive outpatient rehabilitation facility services.

Healthcare facilities exempt from Medicare's prospective payment system (PPS) are reimbursed based on reasonable costs, subject to a limitation on the rate of increase in inpatient costs, determined in accordance with the Tax Equity and Fiscal Responsibility Act (TEFRA). In other words, Medicare inflates a "base-year" cost per discharge by annual TEFRA adjustment factors to establish the current-year cost limit. PPS-exempt facilities include psychiatric, rehabilitation, children's, and certain cancer hospitals, subject to per-discharge limits; outpatient therapy providers; and rural health clinics.

Medicare Reimbursement Improvements

Funds for Future Use

Certainly, no patient financial services professional—or any healthcare organization executive, for that matter—would say that the Medicare payment system is perfect. Fortunately for the healthcare industry's viability, however, the current Medicare program structure does reflect a heightened awareness that healthcare organizations need to generate cash inflows in excess of cash outflows to be able to set aside funds for future growth and for replacement of capital assets (assets having a life of more than one year that are not bought and sold in the ordinary course of business[13]). Under specified conditions, certain funds that a healthcare organization sets aside with trustees or that its board of directors specially designates receive special treatment in the Medicare program: Medicare does not use the generated interest income to reduce otherwise allowable interest income. In addition, interest expense that a provider incurs on funds it borrowed to meet a financial need is an allowable cost, subject to the usual reimbursement rules.

Please note, however, that Medicare makes no specific payment to the healthcare organization or other providers as a "return on investment" or "return on equity." The program expects, for example, that the PPS will allow healthcare facilities to reduce their costs below the PPS payment rate, thereby generating the profits necessary for future growth. PPS profit margins are a regular feature of the Prospective Payment Assessment Commission's reports to Congress.

Capital-related Costs

On August 30, 1991, Health Care Financing Administration (HCFA) released its final rules regarding payment for capital-related costs under Medicare PPS. The September 1, 1992, *Federal Register* reports changes to some details of this system.

Generally, HCFA bases provider payments on a national capital payment rate that it adjusts for geographic differences. HCFA also adjusts for large urban healthcare facilities and facilities that serve a disproportionate share of low-income patients.

Beginning with the first cost-reporting period starting after September 30, 1991, and during the first ten years of this program, the following transition rules apply:

- Healthcare facilities whose base-year costs fall below the national average receive payment on a "fully prospective" basis. Over the ten years, HCFA will blend the hospital-specific capital rate with the federal rate so that the mix is 90 percent hospital-specific and 10 percent federal the first year, with the mix changing by 10 percent each year until 2001, when HCFA will pay the healthcare facility at 100 percent of the federal rate.

- Healthcare facilities whose base-year costs exceed the national average receive payment under the "hold harmless" method. Under this method, and only during the transition, these providers receive 85 percent of their Medicare capital-related costs for "old" capital, plus a portion of the federal rate for their "new" capital.

Specific details regarding Medicare inpatient capital-related payments are in the *Federal Register* of August 30, 1991.

Day-to-Day Expenses

Medicare has become more progressive in addressing the provider's recovery of operating expenses. The program's DRG payments (more on this concept later in the chapter) are designed to cover the full cost of inpatient services, exclusive of pass-through items. Although HCFA receives and settles provider cost reports annually, providers do not actually wait until year-end to accumulate all of the cost, pass-through, and DRG claims. Rather, HCFA makes payments on an interim basis—claim by claim or, in some cases, biweekly lump-sum amounts. These interim payments are then adjusted retrospectively at year-end to the amount actually due the provider, based on its cost report.

Medicare Bad Debts

Another financial concern for any healthcare organization, bad debts, is addressed by the Medicare program. Medicare pays the full amount of bad debts related to Medicare deductible and coinsurance if the claims meet four conditions:

1. Debt must be related to covered services and derived from deductible and/or coinsurance amounts.

2. The provider must be able to establish that it made reasonable collection efforts.

3. The debt was actually uncollectible when the provider claimed it as worthless.

4. The provider exercised sound business judgment in establishing that there was no likelihood of the debt's recovery at any time in the future [42 CFR § 413.80(e)].

In addition, Medicare presumes uncollectibility if, after the healthcare facility makes reasonable collection efforts, a claim remains unpaid after 120 days.

Be aware, however, that HCFA has become very stringent in its audits of Medicare bad debts, and providers must document their efforts at determining any other available insurance coverage.

Addressing Provider Needs and Concerns

A number of professional healthcare associations and government committees are involved in refining Medicare/Medicaid reporting and disbursement procedures. For example, HCFA has an ongoing research and development program for this purpose. Also, in 1983, Congress created the Prospective Payment Assessment Commission (ProPAC) in the same legislation that enacted Medicare's prospective price-setting system. This permanent, independent commission is not an appeals body, nor does it have any regulatory powers. Rather, ProPAC is responsible for making recommendations on the proper maintenance and modifications needed to the prospective payment system. Specifically, Congress charges ProPAC with

- making an annual recommendation to the Secretary of the Department of Health and Human Services on the appropriate annual percentage change in payment for the provider's inpatient discharges;

- consulting with and recommending to the secretary needed changes in the diagnosis-related-group (DRG) classification and relative weighting factors; and

- evaluating any changes the secretary makes to these classifications and weighting factors.[14]

Healthcare industry associations such as the American Hospital Association (AHA) and the Federation of Healthcare Systems (FAHS) have been instrumental in advocating healthcare reforms at the national level. These associations, their member institutions, and allied hospital associations advocated many of the changes that HCFA included in its final rule for incorporating Medicare capital-related payments into the prospective payment system starting in fiscal 1992. The improvements to HCFA's proposed rule, AHA believes, will help alleviate large and potentially inequitable swings in payment had HCFA implemented the proposed rule without modifications. Among AHA's criticisms of the final rule are its administrative burdens and payments eventually based on averages that are inadequate in reflecting local provider circumstances. The association will work with its allied hospital associations to monitor the new rule's implementation of the new capital payment system and its impact on providers.[15]

Although the aforementioned activities contribute to improving the payment system, it is the financial officers of the nation's healthcare organizations who ultimately can resolve the reimbursement dilemma. They must lobby aggressively and protect the financial viability of their own healthcare facilities and that of the industry as a whole. To accomplish these goals, healthcare providers and their financial officers must

- establish charges based on the facility's total financial requirements;

- challenge third-party interpretation of reimbursement regulations when appropriate;

- keep abreast of pending or proposed changes in reimbursement regulations—informative resources include Commerce Clearing House's *CCH Medicare and Medicaid Guide,* the Bureau of National Affairs' *BNA Medicare Reporter,* program memoranda from Medicare fiscal intermediaries, and newsletters produced by Healthcare Financial Management Association (HFMA) and several accounting and consulting firms; and

- become actively involved in professional associations such as AHA, HFMA, the FAHS, and other organizations that are politically active, in an effort to keep viable the institutions comprising the healthcare industry.

In the end, the healthcare organization is not only a business but part of a political process.

Rate Setting

Rate setting is the process a healthcare organization uses to establish the gross prices it will charge all of its patients. However, as the case study illustrates, even though the facility charges all patients the same gross price for services, the patients' third-party insurance companies do not pay the healthcare provider the same amount of cash. Presently, most healthcare organizations establish their prices for services on a prospective basis in that they determine prices before the patient receives any health services. These prospective payment systems can be determined using at least four different methodologies:

1. *Per service,* or "a la carte": the facility charges the patient only for each service purchased or received, i.e., chest X ray, CBC lab test, etc., which have a specific price.

2. *Per diem,* or all-inclusive: the patient is charged one price for each day spent in the healthcare facility, regardless of the amount of services received.

3. *Per case or diagnosis:* the facility charges the patient one amount for the entire hospital stay based upon the type of admitting and/or the discharge diagnosis; Medicare's diagnosis-related-group (DRG) concept is an excellent example. Most prospective payment systems, promoted by the Medicare program in the early 1970s and mandated by the Social Security Amendments of 1983 to encourage more effective healthcare management, were paid by HCFA on a per-diem or per-patient-day basis until October 1, 1983. On this date, HCFA began paying providers on a per-case, or diagnosis-related-group, basis.[16] The DRG system was developed by Yale University for classifying patient admissions into clinically coherent and homogeneous groups with respect to resources used by the provider in delivering healthcare services.[17] There are 492 DRGs, of which 483 are grouped into twenty-five major diagnostic categories (MDCs), broad clinical categories differentiated from all others based on body-system involvement and disease etiology. Two DRGs are for ungroupable cases, and seven cases group to DRGs having no assignment to MDCs.

4. *Per capita:* the patient pays the healthcare provider a periodic (usually monthly) payment for services whether services are received or not; most health maintenance organizations utilize this type of prospective payment arrangement.

With the advent of managed-care or risk-based contracting, healthcare facilities could have one or more of the above types of negotiated payment systems. However, a negotiated plan that utilizes the per-service system is frequently supplemented with some percentage amount as a "discount" from the established price.

The Per-Diem Rate

The per-diem rate is occasionally used in municipal and long-term healthcare facilities. As defined earlier, a single rate per patient day includes all the services the patient receives as part of that unit of time. The following example shows how the healthcare facility determines the per-diem rate.

Medical Center Divisions	Costs
General services	$1,500,000
Financial services	1,000,000
Nursing services	3,000,000
Professional services	2,500,000
Total costs	$8,000,000
Total patient days	20,000
Average cost per patient day	$ 400
Number of admissions	4,000

If the facility bases the per-diem rate upon its number of admissions or diagnoses, the average cost per admission would be computed as follows:

$$\frac{\text{Total Facility Costs}}{\text{Number of Relevant Admissions}} = \text{Average Cost per Admission}$$

or

$$\frac{\$8,000,000}{4,000} = \$2,000$$

The facility must add a provision for profit to this average cost per admission. Using this example, for instance, assume the medical center wants to realize a 25-percent margin above its average cost. We can then compute the selling price as follows:

Average cost per admission	$2,000
25 percent of average cost per admission	$ 500
Selling price	$2,500

Please note, however, that the $500 margin only provides a 20-percent margin above the selling price:

Average cost per admission	$2,000
Markup margin	$ 500
Average selling price	$2,500
Margin percentage of cost	25%
($500 ÷ $2,000)	
Margin percentage of selling price	20%
($500 ÷ $2,500)	

The per-diem rate has these advantages:

- Before admission and/or discharge, the healthcare organization and the patient know the total patient charge amount.

- The charging and accounting systems are relatively easy to understand and compute.

- The charge system facilitates the cash collection process.

- Using this charge system reduces the size of the billing staff.

Some of the disadvantages of the per-diem rate are as follows:

- The rate does not necessarily represent the amount of financial resources needed by the healthcare organization to produce the service.

- The rate does not produce a system conducive to the price sensitivity testing necessary to ensure an organization's profitability.

The Per-Service Rate

Prior to the advent of Medicare's DRG payment system, the per-service system of rate setting was the most common method used in the healthcare industry. The key to per-service rate setting lies in selecting the unit of service to be priced. Units of service may be either macro or micro. The macro unit of service grossly represents the service a patient receives; for example, X ray examination, laboratory test, and operating room care. Even though this statistic has considerable value, it does not adequately represent the amount of resources the healthcare facility used to furnish the service.

The weighted, or micro, unit of service endeavors to establish a series of relative value units (RVUs) for each service. The value management assigns to each RVU is directly proportional to the amount of resources, that is, labor, supplies, and equipment, required by the healthcare facility to provide the service. One of the earliest and most commonly used RVU system is the work-load measurement for laboratory services developed by the College of American Pathologists. Under this system, the healthcare facility can determine a price per RVU and simply multiply this price (charge) by the number of RVUs assigned to each laboratory test. We can compute the RVU cost as follows:

Laboratory Description	Total Cost	Unit Cost
Direct Expenses		
Salaries and Wages	$ 800,000	$ .40
Nonsalary Expenses	600,000	.30
Depreciation	200,000	.10
Total Direct Expenses	$1,600,000	$ .80
Plus: Allocated Costs	800,000	.40
Total Accounting Costs	$2,400,000	$1.20
Plus: Provision for		
(a) Deduction	$ 240,000	$ .12
(b) Profit	240,000	.12
Total Economic Costs	$2,880,000	$1.44
Total Relative Value Units	2,000,000	1

Another example of a weighted unit of measurement, which reflects the mix of micro outputs for various departments, is the Resource Based Relative Value Scale (RBRVS).[18] Developed for HCFA by reseachers at Harvard University, the RBRVS groups the inputs necessary to provide physician services in three categories:

1. physician work

2. practice expenses

3. opportunity costs (this category not included in the RBRVS adopted by HCFA for Medicare patients)[19]

Sensitivity Testing

Whichever rate-setting methodology the healthcare organization adopts, it is important to test its price sensitivity to the third-party payment system. *Sensitivity testing,* an extended variation of break-even analysis, is the process of taking known factors and evaluating them under changing conditions. All but one of the factors in the break-even formula are fixed by either budgetary restrictions or management decisions. The one remaining element in the formula is price. Since price is the only variable factor, it lends itself uniquely to sensitivity testing.[20]

The objective of sensitivity testing is to analyze the impact of price changes on the institution's or the department's operating profit. Armed with this information, management can then best determine which final selling price is most appropriate for a specific service or commodity. In setting the price, there are many considerations. For example, the lowest price may be the most attractive for the market, but it requires the highest volume of sales to break even. Conversely, while the highest price may require fewer units of sales to break even, it may be too expensive for the institution's market. This type of analysis, which can be expanded over a wide price range, serves as a guide to management and assists in making optimal pricing decisions.[21]

Usually, it is not in the provider's best interest to use a common profit margin for all departments. Management should analyze each revenue-producing department to determine the percentage of charges generated by the third-party, cost-based payer. As a general rule, departments that provide the largest portion of services to a cost-based payer should have a narrow profit margin, thereby reducing the amount to be written off by the healthcare organization as a contractual allowance. Conversely, revenue-generating departments with lower utilization by cost-based programs should have a broader profit margin to maximize the cash flow from charge-based patients. The following example illustrates this rate-setting policy.

Assume that Memorial Medical Center's laboratory and radiology departments have identified these operating expenses:

	Laboratory	*Radiology*
Direct Expenses	$1,600,000	$1,600,000
Allocated Costs	800,000	800,000
Total Expenses	$2,400,000	$2,400,000

If a uniform profit margin of 25 percent is applied to the total expenses, the planned profit would be $600,000.

Assume that 60 percent of laboratory services and 30 percent of radiology services were purchased by cost-based programs. The comparative operating statement would be as follows:

	Laboratory	*Radiology*
Cost-based Reimbursement	60%	30%
Revenue:	$3,000,000	$3,000,000
(@ 25% Total Expenses)		
Less: Contractual Allowances	360,000	180,000
Net Revenue	$2,640,000	$2,820,000
Total Expenses	$2,400,000	$2,400,000
Net Profit	$ 240,000	$ 420,000

Monitoring Product and Product-Line Profitability

A healthcare organization's *product line* is a group of healthcare services sharing a common characteristic and/or clientele. Pediatric services, obstetric services, cardiovascular services, and emergency services are all product lines. For example, a "normal delivery" is classified as a product within the obstetric product line. Another example of a product line could be one man aged-care contract that binds the healthcare provider and a purchaser to a negotiated prospective payment system over a period of time, usually one year.

Regardless of the types of products or product lines, it is imperative that management constantly monitor each as to their expense-to-cash ratio. The *expense-to-cash ratio* is the relationship between the total (direct and indirect) expense required by the provider to produce the related services/products and the amount of cash it actually received for the services. For example, assume that a "normal delivery" costs $2,000, and the average cash received for this service/product is $1,900. These totals would produce a negative

TABLE 9–1

RCC Distribution of Gross Patient Charges by Managed-Care Contract

Memorial Medical Center
Anytown, U.S.A.

RCC DISTRIBUTION OF GROSS PATIENT CHARGES BY MANAGED-CARE CONTRACT

For the Three-Month Period Ending September 30, 19x2

Description (1)		HMO–1 (2)	HMO–2 (3)	HMO–3 (4)	HMO–4 (5)	HMO–5 (6)	Total (7)
Routine Nursing	Revenue	$ 520,550	$335,700	$150,630	$245,980	$ 759,650	$2,012,510
	Percent	0.258	0.166	0.074	0.125	0.377	1
Surgery	Revenue	$ 247,890	$127,545	$ 50,560	$112,350	$ 389,650	$ 927,995
	Percent	0.267	0.137	0.055	0.121	0.420	1
Laboratory	Revenue	$ 175,880	$ 67,840	$ 35,650	$ 85,795	$ 325,895	$ 691,060
	Percent	0.254	0.098	0.052	0.124	0.472	1
Radiology	Revenue	$ 130,850	$ 55,895	$ 45,698	$ 58,630	$ 315,950	$ 607,023
	Percent	0.210	0.092	0.075	0.097	0.520	1
Emergency	Revenue	$ 247,830	$ 75,840	$ 36,900	$ 54,680	35,820	$ 451,070
	Percent	0.549	0.168	0.082	0.122	0.079	1
Total	Revenue	$1,323,000	$ 662,820	$319,438	$557,435	$1,826,965	$4,689,658
	Percent	0.282	0.141	0.068	0.118	0.389	1
Number of Discharges		375	146	120	86	340	1,067
Average Gross Charge per Discharge		$ 3,528	$ 4,539	$ 2,661	$ 6,481	$ 5,373	$ 4,395

expense-to-cash ratio of 20:19, or 1.05. This ratio is computed by dividing the amount of cash received by the provider into the total expense ($2,000/ $1,900 = 1.05). Any expense-to-cash ratio that is over 1.00 is classified as a negative ratio. A negative ratio is generally unacceptable unless the healthcare organization is using this service as a "loss leader" to attract the female market segment for other services within the product line and/or its facility. Generally, the net cash inflow should be greater than the total operating expense to produce the service.

Currently, there are two types of products and product lines that all healthcare providers must constantly monitor. These are

1.   managed-care contracts and

2.   diagnosis-related groups.

The following case study is a methodology that patient financial services managers can use in computing the expense-to-cash ratio to either of these groups. The study uses what is referred to as the RCC, or ratio of charges to charges, method of distributing costs to specific products and/or product lines. The RCC method assumes that there is a direct relationship between the gross charge per service and the expense to produce the service. Applying this methodology in table 9–1, the total gross charges of Memorial Medical Center's five HMOs amounted to $4,689,658. This is divided among its producing departments. For example, the total charges used in routine nursing were $2,012,510, of which HMO–1 used $520,550, or 0.258 percent. This percentage is used in table 9–2 to distribute the total routine nursing expenses of $1,955,684, allocating $504,566 as the total expense of producing HMO–1's routine nursing care.

After distributing the total operating expenses to each HMO contract as line 6 of table 9–1 illustrates, the next step is to ultimately determine the profitability of each HMO or product line (table 9–2, line 16). There are many approaches to monitoring the costs of a product or product line; the RCC method is but one.[22] The important point to stress is that each product, i.e., DRG, HMO, etc., must be monitored at least once a month and evaluated by management to determine its profitability. Armed with this knowledge, the healthcare organization will be in a stronger position at the next contract negotiations, and it will realize a positive cash flow.

In summary, it is absolutely necessary to use price sensitivity testing on a departmental as well as on a product-line basis. Always keep in mind that the price the healthcare facility charges should be related to the total cost of producing the service. The ideal healthcare rate-setting policy should emphasize

•   reducing the amount of contractual allowances,

•   maximizing cash inflows to cover all related costs, and

•   obtaining a reasonable profit.

TABLE 9–2

RCC Analysis of Expense and Profitability of Managed-Care Contracts

Memorial Medical Center
Anytown, U.S.A.

RCC ANALYSIS OF EXPENSE AND PROFITABILITY OF MANAGED-CARE CONTRACTS
For the Three-Month Period Ending September 30, 19x2

Line	Description (1)		HMO–1 (2)	HMO–2 (3)	HMO–3 (4)	HMO–4 (5)	HMO–5 (6)	Total (7)
1–A	Routine Nursing	% Revenue	0.258	0.166	0.074	0.125	0.377	1
1–B	Routine Nursing	Expenses*	$ 504,566	$324,643	$144,720	$244,460	$ 737,292	$1,955,684
2–A	Surgery	% Revenue	0.267	0.137	0.055	0.121	0.42	1
2–B	Surgery	Expenses*	$ 300,500	$154,189	$ 61,900	$136,181	$ 472,696	$1,125,469
3–A	Laboratory	% Revenue	0.254	0.098	0.052	0.124	0.472	1
3–B	Laboratory	Expenses*	$ 126,197	$ 48,690	$ 25,835	$ 61,608	$ 234,508	$ 496,840
4–A	Radiology	% Revenue	0.216	0.092	0.075	0.097	0.52	1
4–B	Radiology	Expenses*	$ 98,475	$ 41,943	$ 34,192	$ 44,222	$ 237,070	$ 455,905
5–A	Emergency	% Revenue	0.549	0.168	0.082	0.122	0.079	1
5–B	Emergency	Expenses*	$ 347,239	$106,259	$ 51,864	$ 77,164	$49,967	$ 632,495
6	Total Expenses*		$1,376,979	$675,725	$318,514	$563,637	$1,731,536	$4,666,393
7	Total Discharges		375	146	120	86	340	1,067
8	Average Expense* per Discharge		$ 3,671	$ 4,628	$ 2,654	$ 6,553	$5,092	$ 4,373
9	Average Charge per Discharge		$ 3,528	$ 4,539	$ 2,661	$ 6,481	$ 5,373	$ 4,395
10	Charge-to-Expense* Ratio		0.9607	0.9807	1.0025	0.9888	1.0550	1.0049
11	Total Cash Collected		$1,297,850	$670,439	$325,900	$575,833	$1,946,752	$4,816,774
12	Expense*-to-Cash Ratio		1.0609	1.0078	0.9773	0.9788	0.8894	0.9687
13	Average Charge Allowance per Discharge		$ –143.94	$ –89.25	$ 6.71	$ –72.92	$ 280.24	$ 21.62
14	Average Cash Received per Discharge		$ 3,460.93	$4,592.04	$2,715.83	$6,695.73	$ 5,725.74	$ 4,514.31
15	Average Cash Received/Expense* per Discharge		$ –211.01	$ –36.20	$ 61.54	$ 141.80	$ 632.98	$ 140.93
16	Profitability per HMO Contract: Cash Received – Total Expenses		$ –79,129	$ –5,286	$ 7,385	$ 12,195	$ 215,215	$ 150,381

* Expenses include direct and allocated indirect expenses

Patient financial services managers should be acutely aware of pricing techniques and objectives such as those described, and they should be prepared to assist management in attaining these objectives. They must know their healthcare organization's method of determining prices for services to be able to explain clearly to the troubled or puzzled patient how and why these charges are established.

By being keenly aware of rate-setting techniques, patient financial services managers can better serve the patient as well as the healthcare organization. These managers can no longer afford to sit on the sidelines when rates and reimbursement are being determined; they must be actively involved, especially in the managed-care contracting process.

NOTES

1. Howard J. Berman, Lewis E. Weeks, and Steven F. Kukla, *The Financial Management of Hospitals,* 7th ed. (Ann Arbor, Mich.: Health Administration Press Division of the Foundation of the American College of Healthcare Executives, 1990), 727.
2. James D. Suver, Bruce R. Neumann, and Keith E. Boles, *Management Accounting for Healthcare Organizations,* 3rd ed. (Westchester, Ill.: Healthcare Financial Management Association; Chicago: Pluribus Press, Inc. Division of Teach'em, Inc., 1992), 12.
3. L. Vann Seawell, *Hospital Financial Accounting: Theory and Practice,* 2nd ed. (Westchester, Ill.: Healthcare Financial Management Association, 1987), 167–68.
4. Berman, Weeks, and Kukla, *The Financial Management of Hospitals,* 239.
5. Berman, Weeks, and Kukla, *The Financial Management of Hospitals,* 241.
6. Berman, Weeks, and Kukla, *The Financial Management of Hospitals,* 239.
7. Seawell, *Hospital Financial Accounting,* 167.
8. Peter F. Drucker, *The Frontiers of Management: Where Tomorrow's Decisions Are Being Shaped Today* (New York: Dutton Signet, a division of Penguin Books USA, Inc., 1986), 225.
9. Allen G. Herkimer Jr., *Understanding Hospital Financial Management,* 2nd ed. (Rockville, Md.: Aspen Publishers, Inc., 1986), 423.
10. Herkimer, *Understanding Hospital Financial Management,* 423.
11. Seawell, *Hospital Financial Accounting,* 167.
12. "Medicare Reimbursement," Jack C. Wood, ed., *Topics in Health Care Financing* 1, no. 3 (Spring 1975), 8.
13. Berman, Weeks, and Kukla, *The Financial Management of Hospitals,* 724.
14. *Description and Analysis of Medicare Prospective Price Setting, Including Changes for Year Six,* rev. ed. (Westchester, Ill.; Healthcare Financial Management Association, 1988), 11–12.
15. Group Vice President Bruce McPherson, letter to colleagues, American Hospital Association, Chicago, October 1991.
16. Herkimer, *Understanding Hospital Financial Management,* 3.
17. Herkimer, *Understanding Hospital Financial Management,* 191.
18. Suver, Neumann, and Boles, *Management Accounting for Healthcare Organizations,* 194.
19. Suver, Neumann, and Boles, *Management Accounting for Healthcare Organizations,* 264.
20. Allen G. Herkimer Jr., *Understanding Health Care Budgeting* (Rockville, Md.: Aspen Publishers, Inc., 1989), 150.
21. Herkimer, *Understanding Health Care Budgeting,* 150.
22. Allen G. Herkimer Jr., *Understanding Health Care Accounting* (Rockville, Md.: Aspen Publishers, Inc., 1989), 208–13.

CHAPTER 10

Cash Forecasting and Management

Cash forecasting and management are essential to the completeness of any healthcare organization's budgetary control system—and essential to the organization's financial health. The *cash flow forecast* is a plan for projecting cash inflows and outflows and the resultintg cash balances. Managers and administrators use this information to predict cash shortfalls and excesses and make timely and appropriate corrective decisions.[1] The forecast also serves as the mechanism or instrument that expresses the organization's operating budget and capital expenditure plan in cash terms. Further, since patient financial services managers have the ultimate responsibility for converting their organization's largest single asset—patient accounts receivable—into cash, they need to be involved in cash forecasting and management for the overall institution.[2]

After describing preparations for effective cash forecasting and the process' objectives, chapter 10 will describe four basic components of the cash flow forecast and the two major analyses managers can employ in forecasting. The chapter concludes with a discussion of the functions patient financial services managers can and should perform in preparing and monitoring the forecast.

Laying the Groundwork

The healthcare organization's budgetary control system begins with managers and administrators preparing the organization's operating budget and capital expenditure plan (see chapter 6). Once management develops these financial planning tools, it can begin the cash forecasting and management process.

Management's first step in cash forecasting is analyzing the healthcare organization's monthly income and expense statements to determine cash inflows and outflows. This analysis uses two time-lag factors, which management must compute and monitor:

1. *cash inflow time-lag factor:* the amount of time between the healthcare organization's billing the patient for services and its receipt of the payment.

2. *cash outflow time-lag factor:* the amount of time between the organization's incurring an expense and its disbursement of cash to pay it.

Keep in mind that in reality, cash forecasting converts the organization's accrual system of accounting into a cash accounting statement.

Management can control each time-lag factor with any one of several methods, each of which features varying degrees of efficiency. Later on, this chapter will discuss techniques for matching cash inflows and outflows for the most profitable use of the healthcare organization's resources.

The Purposes of Cash Forecasting and Management

The primary purpose of cash forecasting and management is to assist healthcare managers and administrators in determining whether there will be a sufficient amount of cash coming into the organization to cover its projected expenditures. The forecast helps alert management for the fact that additional funds may be needed to carry out the operating budget and the capital expenditure plan. The process also indicates the existence of surplus operating funds that can be invested, thus allowing the healthcare organization to maximize its cash resources.

A secondary purpose of cash forecasting and management is to help the healthcare organization satisfy the requirement of the Joint Commission on Accreditation of Healthcare Organizations (JCAHO) that the organization's chief executive officer (CEO), consistent with governing board policy, maintain and safeguard appropriate physical resources and use them judiciously to implement organization programs and meet patient needs. JCAHO also prescribes that the CEO be responsible for implementing governing board policy covering the financial management of the healthcare organization. This includes the development of cash inflow budgets.[3]

Effective cash forecasting and management will help ensure that the healthcare organization will have enough cash to

- meet operating needs,

- finance capital expenditures, and

- receive maximum earnings from investments.

Basically, there are at least five ways to increase cash resources:

1. Reduce the amount of current assets, for example, accounts receivable, inventories, prepaid expenses, etc.

2. Increase the amount of current liabilities, for example, accounts payable, notes payable, taxes payable, etc.

3. Increase operating revenues, that is, charges to patients, and reduce operating expenses.

4. Restrict capital expenditures.

5. Take advantage of float.

Management can use these singly or in combination. The first four are self-explanatory; use of float will be discussed later in this chapter.

If the healthcare organization has a reasonably steady or even inflow of cash, its ideal operating cash balance is zero, as illustrated in table 10–1, line 5. A zero balance means that management is indeed using the facility's resources judiciously.

Major Components

The cash forecasting and management process involves the control of five major components:

1. cash inflows

2. cash outflows

3. borrowings and investments

4. float

5. beginning and ending (month's) balance

The healthcare organization's master cash flow forecast statement (see table 10–1) shows cash inflows, cash outflows, and borrowings and investments. Float, on the other hand, is not shown on the statement because it represents cash available only for a very limited time.

Cash Inflows

Patient accounts receivable typically represent a healthcare organization's largest asset and its greatest source of cash inflows. There are two bases management can use to forecast cash from patient revenue:

1. gross charges to patients

2. net charges to patients

The basic distinction between the two is that the forecaster determines the gross amount before adjusting for deductions, such as bad debts, contractual allowances, and courtesy discounts. Net charges result after the forecaster makes these deductions. There are conflicting opinions in the healthcare industry about which forecasting method is better. The author prefers the net charges method, so it will be the approach that this chapter will present.

TABLE 10–1

Master Cash Flow Forecast Statement

Memorial Medical Center
Anytown, U.S.A.

MASTER CASH FLOW FORECAST STATEMENT
For the Budget Year Ending December 31, 19x1
(In Thousands of Dollars)

							Months							
		1	*2*	*3*	*4*	*5*	*6*	*7*	*8*	*9*	*10*	*11*	*12*	*Total*
1.	Beginning Cash Balance	$ 50	$ 0	$ 0	$ 0	$ 0	$ 0	$ 0	$ 0	$ 0	$ 0	$ 0	$ 0	$ 50
2.	Cash inflows													
	a. Net Patient Receivables	$227	$277	$287	$308	$316	$327	$326	$323	$316	$302	$313	$320	$3,642
	b. Other Operating Sources	20	13	16	21	16	14	15	15	14	20	16	26	206
	c. Borrowings (Investments)	(28)	(39)	(26)	(51)	(50)	32	39	(9)	52	(33)	(38)	51	(100)
	d. Total Cash Inflows	$219	$215	$277	$278	$282	$373	$380	$329	$382	$289	$291	$397	$3,748
3.	Total Cash on Hand													
	(line 1 + line 2 = line 3)	$269	$251	$277	$278	$282	$373	$380	$329	$382	$289	$291	$397	$3,748
4.	Cash Outflows													
	a. Salaries, Wages, and Related Expenses	$190	$184	$196	$193	$198	$197	$201	$199	$203	$198	$204	$205	$2,368
	b. Capital Expenditures	5	0	10	0	5	100	100	50	100	10	5	110	495
	c. Noncapital and Nonsalary Expenses	74	67	71	85	79	76	79	80	79	81	82	82	935
	d. Total Cash Outflows	$269	$251	$277	$278	$282	$373	$380	$329	$382	$289	$291	$397	$3,798
5.	Ending Cash Balance													
	(line 3 - line 4 = line 5)	$-0-	$-0-	$-0-	$ -0-	$ -0-	$ -0-	$ -0-	$ -0-	$-0-	$ -0-	$ -0-	$ -0-	$ -0-

Borrowings, or outside financing (for example: loans, mortgages, bonds, and stock issues), constitute the healthcare organization's second largest source of cash inflows. Short-term loan and investment accounts frequently appear in the cash inflow statement as balancing accounts to show additional funds generated from short-term loans or the investment of surplus cash. The cash inflows from borrowings and investments are entered in the master cash flow forecast statement as shown in table 10–1, line 2c.

The remaining cash inflows to the facility usually come from a variety of sources, including the following:

- cafeteria sales
- medical record transcriptions

- investment income
- transfer from other of the organization's funds
- rentals
- vendors
- concessions
- gifts and donations
- other nonpatient revenue

Moreover, some nontaxable healthcare organizations have found fund-raising drives to be an excellent source of cash, while others have not. To gauge whether their facility should undertake a fund-raising drive, healthcare executives must consider the community and its likely response to a campaign for gifts. Certainly, for the taxable healthcare organizations, selling stock is an excellent source of cash.

Cash Outflows

Basically, cash outflows separate into four major classifications:

1. salaries, wages, and related expenses
2. fixed or programmed nonsalary expenses
3. variable nonsalary expenses
4. capital expenditures

A healthcare organization's largest cash outflow is for salaries, wages, and related expenses; for example, Social Security taxes, retirement benefits, and group insurance premiums. Although management usually budgets these expenses on a monthly basis, for cash management purposes they must be planned and monitored according to the frequency and to the time of actual cash disbursement to employees, whether it be weekly, biweekly, or monthly.

Programmed nonsalary expenses are those for which payment is scheduled or programmed for specific times throughout the year. Such expenses include

- insurance premiums,
- capital expenditures,
- mortgage payments,
- short-term loans,
- rentals and leases,
- utilities, and
- training and education.

Except for utilities, programmed expenses represent a fixed amount of money that does not vary regardless of volume of activity. Capital expenditures are handled as a separate line item direct from the capital budget.

Variable nonsalary expenses are operating expenses, for example, food, medical and surgical supplies, and office supplies, that vary in direct proportion to the volume of work.

Capital expenditures represent most of the manageable cash outflow items in terms of time available to disburse cash, and they can usually be delayed without jeopardizing operations. Consequently, management can place a "hold" on purchasing any capital asset until the institution's cash position is more favorable. Conversely, if there is an excess of operating cash, appropriate capital expenditures (investments) probably should be made.[4]

In one way or another, all the expenses or purchases in the healthcare facility's statement of operations and capital expenditure plan appear in its cash flow forecast, except the provision for depreciation. Depreciation is a noncash item that must be included in computing the facility's total operating expenses. Since depreciation is only an accounting procedure to indicate the amortization of a capital purchase, management does not include it in the cash flow forecast. A capital expenditure is recorded in the forecast only when cash is actually paid out, or when the payment of that cash is planned.

Borrowings and Investments

Borrowings and/or investments are usually shown as a "balancing" account in a cash flow forecast. For example, after computing all cash inflows and outflows for the month, the cash forecaster may find that cash inflows are not sufficient to cover cash outflows. In this case, the healthcare organization must borrow the required amount of cash to maintain the necessary planned bank balance. On the other hand, if the cash forecaster finds that cash available to the organization after cash outflows have been taken into account is too great to remain in a noninterest-bearing checking account, the surplus will be invested.

There are two methods commonly used in the healthcare industry for recording these activities. In the first method, the forecaster considers each activity as a separate function or account. Therefore, borrowings would be considered cash inflows and investments would be treated as cash outflows.

The second method considers these two activities as a single line item under cash inflows. If the organization borrows cash, the forecaster would record the amount in the same manner as any other cash inflow. If cash is invested, the amount would be bracketed, as illustrated below:

	January	February	March	Total
Borrowings (Investments)	$10,000	$20,000	($15,000)	$15,000

An advantage of using one line item is that the viewer can readily identify the "balancing" account because it is netted out in the Total column. Moreover, using two line items requires an additional computation.

Float

Float represents an intangible and relatively uncontrollable amount of cash that the healthcare organization can use by taking advantage of cash in transit. Float represents the portion of the bank balance created by the time interval between the drawing of checks on the facility's account and the actual debiting of the account for those checks.

Delays in the collection-payment system resulting from the transportation and processing of checks cause float. However, with the increased use of electronic payment systems as well as deliberate action by the Federal Reserve system, it is a matter of time before float virtually disappears. In the meantime, managers need to understand float and use it to their organization's advantage.[5] For example, if a facility generally has $100,000 in outstanding checks at the time the bank account balance is reconciled to the facility's bank balance, management could use this amount for short-term investments or for paying additional expenses. This example illustrates the *time value of money:* the value of money to be received or to be disbursed is directly related to the timing of its receipt or disbursement.[6]

Nonetheless, proceed with caution when using float—it requires relatively constant and consistent cash flow.

Cash Forecasting Methods

As stated earlier, the healthcare organization's operating budget and capital expenditure plan must be completed before forecasting cash. Only then can management begin the analysis of time-lag factors and amounts of cash inflows and outflows. The two major analyses involved in cash forecasting are

1. cash receipts analysis and

2. cash disbursement analysis.

Cash Receipts Analysis

The first step in cash forecasting is to analyze cash inflows from patient accounts receivable. This analysis involves determining

- the type of paying agent and

- the length of time from the billing date to the time the facility receives payment.

Assume that the analysis of gross charges to patients indicates that the mix of paying agents corresponds to the one shown in table 10–2. Historical cash receipts are then analyzed and time-lag factors are established for each paying agent based on the amount of time it takes to collect cash from that agent for services rendered. Generally, the accounts of most patients are not paid in full with a single payment; rather, the payment period may extend over time. For example, assume that a patient with commercial insurance has a $5,000 account. The payoff schedule might look like this:

Time of Payment	Source of Payment	Amount of Payment	
		(Dollars)	(Percents)
Admissions day	Patient deposit	$ 500	10%
Thirty days after billing	Insurance	3,600	72
Sixty days after billing	Patient	450	9
Ninety days after billing	Patient	450	9
Total		$5,000	100%

The process of analyzing each paying agent's payment schedule is essential, yet extremely time consuming. In addition, these schedules can vary according to outside economic factors, such as inflation and interest rates. For this reason, patient financial services managers should conduct only a statistical sampling of the process instead of using a large amount of hours and resources to do a comprehensive study. The best approach is to do a statistical sampling of payment schedules and time-lag factors every six months purely for verification and control.

The second step in cash forecasting is analyzing cash inflows from gross charges to patients according to the time cash is received. Table 10–3 shows a typical mix of payment schedules and time-lag factors by paying agent.

TABLE 10–2

Percentage Analysis of Gross Charges to Patients by Paying Agent

Memorial Medical Center
Anytown, U.S.A.

Paying Agent	Percentage of Gross Charges
Blue Cross	30%
Medicare	40
Medicaid	10
Commercial Insurance	15
Self-paying and Others	5
Total	100%

TABLE 10–3

Percentage Analysis of Cash Payment Schedules and Time-Lag Factors of Gross Charges to Patients by Paying Agent

Memorial Medical Center
Anytown, U.S.A.

Paying Agent	*Percentage of Payments Schedule Month after Charges Are Generated*							Total Percentage
	1	*2*	*3*	*4*	*5*	*6*	*7*	
Blue Cross	50	30	15	5	—	—	—	100%
Medicare	60	25	10	5	—	—	—	100
Medicaid	10	20	30	20	10	5	5	100
Commercial Insurance	30	40	15	10	5	—	—	100
Self-paying and Others	15	25	25	15	10	5	5	100

Although the table classifies paying agents into major groups, some patient financial services managers might find it beneficial to expand these classifications, especially if some categories include agents with widely different payment systems or schedules. For example, a healthcare organization may be a member of two or more Blue Cross plans, one of which pays the facility prospectively based on patient gross charges, while the other pays the facility based on costs with a retroactive adjustment based at the end of the fiscal period. Another good reason for a more detailed breakdown of paying agents would be the need for closer surveillance of cash inflows in situations in which one commercial insurance company or health maintenance organization dominates its segment of the market.

After payment schedules and time-lag factors have been analyzed by major paying agent, the next step is to determine the net charges to patients by making provisions for contractual allowances and bad debts for each paying agent, as table 10–4 illustrates.

There are, essentially, two different methods for forecasting cash inflows from paying agents. One is the weighted average monthly cash inflow percentage method, which uses the healthcare organization's weighted average for its provision for deductibles when computing net patient revenues.[7] Table 10-5 presents an application of this weighted average concept.

After determining the deductible percentage, management computes the weighted average of monthly collection percentage of the net patient revenue. Let

MC = Weighted monthly collection percentage

R = Paying agent's share of net revenues

$(R \times MC^1)$ = Weighted percentage (first month)

$\Sigma(R \times MC^1)$ = Sum total of weighted percentages (first month)

In this illustration, we can compute the sum of the weighted averages $\Sigma(R \times MC^1)$ for the first month is computed as follows:

TABLE 10–4

Percentage Analysis of Net Patient Charges by Paying Agent

Memorial Medical Center
Anytown, U.S.A.

Paying Agent	Gross Charges	Less: Provision for Deductibles	Net Charges
Blue Cross	100%	10%	90%
Medicare	100	20	80
Medicaid	100	40	60
Commercial Insurance	100	5	95
Self-paying and Others	100	15	85

TABLE 10–5

Analysis and Computation of Weighted Collection Percentage of Patient Charges Collected

Memorial Medical Center
Anytown, U.S.A.

Paying Agent	R Percentage of Total Revenue		Month after Charges Are Generated											
		First		Second		Third		Fourth		Fifth		Sixth		Seventh	
		MC^1	$R{\times}MC^{1*}$	MC^2	$R{\times}MC^2$	MC^3	$R{\times}MC^3$	MC^4	$R{\times}MC^4$	MC^5	$R{\times}MC^5$	MC^6	$R{\times}MC^6$	MC^7	$R{\times}MC^7$
(1)	(2)	(3)	(4)	(5)	(6)	(7)	(8)	(9)	(10)	(11)	(12)	(13)	(14)	(15)	(16)
Blue Cross	30%	50	15.0	30	9.0	15	4.5	5	1.5	—	—	—	—	—	—
Medicare	40	60	24.0	25	10.0	10	4.0	5	2.0	—	—	—	—	—	—
Medicaid	10	10	1.0	20	2.0	30	3.0	20	2.0	10	1.0	5	.5	5	.5
Commercial Insurance	15	30	4.5	40	6.0	15	2.3	10	1.5	5	.8	—	—	—	—
Self-paying and Others	5	15	.8	25	1.2	25	1.2	15	.8	10	.5	5	.2	5	.2
Total $\Sigma(R \times MC)$	100%		45.3		28.2		15.0		7.8		2.3		.7		.7

*Col. 2 × Col. 3 = Col. 4

Paying Agent	$(R \times MC^1)$
Blue Cross	15.0%
Medicare	24.0
Medicaid	1.0
Commercial Insurance	4.5
Self-paying and Others	0.8
Total	45.3%

According to this computation, the weighted average of 45.3 percent is the percentage of monthly net patient charges that the healthcare organization could expect to collect during the first month after discharge, based on the most recent patient accounts payment pattern analysis. Table 10–6 shows a complete cash collection schedule of net patient charges.

The second method used to forecast cash inflows from patient charges is to analyze the cash inflows by individual paying agent. If a computer is available this method is recommended because of its greater accuracy. However, if the cash forecast is to be done manually, the weighted average method is preferable. Table 10–7 depicts an application of the weighted average percentage developed in table 10–6.

Table 10–7 starts with the beginning patient accounts receivable balance of $500,000, which is distributed by the weighted average collection method. Net charges to patients are distributed monthly and totaled for each month as

TABLE 10–6

Weighted Average Cash Collection Schedule of Net Patient Charges

Memorial Medical Center
Anytown, U.S.A.

Month after Charges Are Generated	Weighted Average Collected
1	45.3%
2	28.2
3	15.0
4	7.8
5	2.3
6	.7
7	.7
Total	100.0%

TABLE 10–7

Cash Inflow Analysis of Net Patient Charges

Memorial Medical Center
Anytown, U.S.A.

CASH INFLOW ANALYSIS OF NET PATIENT CHARGES
For the Budget Year Ending December 31, 19x1
(In Thousands of Dollars)

Month	Beginning Net Patient Accounts Receivable Balance	1	2	3	4	5	6	7	8	9	10	11	12	Ending Net Patient Accounts Receivable Balance
		(45.3)	(28.2)	(15.0)	(7.8)	(2.3)	(.7)	(.7)						
	$500	$227	$141	$75	$39	$12	$3	$3						
1	300		136	85	45	23	7	2	$2					
2	280			127	79	42	22	6	2	$2				
3	320				145	90	48	25	8	2	$2			
4	330					149	93	49	27	8	2	$2		
5	340						154	96	51	27	8	2	$2	
6	320							145	90	48	25	8	2	$2
7	315								143	89	47	25	7	4
8	310									140	87	47	24	12
9	290										131	82	44	33
10	325											147	92	86
11	330												149	181
12														310
Total Net Charges to Patients	$3,770													
Cash Inflow from Net Charges	$3,642	$227	$277	$287	$308	$316	$327	$326	$323	$316	$302	$313	$320	
Ending Patient Accounts Receivable Balance														$628

Note: Net charges were distributed using the weighted average collection in table 10–6.

the cash inflows from net patient charges for that month. Any uncollected net charges are accumulated in the far right-hand column to determine the ending patient accounts receivable balance for the period.

The cash inflows from other operating sources, such as cafeteria sales and medical records transcriptions, are then analyzed, as illustrated in table 10–8, and the total is spread on the master cash flow statement (see table 10–1, line 2b). The next step is to enter the cash inflows from net patient receivables in the master cash flow statement (see table 10–1, line 2a). Once these inflows have been recorded, the analysis of cash outflows can begin.

TABLE 10–8

Analysis of Monthly Cash Inflows from Other Operating Sources

Memorial Medical Center
Anytown, U.S.A.

ANALYSIS OF MONTHLY CASH INFLOWS FROM OTHER OPERATING SOURCES
For the Budget Year Ending December 31, 19x1
(In Thousands of Dollars)

| Month | Source | | | Total |
	Cafeteria	Medical Records	Other	
1	$ 10	$ 2	$ 8	$ 20
2	8	1	4	13
3	9	1	6	16
4	11	2	8	21
5	10	1	5	16
6	9	1	4	14
7	8	1	6	15
8	9	2	4	15
9	10	1	3	14
10	9	2	9	20
11	10	2	4	16
12	10	1	15	26
Total	$113	$17	$76	$206

Cash Disbursement Analysis

As stated earlier, even though most healthcare organizations use the accrual accounting system, the analysis of cash outflows must be forecast based strictly on the cash that is actually distributed out of the institution. This is especially important where salaries, wages, and other related expenses are concerned.[8]

Many healthcare organizations maintain a special imprest cash account for the disbursement of payroll checks. This imprest fund maintains a fixed amount, such as $10,000, and is routinely reimbursed from the organization's operating cash account in the exact amount(s) to be disbursed, thus maintaining the original fixed sum. In addition, separate checks may be drawn from the operating fund and deposited in the payroll account to cover taxes and other withholding requirements.[9]

There are many ways a healthcare organization can use imprest payroll accounts. However, some facilities do not use these accounts at all, simply disbursing payroll from the general operating fund. Nevertheless, salaries, wages, and related expenses must appear on the cash flow forecast statement at the time the payroll checks are disbursed.

TABLE 10–9

Analysis of Employee Payroll Check-cashing Process

**Memorial Medical Center
Anytown, U.S.A.**

Number of Days after Issuance	Amount		Employees	
	Dollar	*Percent*	*Number*	*Percent*
1	$21,375	25%	195	30%
2	12,825	15	130	20
3	8,550	10	98	14
4	8,550	10	65	10
5	6,840	8	52	8
6	1,710	2	13	2
7	8,550	10	39	6
8–14	4,275	5	13	2
15–22	4,275	5	13	2
23–30	8,550	10	32	5
Total	$85,500	100%	650	100%

Most healthcare organizations disburse payroll and related expenses in the month in which they are budgeted. Within that month, however, there is a time lag between disbursement of the check to the employee and the cashing of that check. A typical time-lag factor is shown in table 10–9. Note that 30 percent of the organization's employees cash their payroll checks on payday, while 5 percent of the employees cash their checks as long as 23 to 30 days after they are issued. The organization can use this kind of information to make short-term investments by staggering payments from   the general operating fund to the imprest payroll account to cover payroll checks as they are cashed.

For illustration, assume that Memorial Medical Center of Anytown, U.S.A., pays its employees on the first and fifteenth of each month. Also assume that the cash outflows for salaries, wages, and related expenses for Memorial Medical Center's budget year ending December 31, 19x1, are as shown in table 10–10. (These cash outflows are shown on the master cash flow statement in table 10–1, line 4a).

Nonsalary cash outflows can be divided into two major categories of expenditure:

TABLE 10–10

Analysis of Cash Outflow for Salaries, Wages, and Related Expenses

Memorial Medical Center
Anytown, U.S.A.

ANALYSIS OF CASH OUTFLOW FOR SALARIES, WAGES, AND RELATED EXPENSES
For the Budget Year Ending December 31, 19x1
(In Thousands of Dollars)

Month	Payroll Date	Monthly Payroll	Payroll-related Expense	Total Salaries, Wages, and Related Expenses
1	1/1– 1/15	$ 165	$ 25	$ 190
2	2/1– 2/15	160	24	184
3	3/1– 3/15	170	26	196
4	4/1– 4/15	118	25	193
5	5/1– 5/15	172	26	198
6	6/1– 6/15	170	27	197
7	7/1– 7/15	175	26	201
8	8/1– 8/15	173	26	199
9	9/1– 9/15	176	27	203
10	10/1–10/15	172	26	198
11	11/1–11/15	177	27	204
12	12/1–12/15	178	27	205
Total		$2,056	$312	$2,368

1. capital

2. noncapital

Cash outflows for capital expenditures come directly from the organization's capital expenditure plan or capital budget. For illustration, Memorial Medical Center's capital expenditure plan for the budget year ending December 31, 19x1, is shown in table 10–11. (These totals are recorded on the master cash flow statement in table 10–1, line 4b).

Noncapital cash outflows can be classified by several methods. For purposes of this discussion, these expenditures are classified as either

- programmed (fixed), or
- variable.

TABLE 10–11

Summary Analysis of Capital Expenditure Cash Flow Requirements

Memorial Medical Center
Anytown, U.S.A.

SUMMARY ANALYSIS OF CAPITAL EXPENDITURE CASH FLOW REQUIREMENTS
For the Budget Year Ending December 31, 19x1
(In Thousands of Dollars)

Month	Amount Needed
1	$ 5
2	-0-
3	10
4	-0-
5	5
6	100
7	100
8	50
9	100
10	10
11	5
12	110
Total	$495

TABLE 10–12

Payment Priority Classification for Cash Outflows

Memorial Medical Center
Anytown, U.S.A.

Payment Priority	Description of Payment	Payment Schedules from Date of Receipt
A	Payroll, Commission, etc.	Current month
B	Mortgage, Rent, Leases, Utilities, Service Contracts	Current month
C	Foods, Medical and Surgical Supplies, Drugs	30 days (following month)
D	Discount Vendors	30 days (following month)
E	Funded Depreciation, Investments	30 days (following month)
F	Special Vendors	30–59 days (second month)
G	Other Vendors	60–90 days (third month)

TABLE 10–13

Schedule of Noncapital and Nonsalary Cash Outflow Requirements

Memorial Medical Center
Anytown, U.S.A.

SCHEDULE OF NONCAPITAL AND NONSALARY CASH OUTFLOW REQUIREMENTS
(In Thousands of Dollars)

Month	Cash Require-ment	*Days after Receipt of Statement*				
		1–15 Days *A, B = 55%*	*15–30 Days* *C = 10%*	*30 Days* *D, E = 10%*	*30–45 Days* *F = 10%*	*45–90 Days* *G = 15%*
1	$ 70	$39	$7	$7	$7	$10
2	73	40	7	7	7	12
3	78	43	8	8	8	11
4	77	42	8	8	8	11
5	79	43	8	8	8	12
6	75	41	8	8	8	10
7	80	44	8	8	8	12
8	80	44	8	8	8	12
9	82	45	8	8	8	13
10	81	45	8	8	8	12
11	83	46	8	8	8	13
12	82	45	8	8	8	13
Total	$940					

Programmed expenditures are noncapital, nonsalary cash flow requirements, such as

- utilities,
- rent and/or leases,
- insurance, and
- mortgage payments.

In short, these expenses are fixed payments that are essential to provide the facilities and equipment necessary to perform services to patients. Another example of a programmed expense is education and training. The total amount for the annual expenditure is established at the beginning of the budget year, and this amount is programmed to be paid as appropriate training and educational programs occur.

TABLE 10–14

Analysis of Noncapital and Nonsalary Cash Outflows by Priority Classification

Memorial Medical Center
Anytown, U.S.A.

Priority Classification	Payment Schedule from Date of Receipt	Percent of Cash Outflows	Monthly Accumulated Percentage
A	Current month	40%	—%
B	Current month	15	55
C	30 days	10	—
D	30 days	5	—
E	30 days	5	75
F	30–59	10	85
G	60–90 days	15	100%
Total		100%	

Variable noncapital, nonsalary expenses are those cash outflow requirements that usually vary in direct proportion to the volume of work, that is, patient days and outpatient visits.

Setting priorities for individual expenses is a method used by some healthcare organizations to schedule cash outflows. Table 10–12 shows the payment priority classification system Memorial Medical Center uses for all cash outflows. Memorial Medical Center has analyzed its noncapital, nonsalary cash outflows, as shown in table 10–13. The accumulated percentages in the right-hand column of table 10–14 are then applied to the facility's budgeted noncapital and nonsalary expenses shown in table 10–15. The monthly cash outflows for these expenses are then recorded in the master cash flow statement (see table 10–1, line 4c).

At the beginning of the cash forecasting process, the cash balance was $50,000 (see table 10, line 1). During the first month, the total cash inflows shown in table 10–1 were as follows:

Line		
2a	Net Patient Receivables	$227,000
2b	Other Operating Revenue	20,000
	Total Cash Inflows	$247,000

Thus, total cash on hand is $297,000.

TABLE 10–15

Schedule of Noncapital and Nonsalary Cash Outflow Requirements

Memorial Medical Center
Anytown, U.S.A.

SCHEDULE OF NONCAPITAL AND NONSALARY CASH OUTFLOW REQUIREMENTS
For the Budget Year Ending December 31, 19x1
(In Thousands of Dollars)

Month	Beginning Accounts Payable Balance	1	2	3	4	5	6	7	8	9	10	11	12	Ending Accounts Payable Balance
		(.55)	(.75)	(.85)	(1.00)									
	$65	$35	$13	$7	$10									
1	70	$39	14	7	10									
2	73		40	14	7	$12								
3	78			43	16	8	$11							
4	77				42	16	8	$11						
5	79					43	16	8	$12					
6	75						41	16	8	$10				
7	80							44	16	8	$12			
8	80								44	16	8	$12		
9	82									45	16	8	$13	
10	81										45	16	6	$12
11	83											46	16	21
12	82												45	37
Total Net Cash Requirements	$1,005													
Cash Outflow for Expenses	$935	$74	$67	$71	$85	$79	$76	$79	$80	$79	$81	$82	$82	
Ending Accounts Receivable Balance														$70

Total cash outflows were as follows:

Line		
4a	Salaries, Wages, and Related Expenses	$190,000
4b	Capital Expenditures	5,000
4c	Noncapital and Nonsalary Expenses	74,000
4d	Total Cash Outflows	$269,000

Hence, there is a cash net difference or balance of $28,000. Since the medical center had adopted a "zero" cash balance policy, it invested the $28,000 in short-term instruments, leaving a net cash inflow of $219,000 (see table 10–1, line 2d) and a total of $269,000 cash on hand for the month. Checking the borrowings/investments account (see table 10–1, line 2c), the cash forecaster can project the need to either borrow or invest.

During the second month, $39,000 was deposited in the investment account, representing excess cash inflows. During the following three months, the following additions were added to the investment account, for a total of $194,000 in investments:

Month	Amount Deposited
3	$ 26,000
4	51,000
5	50,000
	$127,000

During the sixth month, the shortfall of cash inflows to cash outflows was $32,000; this amount was withdrawn from the investment account. During the seventh month, there was a $39,000 shortfall. The following is a recalculation of the borrowings/investments account at the end of the seventh month:

Month	Deposits	Withdrawals	Balance
1	$28,000		$ 28,000
2	39,000		67,000
3	26,000		93,000
4	51,000		144,000
5	50,000		194,000
6		$32,000	162,000
7		39,000	123,000

The subsequent months' cash flow forecasts were projected in the same manner, that is, using the borrowings/investments account as the "equalizer." The annual result was a total net cash investment of $100,000 (see table 10–1, line 2c). Here is a summary of the budgeted cash inflows and outflows.

Beginning Cash Balance	$ 50,000
Plus:	
Cash Inflows	
Net Patient Accounts Receivable	$3,642,000
Other Operating Sources	206,000
Total Cash Inflows	$3,848,000
Cash on Hand	$3,898,000
Less:	
Cash Outflows	
Salaries, Wages, and Related Expenses	$2,368,000
Capital Expenditures	495,000
Noncapital and Nonsalary Expenses	935,000
Investments	100,000
Total Cash Outflows	$3,898,000
Ending Cash Balance	$ –0–

The Patient Financial Services Managers' Role

The process of cash forecasting is probably one of the most important functions in healthcare financial management. If properly used, the process can be the instrument that will help keep the facility solvent because it will be able to predict cash shortfalls and excesses and take corrective actions, such as

- adjusting patient charges to meet expenses,

- reducing expenses, and

- preparing for borrowings and/or investments.

Patient financial services managers need to play a vital role in this process. The following are some of the functions these managers can and should perform.

Forecast Preparation

1. Analyze patient accounts receivable by paying agent.

2. Identify the time-lag factors for payments by paying agent, especially managed-care contracts, HMOs, etc.

3. Estimate the amount of bad debt writeoffs.

4. Calculate third-party contractual allowances.

5. Estimate the amount of courtesy allowances and other similar deductions from gross patient charges.

Forecast Monitoring

1. Assist in the preparation of the organization's daily cash report (see exhibit 10–1).

2. Maintain close communication between the patient financial services department and the chief financial officer (CFO); alert CFO to any potential trouble spots.

3. Assist in developing the organization's payment terms in all prospective payment plans, i.e., HMO, PPO, etc.

EXHIBIT 10–1
Daily Cash Report Form

Memorial Medical Center
Anytown, U.S.A.

Daily Cash Report

as of _____, 19____

	Today	MONTH TO DATE Actual	Budgeted
1. Beginning Cash Balance	$ _____	$ _____	$ _____
2. Plus:			
Cash Inflows			
a. Net Return Accounts Receivable	$ _____	$ _____	$ _____
b. Other Operating Sources			
c. Borrowings			
d. Total Cash Inflows	$ _____	$ _____	$ _____
3. Total Cash on Hand			
(line 1 + line 2d)	$ _____	$ _____	$ _____
4. Less:			
Cash Outflows			
a. Salaries, Wages, and			
Related Expenses	$ _____	$ _____	$ _____
b. Capital Expenditures			
c. Noncapital and Nonsalary Expenses			
d. Investments			
e. Total Cash Outflows	$ _____	$ _____	$ _____
5. Ending Cash Balance			
(line 3 – line 4e)	$ _____	$ _____	$ _____

4. Maintain close communication with all major third-party payers to expedite payments.

5. Keep abreast of new systems and procedures which might expedite cash payments from all types of payers.

In summary, patient financial services managers are responsible for the effective processing of their healthcare organization's largest single asset, the patient accounts receivable, for cash conversion—cash inflows. And because cash inflows are an integral part of the cash forecasting and management process, patient financial services managers must be involved in this process. If such participation is not the case in their organization, the patient financial services managers had better become involved—to protect the future of their healthcare organization and their position as well.

NOTES

1. Allen G. Herkimer Jr., *Understanding Health Care Budgeting* (Rockville, Md.: Aspen Publishers, Inc., 1989), 176.
2. Herkimer, *Understanding Health Care Budgeting,* 176.
3. 1993 Joint Commission, *Accreditation Manual for Hospitals* (Oakbrook Terrace, Ill.: Joint Commission on Accreditation of Healthcare Organizations, 1992), 41, 44.
4. Allen G. Herkimer Jr., *Understanding Hospital Financial Management,* 2nd ed. (Rockville, Md.: Aspen Publishers, Inc., 1986), 306.
5. Lawrence J. Gitman, *Principles of Managerial Finance,* 6th ed. (New York: HarperCollins Publishers Inc., 1991), 731.
6. John D. Finnerty, *Corporate Financial Analysis: A Comprehensive Guide to Real-World Approaches for Financial Managers* (New York: McGraw-Hill Book Company, 1986), 51.
7. Herkimer, *Understanding Health Care Budgeting,* 167.
8. Herkimer, *Understanding Health Care Budgeting,* 170.
9. Herkimer, *Understanding Health Care Budgeting,* 170.

CHAPTER 11

Analyzing the Financial Statements

Today, healthcare organizations appear to be contending with two opposing forces:

- meeting an increased need for more financial resources

- maintaining financial strength and debt-paying ability to satisfy lenders' criteria

These forces make it absolutely vital for the healthcare organization's financial management team to (1) keep abreast of developments in the external financial and legislative environment that may have an impact on the organization's financial position, and (2) routinely analyze its internal financial position. By constantly analyzing and evaluating these factors, the team can develop a cohesive financial plan that will assure the healthcare organization's financial viability.

As a member of the organization's financial management team, patient financial services managers must assume an appropriate share of this responsibility. Consequently, they must be thoroughly acquainted with techniques for analyzing financial statements, a process known as financial analysis. Financial analysis can assist management in making rational decisions in keeping with the mission, goals, and objectives of the healthcare organization. The purpose of this chapter is to acquaint patient financial services managers with the nature and application of the major ratios or tools used in financial analysis.

Using Financial Ratios

To evaluate the healthcare organization's financial condition and performance, its financial managers need a set of benchmarks or yardsticks. The benchmark most frequently used in financial analysis is known as either a ratio or an index. A ratio relates two segments of financial data, for example, gross and/or net patient accounts receivable and gross and/or net patient revenue, to each other. Analyzing and interpreting sets of ratios should give experienced financial analysts a better understanding of the healthcare facility's

TABLE 11–1

Five-Year Analysis of Patient Accounts Receivable and Revenue

Memorial Medical Center
Anytown, U.S.A.

RATIO ANALYSIS OF GROSS PATIENT ACCOUNTS RECEIVABLE TO GROSS PATIENT REVENUE
For the Five-Year Period Ending September 30, 19x5

Year (a)	Gross Patient Revenue (b)	Gross Patient Accounts Receivable (c)	Ratio (d) (b ÷ c = d)	Percent (e) (c ÷ b = e)
19x1	$3,565,000	$582,400	6.1:1	16.3%
19x2	3,922,500	588,300	6.7:1	15.0
19x3	4,315,700	733,600	5.9:1	17.0
19x4	4,530,300	679,500	6.7:1	15.0
19x5	5,209,845	937,700	5.6:1	18.0

financial condition and performance than they could obtain solely from the financial statements.

Financial analysis involves two types of comparisons. The first method of comparison involves evaluating performance of the healthcare organization according to past, present, and forecasted ratio trends. When these ratios are displayed in a time series chart, as table 11–1 illustrates, the analyst can study the changes and determine whether the financial condition and performance of the healthcare organization has improved or deteriorated over a period of time. For easier interpretation, these data can be displayed in a graph similar to the one that figure 11–1 depicts.

The second method of comparison involves comparing ratios of one healthcare organization with those of another similar organization, or with a regional, state, or national industry average (see table 11–2). Again for ease of interpretation, the graph shown in figure 11–2 displays these data. In analyzing these data, it is important to avoid the assumption that industry averages represent the "gospel truth." On the other hand, the healthcare organization that is substantially out of line with an industry average may well have a weakness in its financial performance. Therefore, the analyst should investigate substantial deviations from the averages and take any necessary corrective measures.

In many situations, it may be necessary to go well beyond reported figures and ratios to properly analyze the healthcare organization's financial condition and performance. For example, table 11–1 indicates that the percentage of gross patient accounts receivable to the gross patient revenue increased from 15.0 percent to 18.0 percent in years 19x4 and 19x5. Such a phenomenon could have any of the following causes:

- change in collection policy

- increase in rates

- slow reimbursement by third-party payer

- change in paying agent mix

FIGURE 11–1

Five-Year Graphic Analysis of Patient Accounts Receivable and Revenue

Memorial Medical Center
Anytown, U.S.A.

PERCENT RATIO OF GROSS PATIENT ACCOUNTS RECEIVABLE TO GROSS PATIENT REVENUE

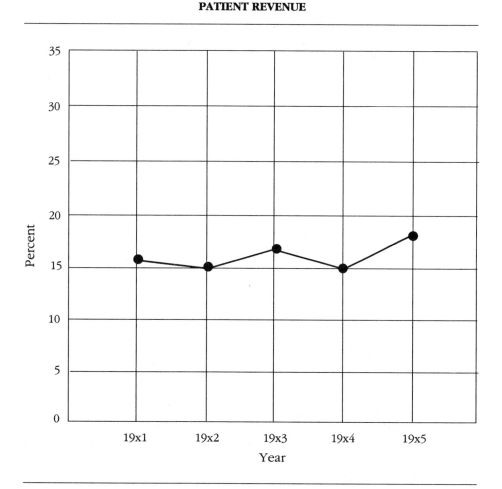

TABLE 11–2
Memorial Medical Center's Average Percentage of Gross Patient Accounts Receivable to Gross Patient Revenue Compared with the Regional Average

Year	Memorial Medical Center	Regional Average	Variance Favorable/(Unfavorable)
19x1	16.3%	15.8%	(.5)%
19x2	15.0	15.4	.4
19x3	17.0	15.9	(1.1)
19x4	15.0	16.0	1.0
19x5	18.0	17.0	(1.0)

These or many other factors could have produced this adverse trend. Investigating and resolving the problem is the responsibility of the patient financial services manager.

A word of caution about the use of industry standards is necessary here: it is important to compare apples with apples, not apples with oranges. Even with industry standards, the analyst must use discretion in interpreting the comparisons.

Ratio Analysis Types

For the purposes of this discussion, financial ratios will be divided into five major categories:

1. liquidity

2. leverage

3. activity

4. profitability

5. profit planning

The first two kinds of ratios are developed from information displayed on the statement of condition, or balance sheet. The three remaining types of ratios are based on information derived from the statement of operations, the income statement, or from both statements. In analyzing the healthcare organization's financial condition, keep in mind that no single ratio or index will give the analyst the total picture. The analyst must therefore consider and evaluate a considerable number of ratios before drawing any final conclusion. Further, the analyst should not limit the analysis to just one year; considering three or more years to identifies trends more clearly. For example,

FIGURE 11–2

Memorial Medical Center's Average Percentage of Gross Patient Accounts Receivable to Gross Patient Revenue Compared with the Regional Average

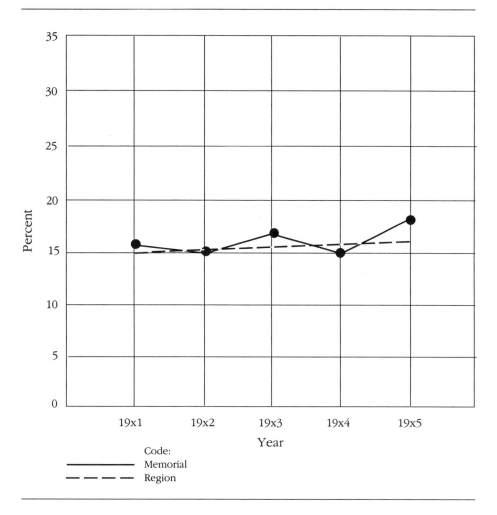

although the data for one year may indicate a rather weak financial position, it may actually reveal a favorable trend when compared with data for previous years.

Liquidity Ratios

Generally, the first concern of the healthcare organization's financial analyst is the institution's liquidity. Liquidity ratios help to identify and evaluate this ability to meet maturing short-term obligations. These ratios compare the facility's current assets with its current liabilities. *Current assets* are assets normally and/or easily converted into cash within one year or less. *Current liabilities,* on the other hand, are debts due within one year or less.

The most commonly used liquidity ratio is the current ratio, which is computed by dividing current liabilities into current assets. Memorial Medical Center's statement of condition (see table 11–3) indicates that current assets for 19x2 include the following:

	Year 19x2
Operating Cash	$ 45,000
Short-Term Investments	175,000
Net Patient Accounts Receivable	1,310,000
Other Receivables	170,000
Inventory	215,000
Prepaid Expenses	85,000
Total Current Assets	$2,000,000

The current liabilities include the following:

Accounts Payable	$ 285,000
Payroll Taxes Payable	350,000
Accrued Payroll Payable	420,000
Due to Third-Party Agencies	445,000
Total Current Liabilities	$1,500,000

Using the current ratio formula:

$$\text{Current Ratio} = \frac{\text{Current Assets}}{\text{Current Liabilities}}$$

We can compute Memorial Medical Center's current ratio as follows:

$$1.33 = \frac{\$2,000,000}{\$1,500,000}$$

In this illustration, Memorial Medical Center has 1.33 times as many current assets as current liabilities. Even though the current ratio is one of the generally accepted measures of liquidity or short-term solvency, its one weakness is that it does not give adequate weight to the fact that $300,000 of the organization's current assets are tied up in inventory and prepaid expenses that cannot be readily converted to cash.

The quick ratio, also known as the acid test ratio, can be used to compensate for this drawback in the current ratio. We can compute the quick ratio by deducting inventories and prepaid expenses from current assets and dividing the balance by current liabilities. Here is the formula:

TABLE 11–3

Comparative Statement of Condition

Memorial Medical Center
Anytown, U.S.A.

COMPARATIVE STATEMENT OF CONDITION
as of September 30, 19x2

	19x2	19x1	Change: Increase/(Decrease) Amount	Percent
ASSETS				
Current Assets				
Operating Cash	$ 45,000	$ 50,000	$ (5,000)	10.0%
Short-Term Investments	$ 175,000	$ 135,000	$ 40,000	29.6
Gross Patient Accounts Receivable	$ 1,485,000	$ 1,363,000	$ 122,000	9.0
Less: Reserves for Uncollectibles	$ 175,000	$ 160,000	$ 15,000	9.4
Net Patient Accounts Receivable	$ 1,310,000	$1,203,000	$ 107,000	8.9
Other Receivables	$ 170,000	$ 150,000	$ 20,000	13.3
Inventory	$ 215,000	$ 195,000	$ 20,000	10.2
Prepaid Expenses	$ 85,000	$ 72,000	$ 13,000	18.0
Total Current Assets	$ 2,000,000	$1,805,000	$ 195,000	10.8
Fixed Assets				
Land	$ 50,000	$ 50,000	$ –0–	0.0
Plant and Equipment	$12,765,000	$11,320,000	$1,445,000	12.8
Less: Accumulated Depreciation	$ 3,930,000	$ 3,750,000	$ 180,000	4.8
Net Plant and Equipment	$ 8,835,000	$7,570,000	$1,265,000	16.7
Total Fixed Assets	$ 8,885,000	$7,620,000	$1,265,000	16.7
Total Assets	$10,885,000	$9,425,000	$1,460,000	15.5
LIABILITIES AND EQUITY				
Current Liabilities				
Accounts Payable	$ 285,000	$ 260,000	$ 25,000	9.6%
Payroll Taxes Payable	$ 350,000	$ 320,000	$ 30,000	9.4
Accrued Payroll Payable	$ 420,000	$ 390,000	$ 30,000	7.7
Short-Term Note Payable	$ –0–	$ 60,000	$ (60,000)	100.0
Due to Third-Party Agencies	$ 445,000	$ 435,000	$ 10,000	2.3
Total Current Liabilities	$ 1,500,000	$1,465,000	$ 35,000	2.4
Fixed Liabilities				
Mortgage Payable	$ 5,790,000	$5,560,000	$ 230,000	4.1
Total Fixed Liabilities	$ 5,790,000	$5,560,000	$ 230,000	4.1
Total Liabilities	$ 7,290,000	$7,025,000	$ 265,000	3.8
Equity				
Beginning Balance	$ 2,400,000	$1,600,000	$ 800,000	50.0
Plus: Operating Profit (Loss)	$ 1,195,000	$ 800,000	$ 395,000	49.4
Ending Balance	$ 3,595,000	$2,400,000	$1,195,000	49.8
Total Equity	$ 3,595,000	$2,400,000	$1,195,000	49.8
Total Liabilities and Equity	$10,885,000	$9,425,000	$1,460,000	15.5

$$\text{Quick Ratio or Acid Test Ratio} = \frac{\text{Current Assets} - (\text{Inventory} + \text{Prepaid Expenses})}{\text{Current Liabilities}}$$

or

$$1.13 = \frac{\$1,700,000}{\$1,500,000}$$

The analyst will also see that $1,310,000 of the $1,700,000 remaining current assets are tied up in patient accounts receivable, and an additional $170,000 in other receivables. The following is a distribution analysis of the current assets, excluding inventories and prepaid expenses:

	Amount	Percent
Operating Cash	$ 45,000	2.65
Short-Term Investments	175,000	10.29
Net Patient Accounts Receivable	1,310,000	77.06
Other Receivables	170,000	10.00
Net Current Assets	$1,700,000	100.00

Since the receivables represent such a significant share of the healthcare organization's current assets, this chapter will present a special set of ratios later.

Leverage Ratios

Leverage ratios, which measure the equity generated by the healthcare organization compared with the financing provided by the organization's creditors, have a number of implications. First, creditors look to the equity or owner-supplied funds to provide a margin of safety. If the owners provide only a small proportion of the total financing, the facility's financial risks are borne mainly by the creditors. Second, by raising funds through borrowing, the organization gains the benefit of maintaining control with limited investment. Third, if the organization earns more on the borrowed funds than it pays in interest, the return to the owners is increased. For example, if assets earn 14 percent and debt costs 12 percent, the 2-percent differential accrues to the facility's benefit. Of course, leverage works both ways: if the return on assets falls to 10 percent, for example, the differential between that figure and the cost of debt must be covered by the facility's equity or total profits. In the first instance, where assets earn more than debt costs, leverage is favorable; in the second, it is unfavorable.

Generally, leverage is evaluated two ways. The first method involves examining statement of condition (balance sheet) ratios and determining the extent to which borrowed funds have been used to finance the organization. The second approach measures the risks of debt with income statement profit and loss ratios designed to determine the number of times fixed charges are covered by operating profits.

The debt ratio measures the percentage of total assets that has been provided by the organization's creditors. Total debt includes current liabilities as well as long-term obligations. Creditors prefer moderate debt ratios because the lower the ratio, the greater the protection for creditors against losses in the event of liquidation. The formula for the debt ratio is

$$\text{Debt Ratio} = \frac{\text{Total Liabilities (Debt)}}{\text{Total Assets}}$$

or

$$66.97\% = \frac{\$7,290,000}{\$10,885,000}$$

In this case, Memorial Medical Center has financed 66.97 percent of its assets through debt, which represents a substantial amount of indebtedness. In all probability, prospective lenders would be reluctant to loan any more money to the facility. If the organization's debt ratio were 50 percent or less, it would be in a much stronger position to borrow additional money.

The times interest earned ratio measures the extent to which the healthcare organization's profits can decline before it will lose the ability to meet its annual interest costs. Failure to meet interest expense could bring legal action from the organization's creditors and possible bankruptcy.

The statement of operations for Memorial Medical Center (table 11–4) provides the profit and interest expense data necessary to compute the times interest earned ratio. The formula for the times interest earned ratio is

$$\text{Times Interest Earned Ratio} = \frac{\text{Profit before Taxes} + \text{Interest Expense}}{\text{Interest Expense}}$$

or

$$= \frac{\$1,194,910 + \$492,150}{\$492,150}$$

or

$$3.43 \text{ times} = \frac{\$1{,}687{,}060}{\$\ 492{,}150}$$

In this illustration, the medical center's gross income or profit available to service the $492,150 interest expense is $1,687,060, so the interest expense is covered only 3.43 times. If the industry average were 7.0 times, the organization would be covering its interest expense with a minimal margin of safety; thus, it would be likely to have a low credit rating.

Fixed-charges coverage analysis determines the number of times fixed charges are covered by the facility's profit. Fixed charges include such items as interest, lease payments, rent, and sinking fund requirements. This ratio is more revealing than the times interest earned ratio because it includes other fixed costs that the organization must meet to stay in business. The formula for fixed-charges coverage is

$$\text{Fixed-Charges Coverage} = \frac{\text{Operating Profit}}{\text{Interest} + \text{Rent} + \text{Leases} + \text{Other Fixed Charges}}$$

or

$$= \frac{\$1{,}194{,}910}{\$492{,}150 + \$205{,}000}$$

or

$$1.7 \text{ times} = \frac{\$1{,}195{,}000}{\$697{,}150}$$

As was the case with the times interest earned ratio, the fixed-charges coverage ratio is substantially low. If the industry average is 3.5 times, a potential lender would probably rate Memorial Medical Center as a low credit risk.

Activity Ratios

Activity ratios measure how efficiently the healthcare organization is using its assets. Generally, the term *turnover rate* means the number of times a particular asset is replenished or turned over in one year. This ratio is frequently used to measure how efficiently the organization is handling its inventory and accounts receivable. One method used to compute the turnover rate for these two assets is as follows:

TABLE 11–4

Comparative Statement of Operations

Memorial Medical Center
Anytown, U.S.A.

COMPARATIVE STATEMENT OF OPERATIONS
For Years Ending September 30, 19x2 and 19x1

	19x2		19x1		Change	
	Amount	*Percent*	*Amount*	*Percent*	*Amount*	*Percent*
Volume						
Inpatient Days	28,567		28,564		12	0.1
Inpatient Admissions	3,402		3,173		229	7.2
Outpatient Visits	11,029		9,840		1,189	12.1
Revenue						
Gross Charges:						
Inpatient Services	$8,172,900	95.0	$7,309,620	95.5	$863,280	11.8
Outpatient Services	430,150	5.0	344,430	4.5	85,720	24.9
Gross Patient Charges	$8,603,050	100.0	$7,654,050	100.0	$949,000	12.4
Less: Provision for Bad						
Debts and Allowances	2,026,650	24.1	1,744,800	22.8	281,850	19.0
Net Patient Charges	$6,526,400	75.9	$5,909,250	77.2	$667,150	10.4
Other Operating Revenue	270,000	3.1	214,000	2.8	56,000	26.2
Total Revenue	$6,796,400	79.0	$6,123,250	80.0	$723,150	11.0
Expenses						
Administrative and Household	$ 924,250	* 10.8	$ 964,700	* 12.6	$(40,450)	(4.2)
Employee Health and Welfare	481,720	5.6	431,180	5.6	50,540	11.7
General Professional Care	1,938,080	22.5	1,804,580	23.6	133,500	7.4
Auxiliary Services	1,327,530	* 15.4	1,229,670	* 16.0	97,860	8.0
Ambulatory Services	257,760	3.0	255,520	3.3	2,150	0.8
Depreciation	180,000	2.1	165,000	2.2	15,000	9.1
Interest Expense	492,150	5.7	472,600	6.2	19,550	4.1
Total Expenses	$5,601,490	65.1	$5,323,250	69.5	$278,150	5.2
Profit (Loss)	$1,194,910	13.9	$ 800,000	10.5	$445,000	49.3

*Includes $205,000 and $195,000 in lease expenses for the years 19x2 and 19x1, respectively.

$$\text{Inventory Turnover to Charges} = \frac{\text{Gross Charges}}{\text{Inventory}}$$

or

$$40.01 \text{ times} = \frac{\$8,603,050}{\$215,000}$$

Here is another way to measure inventory turnover:

$$\text{Inventory Turnover to Purchases} = \frac{\text{Purchases}}{\text{Inventory}}$$

Assume that during the year 19x2, Memorial Medical Center purchased $1,935,000 worth of stock and supplies that were processed through its inventory system. The annual inventory turnover rate would be computed as follows:

$$9.00 \text{ times} = \frac{\$1,935,000}{\$215,000}$$

Generally, the more frequently an inventory turns over, the greater the efficiency. However, an inventory could have such a high turnover rate that the organization is constantly out of stock, and reorder costs could be substantially high; hence, a lower turnover rate might actually be more economical.

Fixed asset turnover is another ratio that is frequently used to evaluate the use of the organization's fixed assets compared with its gross charges. The formula for the fixed asset turnover ratio is

$$\text{Fixed Assets Turnover (Gross Charges)} = \frac{\text{Gross Charges to Patients}}{\text{Fixed Assets}}$$

or

$$0.97 \text{ times} = \frac{\$8,603,050}{\$8,885,000}$$

This formula can also be applied to the healthcare organization's net charges to patients:

$$\text{Fixed Assets Turnover (Net)} = \frac{\text{Net Charges to Patients}}{\text{Fixed Assets}}$$

or

$$0.73 \text{ times} = \frac{\$6,526,400}{\$8,885,000}$$

The total asset turnover ratio compares the organization's total assets with either the gross or net charges to patients:

$$\text{Total Assets Turnover (Gross)} = \frac{\text{Gross Charges to Patients}}{\text{Total Assets}}$$

or

$$0.79 \text{ times} = \frac{\$8,603,050}{\$10,885,000}$$

$$\text{Total Assets Turnover (Net)} = \frac{\text{Net Charges to Patients}}{\text{Total Assets}}$$

or

$$0.60 \text{ times} = \frac{\$6,526,400}{\$10,885,000}$$

Accounts receivable turnover is another activity ratio type that this chapter will cover in more detail later.

Profitability Ratios

Profitability ratios measure the healthcare organization's overall effectiveness in terms of generating profits compared with the facility's revenue and investment. Since profitability ratios can be calculated for either gross or net charges to patients, the following examples will illustrate both types of ratios. When a healthcare organization is required to pay income taxes, the net profit after taxes should always be part of the equation. The formulas are as follows:

$$\text{Profit Margin on Gross Charges} = \frac{\text{Net Profit after Taxes}}{\text{Gross Charges to Patients}}$$

or

$$13.89\% = \frac{\$1,194,910}{\$8,603,050}$$

$$\text{Profit Margin on Net Charges} = \frac{\text{Net Profit after Taxes}}{\text{Net Charges to Patients}}$$

or

$$18.31\% = \frac{\$1,194,910}{\$6,526,400}$$

The profit margin ratio relates the organization's net profit to either gross or net charges to patients. The resulting percentage indicates to management the degree of protection it has from falling charges or rising costs. The higher the percentage or margin, the less risk there is of losses due to reduced income or volume.

The return on total assets ratio compares the healthcare organization's profit after taxes with its total assets. The formula for this ratio is

$$\text{Return on Total Assets} = \frac{\text{Net Profit after Taxes}}{\text{Total Assets}}$$

or

$$10.98\% = \frac{\$1,194,910}{\$10,885,000}$$

The return on net worth or equity ratio measures the net profit after taxes compared with the organization's total net worth or owner's equity. The formula for this ratio is

$$\text{Return on Net Worth (Equity)} = \frac{\text{Net Profit after Taxes}}{\text{Net Worth}}$$

or

$$33.24\% = \frac{\$1,194,910}{\$3,595,000}$$

This ratio gives management a benchmark for comparing what the healthcare organization is earning with what it might obtain from other forms of investment (opportunity costs), such as money market funds and new business.

Profit-planning Ratios

Break-even analysis ratios determine profit for specific time periods, volumes, prices (net income), and patient mixes. Before a break-even analysis can be made, the analyst must separate all the organization's costs into fixed and variable costs. In addition, components known as contribution and the contribution margin are also incorporated into break-even analysis. *Contri-*

bution is the dollar difference between the net price and the variable cost for a unit of service. The *contribution margin* is the difference, expressed as a percentage, between the net price or rate. For example, assume that the average net price (after provision for bad debts and allowances) for a one-day patient stay is $250. Assume further that the variable expense is $150. Computing the contribution and the contribution margin would be as follows:

	Amount	*Percent*
Average daily net price per patient day	$250.00	100.0%
Average variable cost per patient day	150.00	60.0
Average contribution per patient day	$100.00	
Average contribution margin per patient day		40.0%

The break-even analysis identifies the point at which total revenue equals total expense plus the desired profit margin.

Using the data given above, assume that the facility's average daily fixed costs are $15,000. Further assume that the organization has targeted an average daily profit of $3,000. To accomplish these results, the facility's daily break-even census would be as follows:

	Per Patient Day	*Proof*
Average daily net price per patient day	$250.00	$45,000
Average daily variable cost per patient day	150.00	27,000
Average contribution per patient day	$100.00	$18,000
Average daily fixed costs per calendar day	$15,000	$15,000
Target average daily net profit	$ 3,000	
Average daily fixed costs and profit	$18,000	
Break-even census:		
$18,000 ÷ $100	180 patient days	
Net profit (loss) (with $3,000 profit)		$3,000

The arithmetic method is one approach to computing the organization's break-even point; another approach is to use formulas, such as the following:

$$\text{Break-Even Point in Units of Service} = \frac{\text{Fixed Costs} + \text{Net Profit}}{\text{Contribution}}$$

or

$$= \frac{\$15{,}000 + \$3{,}000}{\$100}$$

or

$$180 \text{ units} = \frac{\$18{,}000}{\$100}$$

The analyst could compute the break-even net patient revenue using the following formula. Note that the divisor changes from the contribution to the contribution margin.

$$\text{Break-Even Point in Dollars (Net Charges)} = \frac{\$15{,}000 + \$3{,}000}{0.40}$$

or

$$\$45{,}000 = \frac{\$18{,}000}{0.40}$$

Another application of break-even analysis is determination of the margin of safety, that is, the percentage by which net patient revenue can decline before the healthcare organization experiences a loss. This percentage is a dramatic way of demonstrating to management how close the net patient revenue level is to the break-even point (excluding profit).

Using the following data, we can compute the organization's margin of safety as follows:

Total net patient revenue	$45,000
Contribution margin	40%
Contribution	$18,000
Break-even patient revenue	
(without profit)	$37,500
Profit	$ 3,000

$$\text{Margin of Safety} = \frac{\text{Profit}}{\text{Contribution}}$$

or

$$16.67\% = \frac{\$3{,}000}{\$18{,}000}$$

and

$$\text{Margin of Safety} = \frac{\text{Net Patient Revenue} - \text{Break-Even Net Revenue}}{\text{Net Patient Revenue}}$$

or

$$= \frac{\$45,000 - \$37,500}{\$45,000}$$

or

$$16.67\% = \frac{\$7,500}{\$45,000}$$

Thus, net patient revenue of $45,000 could decline 16.67 percent (or $7,500) to $37,500 before the organization would experience an operating loss.

To prove this analysis, the analyst can use the following procedure:

	Target Plan		**Safety Test**	
	Amount	*Percent*	*Amount*	*Percent*
Net patient revenue	$45,000	100.0%	$37,500	100.0%
Variable expenses	27,000	60.0	22,500	60.0
Contribution	$18,000	40.0%	$15,000	40.0%
Fixed costs	15,000		15,000	
Profit	$ 3,000		–0–	

Measuring Liquidity of Patient Accounts Receivable

Excluding fixed assets and equipment, the patient accounts receivable represent most healthcare organizations' largest single asset. To regard all receivables as liquid when in fact a sizable portion of them may be past due and/or uncollectible overstates the liquidity of the organization. Receivables are liquid assets only to the extent that the organization can collect them within a reasonable amount of time. For this reason, it is imperative that the organization establish an appropriate policy to take into account uncollectible accounts and contractual allowances. While patient accounts receivable may be analyzed as either gross or net, the most realistic approach is to base the analysis on net patient accounts receivable. However, in the following analysis of Memorial Medical Center's patient accounts receivable, both methods will be used.

The most commonly used accounts receivable analysis is the number of days of average daily revenue uncollected or the average collection period ratio. This ratio is computed as follows:

		Gross Patient Accounts Receivable	Net Patient Accounts Receivable
1.	Annual charges to patients	$8,603,050	$6,526,400
2.	Number of calendar days	365	365
3.	Average daily charges (line 1 ÷ line 2)	$ 23,570	$ 17,880
4.	Patient accounts receivable	$1,485,000	$1,310,000
5.	Average collection period (line 4 ÷ line 3)	63.0	73.3

Accounts Receivable Turnover Rate

Another ratio frequently used to analyze patient accounts receivable is the turnover rate. The following is the computation of Memorial Medical Center's accounts receivable turnover rate:

		Gross Patient Accounts Receivable	Net Patient Accounts Receivable
1.	Total annual patient charges	$8,603,050	$6,526,400
2.	Patient accounts receivable	$1,485,000	$1,310,000
3.	Accounts receivable turnover rate (line ÷ line 2)	5.8 times	5.0 times

The cardinal rule in analyzing patient accounts receivable is to always compare gross charges with gross receivables and net patient revenue with net receivables. Never compare gross charges to net receivables or vice versa.

Patient Receivables to Charges

Analyzing patient accounts receivable is also possible with the receivables-to-charges ratio. It is calculated as follows:

		Gross Patient Accounts Receivable	Net Patient Accounts Receivable
1.	Patient accounts receivable	$1,485,000	$1,310,000
2.	Annual patient charges	$8,603,050	$6,526,400
3.	Receivables percent of charges (line 1 ÷ line 2)	17.26%	20.1%

Patient Receivables to Current and Total Assets

While the receivables-to-charges ratio compares the patient accounts receivable and patient account charges, the following analyses compare the receivables with both the healthcare organization's current and total assets:

		Gross Patient Accounts Receivable	Net Patient Accounts Receivable
1.	Patient accounts receivable	$1,485,000	$1,410,000
2.	Current assets	$2,000,000	$2,000,000
3.	Percent of current assets (line 1 ÷ line 2)	74.3%	70.5%

		Gross Patient Accounts Receivable	Net Patient Accounts Receivable
1.	Patient accounts receivable	$ 1,485,000	$1,310,000
2.	Total assets	$10,885,000	$9,425,000
3.	Percent of total assets (line 1 ÷ line 2)	13.6%	13.9%

Patient Receivables to Equity

While the preceding analyses identify the percentage of the healthcare organization's assets tied up in patient accounts receivable, the following ratio computes the relationship of the healthcare organization's net worth or equity to its patient accounts receivable:

		Gross Patient Accounts Receivable	Net Patient Accounts Receivable
1.	Patient accounts receivable	$1,485,000	$1,310,000
2.	Net worth (equity)	$3,595,000	$3,595,000
3.	Percent of net worth (line 1 ÷ line 2)	41.3%	36.4%

We could also express the ratio of patient accounts receivable to equity as (a) 1:2.4 (gross patient accounts receivable), and (b) 1:2.7 (net patient accounts receivable).

Opportunity Costs

Finally, the patient accounts receivable can be evaluated by computing the opportunity costs the organization experiences by having its assets tied up in patient accounts receivable when they could be invested in a money market fund or other interest-bearing investment account. This opportunity cost is computed in the following manner:

		Gross Patient Accounts Receivable	Net Patient Accounts Receivable
1.	Patient accounts receivable	$1,485,000	$1,310,000
2.	Current rate of interest on money market funds or desired rate of return on investment	15%	15%
3.	Total opportunity costs per year (line 1 × line 2)	$ 222,750	$ 196,500

If the average collection periods computed previously of 63.0 and 73.3 days were reduced by 10 days, the facility's patient accounts receivable would reflect this improved collection efficiency:

		Gross Patient Accounts Receivable	Net Patient Accounts Receivable
1.	Patient accounts receivable	$1,485,000	$1,310,000
2.	Average daily charges	$ 23,570	$ 17,880
3.	Target reduction of number of days	10	10
4.	Amount to be reduced (line 2 × line 3)	$ 235,700	$ 178,800
5.	Current rate of interest on money market funds	15%	15%
6.	Opportunity savings per year (line 4 × line 5)	$ 35,355	$ 26,820

In this illustration, Memorial Medical Center gains a one-time increase in working capital of $235,700 (gross) or $178,880 (net), as well as the opportunity to earn $35,355 (gross) or $26,820 (net) by investing in a money market fund.

Other Performance Analyses

Statement of Condition (Balance Sheet)

The statement of condition, also referred to as a balance sheet, in table 11–3 illustrated the necessity of analyzing financial data from more than one year.

If the analyst only has data for one year, there is absolutely no basis for evaluating any increases or decreases. The illustrated statement displays results for two years side by side, and identifies the dollar and percent change from the first year to the second. These changes are summarized in the statement of changes in financial position in table 11–5.

TABLE 11–5
Statement of Changes in Financial Position

Memorial Medical Center
Anytown, U.S.A.

STATEMENT OF CHANGES IN FINANCIAL POSITION
From September 30, 19x1 to September 30, 19x2

Funds Provided by:		
Net Operating Profit	$1,194,910	
Depreciation	180,000	
Total Funds Provided from Operations	$1,374,910	
Funds Applied to:		
Purchase of Plant and Equipment	$1,445,000	
Increase of Mortgage Payable	(230,090)	
Increase in Working Capital (see below)	160,000	
Total Funds Applied from Operations	$1,374,910	

Changes in Working Capital

Uses:		
Decrease in Operating Cash	$ (5,000)	
Increase in Short-Term Investments	40,000	
Increase in Net Accounts Receivable	107,000	
Increase in Other Receivables	20,000	
Increase in Inventory	20,000	
Increase in Prepaid Expenses	$ 13,000	
Net Uses of Working Capital		$195,000
Sources:		
Increase in Accounts Payable	$ 25,000	
Increase in Payroll Payable	30,000	
Increase in Accrued Payroll Payable	30,000	
Decrease in Short-Term Note Payable	(60,000)	
Increase in Amount Due to Third Party	10,000	
Net Sources of Working Capital		$ 35,000
Net Increase in Working Capital		$160,000

Statement of Changes in Financial Position

The statement of changes in financial position identifies the specific changes, uses, and sources of working capital, as well as how the healthcare organization's income was provided and how it was applied. Remember the following formula as a method of showing the source of funds:

$$\text{Cash Flow} = \text{Net Operating Profits} + \text{Depreciation}$$

Net operating profit plus any noncash expenses such as depreciation is the only source of funds, other than borrowing of some kind. Of course, the healthcare organization cannot maintain its viability and grow without profit.

Statement of Operations

The statement of operations in table 11–4 is also based on two years' data. In studying the illustration, note that each year's dollar operatintg results are analyzed as a percentage of the organization's gross patient charges. This approach enables the analyst to compare the change in either revenue or expense mix. For example, outpatient revenue increased as a percentage of gross patient charges from 4.5 percent in 19x1 to 5.0 percent in 19x2, and administrative and household expenses declined from 12.6 percent in 19x1 to 10.8 percent in 19x2. As in the statement of condition, the statement of operations shows changes in both dollars and percentages.

Employee Turnover Rate

Not all performance ratios are generated using information from a healthcare facility's financial statements. For example, the employee turnover rate helps the patient financial services managers to evaluate their supervisors' managerial skills in addition to their own. The employee turnover rate, expressed either as a number or as a percentage, is computed in a manner similar to the accounts receivable or inventory turnover rates:

$$\frac{\text{Beginning Staff} + \text{New Hires}}{\text{Number of Staff End of Year}} = \text{Employee Turnover Rate}$$

This ratio produces the number of times or the percentage of times the employee staff turns over during one year. Whereas a high turnover rate is desirable in the management of inventory and accounts receivable, a low turnover rate is, generally, the most acceptable rate for employees. High employee turnover is expensive. Related costs include recruitment, applicant screening, new employee processing, training and cross-training, low productivity, and many other related expenses. The following is an example of how the patient financial services manager of Memorial Medical Center could analyze the turnover costs of the patient service representative teams:

Description	Team 1	Team 2	Team 3	Team 4	Team 5
1. Beginning staff level	3	3	3	3	4
2. New hires during year	3	1	2	0	2
3. Total employees managed (line 1 + line 2)	6	4	5	3	6
4. Ending staff level	3	3	3	3	3
5. Employee turnover rate (line 3 ÷ line 4)	2.00	1.33	1.67	1.00	2.00

In this example, Team 4 has the lowest employee turnover rate, whereas Team 1 has the highest; the total team average turnover rate is 1.67. Using this information, the patient financial services manager can examine the weaknesses and strengths of each patient service representative team leader and take the appropriate corrective actions; i.e., share the strengths and weaknesses in a focus group setting.

In a recent survey, the average staff turnover rate in patient financial services departments was 9.3%.[1] Using this average employee turnover rate and the other relevant data, we can calculate the annual cost of employee turnover:

1.	Average number of employees	40
2.	Average turnover rate	9.3%
3.	Average cost per employee turnover	$5,000
4.	Annual number of employees turned over (line 1 × line 2 = line 4)	3.72
5.	Annual cost of employee turnover (line 3 × line 4 = line 5)	$18,600

The average annual cost of employee turnover is just another method management can use to evaluate the effectiveness of a patient financial services manager. The key objective is to be very selective in the hiring process. But once the applicant is hired, it is the manager's and supervisors' responsibility to adequately train all departmental employees to improve productivity and morale, thereby minimizing the employee turnover rate.

To summarize, analyzing financial statements calls for some basis for comparing current data. The following information represents some of the bases that can be used for comparing current operating results:

- budget or financial plan
- actual results for the previous month or year

- national, regional, or special industry indexes

The important issue to keep in mind is that a single accounting period's financial or production results are virtually meaningless unless they can be compared with something. The types of financial analyses, ratios, and statements that analysts use for such comparisons are limited only by their imagination. Regardless of what methods are used, intelligent comparisons and analyses that lead to appropriate management decisions and corrective action are vital to the healthcare organization's future.

NOTE

1. Healthcare Financial Management Association, 1991 Patient Financial Services Survey (Westchester, Ill: HFMA, 1991).

CHAPTER 12

Internal Audit and Control of Receivables

In the past, many of the managerial tools typically used by executives in the manufacturing industry were considered by healthcare executives to be impractical for application to *their* industry. Today, however, budgeting, cost accounting, productivity measurement, performance planning, and strategic planning are all examples of managerial tools that healthcare executives have embraced enthusiastically. They have found these concepts to be vital to their organization's effective, efficient operation.

Central to this change in opinion is that as healthcare institutions and systems grew in size and complexity, the gap between their administrative-financial departments and their professional services departments widened. This phenomenon required healthcare management teams to reevaluate their technological and managerial tools. On-line, real-time data processing systems, operations research, focus groups, management by objectives, management engineering, simulation analysis, and marketing are among the concepts healthcare organizations began using to increase their organization's productivity and profitability.

Each of these tools depends on financial and statistical data of unquestionable integrity. Because healthcare facilities operate in a more complex environment these days, management and trustees need to make prudent, informed decisions derived from accurate, timely financial information that is not later subject to change.[1] Therefore, healthcare executives must develop and implement an internal audit and control structure to guarantee that this information is accurate and valid.

Furthermore, modern healthcare management requires timely and accurate reports to properly analyze and control the activities for which it is responsible. These reports' timeliness depends on the sophistication and efficiency of the system used to process the data. The reports' accuracy hinges on the extent to which employees adhere to their healthcare organization's established procedures. Patient financial services managers can employ internal audit and control to ensure the integrity of their management information and help protect their organization's assets.

This chapter will address effective internal audit and control objectives and techniques to assist patient financial services managers in evaluating the adequacy of their department's and organization's controls. Chapter 12 ends with practical know-how for managing patient accounts receivable, the single most important factor in the healthcare organization's financial success.

Internal Audit

In its *Statement of Responsibilities of Internal Auditing,* the Institute of Internal Auditors defines *internal auditing* as

> an independent appraisal function established within an organization to examine and evaluate its activities as a service to the organization. The objective of internal auditing is to assist members of the organization in the effective discharge of their responsibilities. To this end, internal auditing furnishes them with analyses, appraisals, recommendations, counsel, and information concerning the activities reviewed. The audit objective includes promoting effective control at reasonable cost. The members of the organization assisted by internal auditing include those in management and the board of directors.[2]

Thus, the internal audit's scope extends far beyond mere number-checking to serve as a managerial tool that appraises all activities within the healthcare organization, thereby promoting the attainment of the organization's objectives.[3]

The institute's statement also includes a description of the activities appropriate to the scope of an internal audit function:

- reviewing the reliability and integrity of financial and operating information and the means used to identify, measure, classify, and report such information

- reviewing the systems established to ensure compliance with those policies, plans, procedures, laws, and regulations that could have a significant impact on operations and reports and determining whether the organization is in compliance

- reviewing the means of safeguarding assets and, as appropriate, verifying the existence of such assets

- appraising the economy and efficiency with which resources are employed

- reviewing operations or programs to ascertain whether results are consistent with established objectives and goals and whether the operations or programs are being carried out as planned[4]

In effect, the internal auditor is the person monitoring the organization's internal control system, assuring that it is not only functioning but also functioning properly.[5]

A key element of an effective internal audit is the element of surprise. The very existence of an internal audit program and the realization that all activities within the organization are subject to scrutiny by an independent party encourages accuracy and compliance with established procedures.

Usually, the internal auditor reports directly to executive management, for example, the chief financial officer, the chief operating officer, or the chief executive officer.[6] In some cases, this auditor reports to the chairman of the governing board. This reporting pattern gives the internal audit staff members considerable independence from those whose work they audit. Independence of the internal audit function is further enhanced by correlating it with the audit work of the healthcare organization's external auditor. In the resulting integrated audit program, the work of the internal auditor and the external auditor complements and supplements each other's somewhat parallel efforts.[7] An integrated audit program becomes even more important as the healthcare organization's work volume grows, as management expands the scope of the audit program, and as the facility makes increasing use of sophisticated technology.

Internal Control

Internal control consists of a group of accounting systems and procedures that serve as systematic, automatic safeguards to protect the integrity of the healthcare organization's accounting information. It also assists the organization's management team by building automatic devices into the management information system to ensure compliance with established policies, systems, and procedures. Moreover, an internal control program aids management in keeping policies and procedures current and in documenting all changes to them.

A good internal control system provides the healthcare organization with other benefits as well:

- It provides management with information that is up-to-date, reliable, and accurate.

- It reduces the risk of losing assets and resources through errors or misappropriations.

- It promotes operational efficiency by, among other things, reducing the likelihood of errors.

- It gives employees definite guidelines on policies and procedures.[8]

An effective internal control system has four fundamental elements:

1. *Separation of duties.* No individual or department should account for its own activities or report on the results of its own operations. Stated simply, no one function should be contained or controlled by one person.

2. *Organizational structure.* Responsibility and accountability must be well documented and defined by using an organizational chart and job descriptions that include specific measurements or expectations of acceptable performance.

3. *Sound policies and procedures.* The healthcare organization's goals and objectives must be well defined, and the governing board must establish, document, and communicate corresponding policies to those employees who are responsible for carrying them out.

4. *Adequate staff of trained personnel.* The healthcare organization must retain only employees who are well trained and knowledgeable about current practice in their profession or trade to ensure proper administration of the organization's operations. An effective inservice education program for *all* employees can help ensure an enlightened and knowledgeable staff. The program's objective should be a competent, reliable, and stable staff capable of quality work and high productivity.

Clearly, internal control covers all elements of management. As Seawell points out, many healthcare executives give undue emphasis to the accounting aspect of internal control. The broader concept of internal control, he says, is composed of administrative controls and accounting controls. Administrative controls consist of those methods and measures in the organization's internal control system that essentially focus on improving the efficiency with which the organization's employees perform activities; they also secure a high degree of compliance with established managerial policies. These controls relate only indirectly to the accounting records. Accounting controls, on the other hand, are primarily for the purposes of safeguarding the organization's assets and to assure a high degree of reliability in the information generated by the accounting process. Certainly, Seawell concludes, the facility's managers and accountants are obligated to protect their organization from the financial dangers of error and fraud, but he emphasizes that internal control dollars can often be invested more productively in administrative controls to eliminate the waste stemming from operational inefficency.[9]

To summarize, internal audit and internal control are management tools that focus primarily on people and systems. These tools are concerned with how well employees

- follow prescribed procedures,

- organize themselves for control purposes, and

- develop themselves professionally.

In light of changes in the healthcare environment such as modifications to Medicare and other third-party payment systems, the rapid growth in risk contracting, reduced inpatient utilization, and costs rising faster than revenues, it is critical that all healthcare organizations review their internal control programs and remedy any deficiencies. In some cases, organizations have not challenged the adequacy or the effectiveness of their internal control systems in several years. They may find that their current systems no longer suffice.[10]

Financial vs. Operational Auditing

The financial audit tests the integrity of the healthcare organization's accounting and statistical records. Through a planned process that includes a variety of sampling, verification, and testing techniques, the internal and/or the external auditor can evaluate the records' creditability. With the auditor's assurance of this creditability, management can make decisions with the confidence that the database it uses is sound.

While the financial audit concerns itself primarily with financial data, the operational audit concentrates on systems in an effort to spot weaknesses. As a representative of management, the operational auditor investigates activities to determine whether departments have a clear understanding of organizational and departmental objectives. This audit is also intended to verify whether departments

- obtain competitive bids from suppliers,
- match packing slips against purchase orders and suppliers' invoices,
- prenumber all forms and checks,
- maintain individual records of all capital assets,
- separate custodial and record-keeping responsibilities,
- require dual signatures on checks, and
- reconcile general and subsidiary ledgers.[11]

The operational audit ensures the effectiveness of the healthcare organization's operational systems, as well as their conformity to management goals and objectives.

External vs. Internal Auditing

Accuracy is the primary concern of both the external auditor and the internal auditor. The internal auditor conducts ongoing testing and evaluation of systems, procedures, and records; the external auditor provides the public and the governing board with an annual statement of opinion on the validity of the fiscal-year statements. In addition, the external independent public auditor

- appraises internal control systems and

- compares the healthcare organization's effectiveness and operations with those of similar institutions.

One of the most valuable services the external auditor performs for the healthcare organization is the management letter, which outlines any major weaknesses discovered during the audit process. Generally, the external audit and the internal audit processes are integrated into a set of complementary procedures. These procedures are effective, continuous devices for testing the accuracy of the healthcare organization's records and systems at reasonable cost and with minimal duplication of effort.

All accounting and operating systems and subsystems have three basic control points:

1. entry,

2. processing, and

3. exit.

The fundamental principle of internal control is the separation or segregation of duties, so no individual has complete control over all three basic control points.

Accounting information requires that precontrolled methods be used to ensure that every transaction is properly recorded. Prenumbered cash receipts and prenumbered checks are the simplest examples of such methods. They are intended to make certain that all transactions are recorded and in proper order.[12]

An example of entry-point control is the midnight census. Most healthcare facilities have a fixed bed capacity that is not normally exceeded. Therefore, the number of in-house patients and the revenue they represent, for accounting purposes, cannot be greater than the number recorded in the census report. To put it another way, a financial record must be established and revenue recorded for every patient listed on the census report.

The vital point to remember about entry-point control is that all entry-point data must be documented through cash register tapes, admitting logs, and so forth. These data comprise evidence for internal and external audits.

Central to processing-point control is monitoring the recording and summarizing of accounting transactions to make sure they are complete and in balance. For example, the general accounting department should review the accounts receivable general ledger account and ensure that in the aggregate all transactions have been accounted for properly. General accounting also determines that the general ledger account balance equals the subsidiary account balance.[13]

Exit-point control requires extensive review of accounting transaction results to determine whether they have been appropriately documented. For example, a patient's medical record should contain the following:

- doctor's request for healthcare services

- nurse's report of rendering services

- medical reports of rendering ancillary department services

Each of these modes of service should be recorded and charged to the patient's financial record as they are performed.

Other examples of exit-point control are financial ratios and predetermined performance standards, such as number of days of average daily revenue uncollected.

As mentioned earlier, it is essential that no individual controls all control points in any healthcare system. If one person controls every point, the possibility of fraud and abuse is increased. Although detecting fraud and abuse is not the chief intent of external or internal auditing, the audit process may uncover one or the other.

Patient Financial Services Audit Instrument

Through the use of an audit survey instrument, the internal auditor can informally examine any department or function in the healthcare organization. The audit instrument should be relatively consistent from one audit period to another. On the other hand, it should also be flexible enough to adjust for the elimination of obsolete functions or systems or for the addition of new ones. In addition, the audit instrument should serve as a reference point from one audit to another so that improvements or weaknesses within the audited area can be tracked.

Exhibit 12–1 shows an audit instrument for the patient financial services department that can be modified for any healthcare facility. Its design is such that any "no" answer signals the need for further investigation and possible corrective action by management. Answering the questions in this audit instrument, and exception report, marks the beginning of the internal audit process. The internal auditor must verify by observation and testing that the policies, systems, and procedures established by management are, in fact, carried out. After completing the audit survey, the internal auditor is responsible for summarizing the findings in a management letter that covers at least the following areas:

- audit approach or methodology used

- findings, including major strengths and weaknesses

- areas in which corrective measures need to be taken

- recommendations for improvement

- conclusion

Once the management report has been completed, with appropriate supporting documentation and work papers, the internal auditor should discuss the report with appropriate members of the healthcare organization's management team. Ideally, the auditor's findings and recommendations should be discussed in advance with the persons responsible for the trouble areas and who might be directly affected by the auditor's recommendations. In this way, Seawell advises, employees may come to view internal auditing as a helpful, constructive function rather than a force to be distrusted and feared. Just as important, the fact that the internal audit function is being taken seriously and supported by top management personnel should be clearly evident to the healthcare organization's employees, he concludes.[14]

Billing Audits

Billing audits, either concurrent or retrospective, compare charge data from a healthcare provider's bill with the provider's corresponding health record of a patient's medical/clinical occurrence. The purpose of these audits is to determine whether all medical and health services recorded on the patient's bill agree with the patient's health record. These audits are generally performed to determine, but are not limited to, the following:

- the necessity to bill or rebill a payer for charges that were not originally included on the healthcare provider's initial bill

- the necessity to make corrections for items or services that were not correctly and appropriately documented

- the necessity to either routinely or spontaneously verify the billing operating system for accuracy and documentation to improve the system

Billing audits generally require documentation from or review of the patient's health record and similar clinical records, as well as the patient's corresponding financial bill for services. One of the most helpful auditing tools for determining the efficiency of a healthcare provider's billing system is to flowchart the process as it is being conducted and compare with a flowchart designated by the healthcare provider's policies, systems, and procedures manual. The policies and procedures manual should incorporate all state and federal regulations concerning patient record use and disclosures to protect the confidentiality of the patient's health and financial records at all times.

EXHIBIT 12–1

Patient Financial Services Audit Instrument Form

Memorial Medical Center
Anytown, U.S.A.

PATIENT FINANCIAL SERVICES DEPARTMENT
AUDIT INSTRUMENT

For the Period Ending _____ 19____

Audited by _____   Date _____ 19____

YES	NO		ORGANIZATION
_____	_____	1.	Does the department have an organizational chart?
_____	_____	2.	Does each employee have a job description? If yes, when were the job descriptions last reviewed and updated?
_____	_____	3.	Does each position have established performance standards? If yes, when were the performance standards last reviewed and updated?
_____	_____	4.	Is each employee classified in a labor grade, and are his/her wages in line with those of similar positions in the rest of the healthcare organization? If yes, when were the labor grades last reviewed and updated?
_____	_____	5.	Does the department monitor employee turnover rates for each position? If yes, what is the employee turnover rate for each position?

Position	*Annual Turnover Rate*
_____	_____
_____	_____
_____	_____
_____	_____

YES	NO		
_____	_____	6.	Are employee production units well defined and capable of being audited? If yes, describe how they are defined and audited:
_____	_____	7.	Does the department conduct in-service education programs? If yes, describe them:
_____	_____	8.	Does the patient financial services manager report to the chief financial officer? If no, to whom does he/she report:

EXHIBIT 12–1 *continued*

YES	NO		ACCOUNTING CONTROL
_____	_____	1.	Are all patient accounts receivable subsidiary records reconciled at least monthly?
_____	_____	2a.	Are all patient accounts receivable records aged at least monthly?
_____	_____	2b.	Are they aged by paying agent?
_____	_____	3.	Are monthly statements mailed to *all* debtors? If no, why not?

_____

_____

4. Are patient accounts that are written off because of

_____	_____	a.	bad debts
_____	_____	b.	courtesy discounts
_____	_____	c.	refunds
_____	_____	d.	other adjustments

authorized by appropriate individuals before posting? If yes, who authorizes

1. bad debts? _____

2. courtesy discounts? _____

3. refunds? _____

4. other adjustments? (Describe these adjustments)

_____

_____

_____	_____	5.	Are bad debts adequately monitored after they have been written off? If yes, describe the monitoring process:

_____

_____

_____	_____	6.	Are all credits to expense recorded and processed through accounts receivable?
_____	_____	a.	sales to employees
_____	_____	b.	medical record transcriptions
_____	_____	c.	sale of obsolete equipment
_____	_____	d.	sale of scrap and waste
_____	_____	7.	Are patient accounts receivable confirmed by either the internal or external auditor directly and routinely?
_____	_____	8.	Are disputed patient accounts receivable reviewed by someone other than an accounts receivable clerk? If yes, who reviews disputed accounts? _____

BUDGETS AND REPORTS

1. Does the department have

_____	_____	a.	a one-year operating budget?
_____	_____	b.	a three-year capital expenditure plan?
_____	_____	2.	Are the department's section heads and supervisors involved in the development of these budgets?
_____	_____	3.	Does the patient financial services manager assist in the development of the organization's cash flow forecast?
_____	_____	4.	Is actual performance compared with the department's budgets at least monthly?

EXHIBIT 12–1 *continued*

YES	NO	
		5. Are the following financial statements prepared and reviewed by appropriate members of management every month?
_____	_____	a. statement of condition
_____	_____	b. statement of operations
_____	_____	c. statement of financial changes
_____	_____	d. cash flow statement

COLLECTION ACCOUNTS

YES	NO	
_____	_____	1. Are aged trial balances of agency accounts reviewed monthly?
_____	_____	2. Does the healthcare organization use more than one collection agent?
_____	_____	3. Does the healthcare organization have a written agreement that the agent will return accounts with no payments in six months to the facility?
_____	_____	4. Are the net agent collection costs computed at least quarterly and compared by agent?

ADMITTING

YES	NO	
		1. Does the healthcare organization require prepayment for
_____	_____	a. inpatient; amount $ _____ ?
_____	_____	b. outpatient; amount $ _____ ?
_____	_____	c. emergency; amount $ _____ ?
		2. Does the healthcare organization have separate admitting offices for
_____	_____	a. inpatient?
_____	_____	b. outpatient?
_____	_____	c.. emergency?
		3. Do admitting office personnel report directly to the patient financial services manager
_____	_____	a. inpatient?
_____	_____	b. outpatient?
_____	_____	c. emergency?
_____	_____	4. Does the healthcare organization use patient identification and/or courtesy cards?

MAIL RECEIPTS

YES	NO	
_____	_____	1. Are *all* mail receipts opened and listed by someone outside of the patient financial services department? If so, who performs these functions? _____
		2. Are copies of the listed mail receipts distributed to the following persons:
_____	_____	a. chief executive officer?
_____	_____	b. chief financial officer?
_____	_____	c. patient financial services manager?
_____	_____	d. cashier?
_____	_____	3. Are checks immediately stamped "for deposit only"?
_____	_____	4. Does the healthcare organization use a bank lockbox for processing mail receipts?

EXHIBIT 12–1 *continued*

YES	NO	

SYSTEMS AND PROCEDURES

_____ _____ 1. Does the department have a manual of standard operating procedures? If yes, when was it last reviewed and updated? _____

_____ _____ 2. Does the department have flowcharts of all its major systems and subsystems?

_____ _____ 3. Are completed sample copies of all forms used included in the standard operating procedures manual?

_____ _____ 4. Does the department have a forms control system?

BILLING AND COLLECTION

1. Does the healthcare organization have a written billing and collection policy that includes

_____ _____ a. exact billing schedules?

_____ _____ b. criteria for a delinquent account?

_____ _____ c. authorized collection actions and procedures?

2. Does the healthcare organization use authorized

_____ _____ a. promissory notes?

_____ _____ b. credit cards?

_____ _____ c. installment contracts?

_____ _____ 3. Are *all* unpaid patient accounts receivable routinely, regularly, and independently mailed to debtors?

PATIENT CHARGES

_____ _____ 1. Does the department have a published list of all charges set by the healthcare organization?

_____ _____ 2. Are department personnel knowledgeable enough to explain to patients how the healthcare organization establishes its charges?

_____ _____ 3. Are patient charges checked against patient medical records to assure that *no* charges are lost?

_____ _____ 4. Is the rates structure designed to cover all the healthcare organization's financial requirements, including bad debts, allowances, capital, growth, and profit?

_____ _____ 5. Are patient charges recorded on a multicharge card to ensure control distribution?

_____ _____ 6. Are all patient charges recorded on separate patient account subsidiary ledger files?

_____ _____ 7. Are patient charges posted by an individual who does not generate the charges?

_____ _____ 8. Are patient charges posted by an individual who does not have responsibility of cash receipts?

CASH PROCESSING

_____ _____ 1. Are *all* cash receipts deposited on the day they are received?

_____ _____ 2. Are unidentified cash receipts credited to a special account and immediately deposited?

_____ _____ 3. Does the healthcare organization have a centralized cashiering system?

_____ _____ 4. Does *each* cashier have a separate cash box and imprest fund?

_____ _____ 5. Are the cashier's work areas isolated from the hospital personnel?

_____ _____ 6. Do the cashier areas have a "silent alarm" system?

EXHIBIT 12–1 *continued*

YES	NO	
_____	_____	7. Does the healthcare organization use a fireproof safe to store undeposited cash and valuables?
_____	_____	8. Are cash receipts recorded by someone other than the individual who receives the cash?

MAIL RETURNS

YES	NO	
_____	_____	1. Is there an established, written procedure for handling mail returns?
_____	_____	2. Have corrective measures been taken to reduce the number of mail returns? If yes, describe these measures:

_____

_____

_____

INSUFFICIENT FUNDS

YES	NO	
_____	_____	1. Does the healthcare organization have a written policy for handling patient checks that have been returned as "insufficient funds" checks? Describe the policy:

_____

_____

_____

IN-HOUSE ACCOUNTS

YES	NO	
_____	_____	1. Do *all* inpatients receive a weekly statement showing the amount they owe while they are still in the healthcare facility? If yes, describe the method used to collect this amount:

_____

_____

_____

YES	NO	
_____	_____	2. Do representatives of the department visit patients in the healthcare facility to firm up patient payment agreements?
_____	_____	3. Does the department use a long-story (30 days or more) report?
_____	_____	4. Are third-party guarantors billed on an interim basis for accounts that have been classified as "long stays"?

PETTY CASH

YES	NO	
_____	_____	1. Does the department use an imprest petty cash fund? If yes, what is the amount? $_____
_____	_____	2. Is only *one* person responsible for the petty cash fund?
_____	_____	3. Does the healthcare organization conduct "spot audits" of the petty cash fund? If yes, how frequently? _____
_____	_____	4. Are all petty cash fund disbursements supported by authorized documents and receipts?
_____	_____	5. Are *all* cashiers and other personnel responsible for handling cash and valuables bonded?

PATIENT REFUNDS

YES	NO	
_____	_____	1. Are all patient refunds drawn from a separate imprest bank account?
_____	_____	2. Is each patient refund authorized by an appropriately designated individual? If yes, who authorizes them?

_____

EXHIBIT 12–1 *continued*

YES	NO	
————	————	3. Are the patient refunds documented with a photocopy of the original supporting patient financial statement?
————	————	4. Is the refund bank account reconciled by someone other than the individual who issues or signs checks?

MANAGED-CARE CONTRACTS

YES	NO	
————	————	1. Is the patient financial services manager involved in the managed-care contract negotiations?
————	————	2. Is a cost/cash flow analysis performed on *each* contract at least once a month?
————	————	3. Does the managed-care account executive report every month directly with the patient financial services manager concerning the cost/cash flow analysis of each contract?
————	————	4. Is each managed-care contract reconciled at least once a month?
————	————	5. Is each managed-care contract's incurred-but-not-reported (IBNR) accounts reconciled every month?

MEDICARE AND OTHER THIRD-PARTY PAYERS

YES	NO	
————	————	1. Has the cost of *each* diagnosis-related group (DRG) been established? If so, when was this computation last made? _____
————	————	2. Is there a monthly comparison of DRG cost/cash flow analysis made for *each* DRG?
		3. Is there a similar cost/cash flow analysis made for
————	————	a. Medicaid
————	————	b. Blue Cross
————	————	c. Blue Shield
————	————	d. Others (name) _____

ACCOUNTS RECEIVABLE

YES	NO	
————	————	1. Do admission or registration procedures ensure that complete and accurate accounts receivable and collection information is gathered, including such documents as signed authorization for admission, patient or guarantor credit and billing information, and/or insurance coverage and assignment?
————	————	2. Do procedures provide reasonable assurance that services rendered to patient are medically necessary?
————	————	3. Is a complete medical record prepared, including the physician's discharge summary and the physician's statement attesting to the description of the principal diagnosis and other clinical information?
————	————	4. Are there procedures to ensure that amounts due from third-party payers for individual accounts are properly supported?
————	————	5. Do procedures exist that ensure the proper recording of cash receipts?
————	————	6. Do procedures exist that ensure charity care balances are identified and excluded from gross receivables?
————	————	7. Are numeric or other controls over individual patient accounts maintained?
————	————	8. Are there procedures that ensure that detailed accounts receivable records are routinely compared with general ledger control accounts and third-party payers' logs?

EXHIBIT 12–1 *continued*

YES	NO	
____	____	9. Are there procedures that require any differences identified in question number 8 to be investigated and reconciled, and, if necessary, adjustments of errors are made promptly?
____	____	10. Are allowances for uncollectibles and contractual and other adjustments periodically reviewed by management to ensure that receivables are reported at estimated net realizable value?
____	____	11. Are writeoffs and allowances for uncollectibles identified and approved in accordance with the organization's established policy?
____	____	12. Are medical records information results in proper DRG assignments for the Medicare prospective payment system (PPS) and/or similar state to other third-party payment systems?
____	____	13. Are medical records personnel properly trained and supervised to provide for the appropriate DRG coding?
____	____	14. Are procedures in place that ensure prompt coding of Medicare and other similar patient data?
____	____	15. Are medical records (primarily for Medicare patients) subject to a second independent coding review?

AMBULATORY ACCOUNTS RECEIVABLE

YES	NO	
____	____	1. Is there a procedure for the accumulation of charges into one (unit) patient account receivable for each patient's multiple ambulatory visits?
____	____	2. Are multiple-ambulatory-visit accounts receivable routinely mailed at least once a month?

3. If the patient unit account system is not used, explain how a chronic patient's multiple accounts are tracked and billed.

_____

_____

_____

4. If the patient unit account system is not used, explain how payments on the account(s) are credited. _____

_____

_____

_____

5. Explain how multiple accounts receivable are aged. _____

_____

_____

_____

6. Explain the admitting system used for recurring admissions. _____

_____

_____

_____

7. Explain the process used to verify insurance coverage for recurring admissions. _____

_____

_____

EXHIBIT 12–1 *continued*

YES	NO		ESTIMATED THIRD-PARTY SETTLEMENTS
_____	_____	1.	Are there procedures that ensure that estimated third-party settlements are determined in accordance with the reimbursements and rate-setting methodologies applicable to the organization?
_____	_____	2.	Are there procedures that ensure that estimated third-party settlements are accurately calculated and reported?
_____	_____	3.	Are interfund borrowings approved by the governing board, and are they periodically evaluated for collectibility?

The *National Health Care Billing Audit Guidelines* identify the following as necessary qualifications or knowledge for all persons performing billing audits as well as for those persons functioning as provider audit coordinators:

- format and content of health record as well as other forms of medical/clinical documentation

- generally accepted auditing principles and practices as they may apply to billing audits

- coding, including ICD-9-CM, CPT, HCPCS, and medical terminology

- billing claims forms, including the UB-93 and the HCFA 1500, and charging and billing procedures

- all state and federal regulations concerning the use, disclosure, and confidentiality of all patient records

- specific critical-care units, specialty areas, and/or ancillary units involved in a particular audit[15]

Finally, the purpose of the provider's health record is to document its patients' diagnoses, treatments, and outcomes. The provider's corresponding patient bills translate these services into charges so that the facility may recover expenses. The patient's health records are generally viewed as the documentation criteria for verifying charges made for services rendered. If the audit uncovers any irregularity, it is the auditor's responsibility to determine the reasons for the inconsistency and make recommendations to management for systems improvement.

Flowcharting

From the information secured by observation and questionnaires, the internal auditor can develop flowcharts of internal control procedures.[16] Flowcharting is one of the most useful techniques for documenting or analyzing systems or procedures because it illustrates a complete system. According to Seawell, flowcharting an actual situation is an effective method for

- determining how a particular system actually works,

- evaluating the effectiveness of the existing internal control procedures,

- developing more effective procedures, and

- instructing employees of their individual duties in relation to the total system.

External auditors, he adds, also make extensive use of flowcharts to obtain a comprehensive picture of a client's internal control program.[17]

We can use the following narrative description of the requisition and processing of a three-piece patient charge card to illustrate how flowcharting simplifies the description.

Case Study

The attending physician requisitions a specific pharmaceutical in the patient's medical chart. The attending charge nurse reads the doctor's order and requisitions the drugs via the use of a three-piece pharmacy charge requisition card. The charge card is carried by messenger to the pharmacy. The pharmacist fills the order, prices the cards, and sends the requested drug to the nursing station via messenger. The messenger also returns one portion of the charge card to the nursing station, while the pharmacist keeps one copy and sends a hard copy to the data processing department via messenger. The nurse administers the drug to the patient and confirms this in the nurse's notes section of the patient's medical chart. The data processing department posts the charge for the drug on the patient's financial record. After discharge, the patient financial services department receives copies of all charges and bills the patient accordingly. The account is stored in the patient accounts receivable file.

Figure 12–1 shows symbols that are used in flowcharting; the flowchart of the aforementioned procedure is illustrated in figure 12–2. This is an example of one of the many methods of flowcharting. Two others are the Program Evaluation and Review Technique (PERT) and the Gantt method, which generally are used to plan projects containing many interrelated tasks that lead to the project's completion if performed in a given sequence. PERT, also referred to as the Critical Path Method (CPM), is useful in planning and scheduling the sequence of individual tasks and in reviewing the project as a whole.[18]

Although PERT charting uses lines to indicate the work flow, the lines' length in no way represents the length of time required to perform interdependent tasks. As a result, the average user has difficulty visualizing time

FIGURE 12–1
Symbols Used in Flowcharting

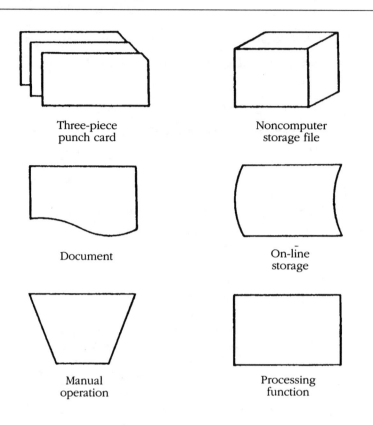

Three-piece
punch card

Noncomputer
storage file

Document

On-line
storage

Manual
operation

Processing
function

relationships in a PERT network diagram. On the other hand, the Gantt chart, named after the person who conceived the idea of plotting tasks instead of time, shows how long a task takes, its earliest starting time (EST), and its latest starting time (LST).[19] Another key difference between PERT and Gantt charting is that PERT charting requires the planner to start at the end of the project and work back to the first task, while Gantt charting requires the planner to start with the first task and identify each task in sequence until the final task is identified. To illustrate the use of these two flowcharting methods, assume that the patient financial services manager wants to implement a healthcare courtesy card system to facilitate patient admission and cash collection.

Project: Implement a healthcare patient courtesy card system for all inpatients and outpatients of Memorial Medical Center, Anytown, U.S.A.

FIGURE 12–2
Flowchart of Patient Charge System

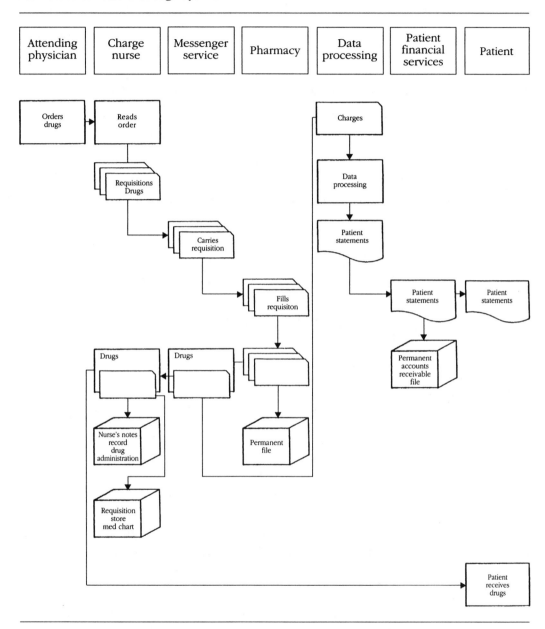

| Attending physician | Charge nurse | Messenger service | Pharmacy | Data processing | Patient financial services | Patient |

Tasks: The following tasks have been identified as primary components necessary for completion of the project. (*Note:* The project being illustrated would include more required tasks than are cited in the example, but the number of tasks in the illustrated case has been condensed for ease of understanding.)

1. Locate space for system.
2. Recruit and hire supervisor.
3. Select and order equipment.
4. Prepare site.
5. Install equipment.
6. Recruit and hire support personnel.
7. Train personnel.
8. Develop and conduct publicity campaign.
9. Test system.

Steps:

1. Identify key words in each task to serve as task indicators in charting (see table 12–1).

2. Estimate how much time will be required to complete each task. (*Note:* Time can be measured in hours, days, weeks, or months, but time estimates should be consistent throughout the flowcharting process.)

3. Identify which tasks must be completed (predecessor tasks) before each task can begin.

4. Start the network at the end of the project by identifying the last event as the end (see figure 12–3).

5. Plot the predecessor tasks to the final tasks as follows:

Install	5		
Train	7	9	End
Publicity	8		

6. Plot other tasks, as illustrated in figure 12–3.

7. To determine the maximum time required to complete the project, locate the start by dividing the circle in half and placing a zero in the left half, as illustrated in figure 12–4.

START	=	0

8. Beginning with the Start circle, add the time required to complete Task 1, and place this number in the left half of the circle for Task 1, as follows:

1	=	1
SPACE	Start:	0 weeks
	Space:	1 week
	Total:	1 week

Continue toward the End circle in this manner, adding the number of weeks required for each task. For example:

3	=	5
EQUIPMENT	Space:	1 week
	Equipment:	4 weeks
	Total:	5 weeks

TABLE 12–1
PERT Network of Tasks for Implementation of Patient Courtesy Card System

Memorial Medical Center
Anytown, U.S.A.

Task		Completion Time	
Number	*Description*	*(Weeks)*	*Predecessor Tasks*
1	Space	1	—
2	Supervisor	4	—
3	Equipment	4	1
4	Preparation	4	3
5	Install	1	4
6	Personnel	4	2
7	Train	2	6
8	Publicity	6	—
9	Final	2	5, 7, 8

FIGURE 12–3
PERT Network for Implementation of Patient Courtesy Card System

Memorial Medical Center
Anytown, U.S.A.

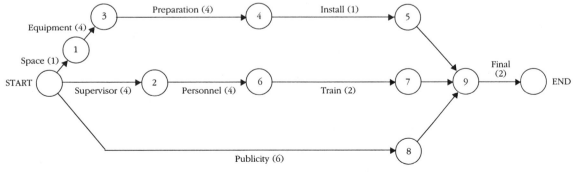

FIGURE 12–4

PERT Network for Earliest Starting Times for Patient Courtesy Card System

Memorial Medical Center
Anytown, U.S.A.

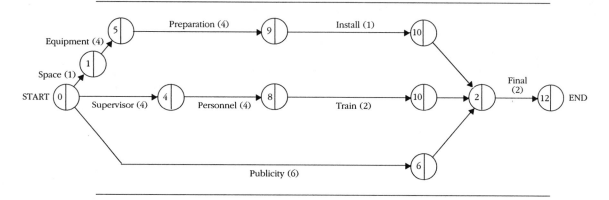

4	=	9
PREPARATION	Space:	1 week
	Equipment	4 weeks
	Preparation:	4 weeks
	Total:	9 weeks

5	=	10
INSTALL	Space:	1 week
	Equipment:	4 weeks
	Preparation:	4 weeks
	Install:	1 week
	Total:	10 weeks

Accordingly, the following time schedules are developed for the Personnel series of tasks:

Task Number	Description	Time Required	Accumulated Time
2	Hire supervisor	4 weeks	4 weeks
6	Recruit personnel	4 weeks	8 weeks
7	Train personnel	2 weeks	10 weeks

Publicity requires six weeks, indicated in the following manner:

8   =   6
PUBLICITY

The final testing task requires two weeks; thus, at the end, total project time is accumulated as follows:

END   =   12

> Maximum weeks for predecessors is 10 weeks plus 2 weeks, totaling 12 weeks for project.

Figure 12–4 illustrates the EST and shows that 12 weeks is the minimum amount of time for completion of the project. If the LST for the end is 12 weeks, the final task, Number 9, must be completed in 10 weeks because completing the final task requires 2 weeks. As shown in figure 12–5, the EST is placed in the left half of each circle; the LST is placed in the right half of each circle.

The slack time for each task is computed by subtracting the LST from the EST. The critical path is the sequence of tasks with no slack time. An excellent example is the publicity task:

Latest starting time: 4 weeks
Earliest starting time: 0 weeks
Slack time: 4 weeks

There are two critical paths in our example:

Number	Task Description	Weeks	Number	Task Description	Weeks
1	Space	1	2	Supervisor	4
3	Equipment	4	6	Personnel	4
4	Preparation	4	7	Train	2
5	Install	1			
	Total weeks	10		Total Weeks	10

Although the PERT flowcharting system has proven to be very effective for professional project planners, it can be confusing and difficult to understand for many laypersons. Its primary flaw lies in the fact that lines in a PERT chart do not represent the length of time required to complete a given task. Consequently, it is very difficult to visualize the relationship of times required to perform the series of tasks that make up the total project.

FIGURE 12–5

PERT Network for Latest Starting Times for Patient Courtesy Card System

Memorial Medical Center
Anytown, U.S.A.

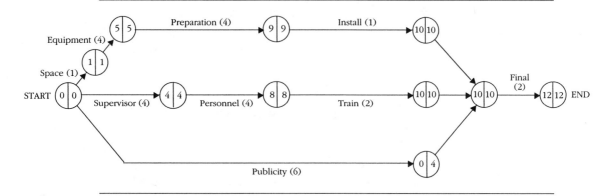

The Gantt chart, on the other hand, displays the tasks that make up a project in a sequential order and shows the amount of time required to perform each task. In a Gantt chart, the length of the time lines corresponds to the amount of time required to complete each task. Figure 12–6 illustrates the way in which a Gantt chart shows these required times.

A Gantt chart is constructed in terms of relevant time frames such as hours, days, weeks, months, or years. In figure 12–6, weeks have been selected as the relevant time frame for the project. Note that tasks have been assigned numbers and briefly described. The numbering system used in a Gantt chart should be designed to facilitate the identification of subtasks. For example:

    1.0 Locate space for system.
        1.1 Determine area required.
        1.2 Determine utilities required.
        1.3 Determine most desirable location.
        1.4 Identify alternative sites.
        1.5 Review alternatives.
        1.6 Select site.
    2.0 Recruit and hire supervisor.

Each task, and its subtasks, is listed in the order in which it is most likely to be implemented. On a bar graph, the time required for each task is blocked in, and the position of the block on the chart shows the starting and ending time for the task. After all tasks and subtasks have been listed and plotted on the chart, a solid block triangle is placed on the graph to indicate the project's completion point. If project planners want interim checkpoints at specific

FIGURE 12–6

Gantt Chart for Implementation of Patient Courtesy Card System

Memorial Medical Center
Anytown, U.S.A.

WEEKS

TASK		

Number	Description	

Weeks: 1 2 3 4 5 6 7 8 9 10 11 12 13 14

Number	Description
1.0	Locate space for system
2.0	Recruit and hire supervisor
3.0	Select and order equipment
4.0	Prepare site
5.0	Install equipment
6.0	Recruit and hire support personnel
7.0	Train personnel
8.0	Develop and conduct publicity campaign
9.0	Test system
10.0	Implement

times, they put an open or white triangle at the places on the graph where checkpoints will occur.

This discussion of flowcharting has acquainted the patient financial services managers with the common techniques used in analyzing existing control systems and in designing or revising systems. Mastering flowcharting techniques can help the managers improve the internal control of patient accounts receivable.

Managing Accounts Receivable

Because a healthcare facility is a community resource—a facility cannot refuse care to a patient unable to pay in full immediately upon discharge—and because it is virtually impossible to deal with third-party payers on a cash-and-carry basis, healthcare organizations are by necessity in the credit business. Even the well-managed facility typically holds about 25 percent of its total assets and 75 percent of its current assets in accounts receivable.[20]

Moreover, a facility's extension of credit only results in additional operating costs, whereas a commercial firm can use the availability of credit as a mechanism for increasing sales and profits.[21]

The patient financial services department's primary goal, then, is to maintain the working capital necessary to finance the healthcare organization's accounts receivable at a realistic minimum. Accordingly, effective management of patient accounts receivable is the single most important factor in the organization's financial success.

Payer Classifications

Generally, healthcare patients fall under one of two major categories in terms of who pays for their care:

1. self-paying

2. third party

The self-paying patients either have no insurance coverage, are totally responsible for paying their healthcare bill, or must pay the balance of the cost of their care after the third party has paid its share. A third-party payer can be an individual, an agency, an insurance company, or some type of prepaid plan that is obligated to pay all or part of a patient's healthcare bill. Payment systems used by third-party payers are usually based on the hospital's costs, charges, or a combination of the two. Some Blue Cross plans and most commercial insurance companies pay the healthcare organization either its full charges or a percentage of full charges, and the patient is responsible for the balance. Other Blue Cross plans, Medicare, and Medicaid pay the hospital according to individualized formulas based on a healthcare organization's costs, "reasonable costs," or "allowable costs." There is also frequently either a deductible and/or coinsurance portion that the patient must pay. Moreover, there is usually a contractual allowance (the difference between the published charge and net cash received) for which the healthcare organization has no recourse to the patient. Thus, the healthcare organization must absorb the difference.

Through proper admitting and discharge procedures, patient financial services managers can maximize cash inflow and minimize contractual allowances. Management's objective revolves around controlling costs by reducing the time and length of the accounts receivable cycle, which consists of four major phases:

1. The patient makes contact with the healthcare organization to deliver a product and/or service.

2. The organization delivers the requested product and/or service.

3. The organization sends a bill to the patient or third-party payer.

4. The organization receives the payment and deposits it.

As Hy points out, the longer it takes the organization to complete this cycle, the larger the amount of its cash tied up in accounts receivable; and the larger the amount of cash tied up, the higher the carrying, opportunity, collection, and delinquent and default costs.[22]

Payment Systems

Basically, there are two payment systems in the healthcare industry: prospective and retrospective. Under prospective payment, the healthcare organization and the purchaser of services determine in advance the amount the organization will charge the purchaser for a specified period of time. A substantial number of Blue Cross plans and state agencies pay healthcare organizations under prospective payment systems. Another variation of prospective reimbursement is capitation funding, whereby the organization agrees to deliver the needed products and/or services for a fixed per-capita amount per period. Healthcare maintenance organizations operate under such funding.[23]

Until 1972, when the Social Security Amendments in Public Law 92–603 were enacted, the Medicare/Medicaid program's virtually universal retrospective payment systems, that is, reimbursement, represented what amounted to a blank check for healthcare providers. The original retrospective reimbursement system allowed healthcare providers to spend money to provide services for third-party subscribers. After the fiscal year ended and the provider audited these expenditures, it computed the total costs for each third party. If the healthcare organization had spent more than it had been paid by the third party in the interim, the third party gave the organization additional money. If final costs were less than these interim payments, the organization returned the difference to the third party.

Under this system, many healthcare organizations were, in effect, being paid by the third party for underutilization. Providers paid very little attention to the relationship of their charges and their costs. By introducing payment based on the lesser of charge or costs, Public Law 92–603 changed that. The payment of the lesser of costs or charges requires a healthcare organization to keep its total charges above the third party's share of reimbursable costs. Otherwise, it will be paid only charges.

Segmentation of Patient Accounts Receivable

Market segmentation, a common technique of market analysis, identifies relevant characteristics of a population to be served and divides them into groups and subgroups. Each group's demands and needs are identified, and advertising and marketing campaigns that appeal to those specific needs are designed. Patient financial services managers can apply this technique to the management of patient accounts receivable through the use of a matrix or grid. This procedure will enable managers to maximize cash inflow and minimize contractual allowances.

The first step in segmenting patient accounts receivable is to divide the total account file into a minimum of six major classifications:

1. unbilled in-house accounts

2. unbilled discharged inpatient accounts

3. unbilled outpatient accounts

4. billed in-house accounts

5. billed discharged inpatient accounts

6. billed outpatient accounts

The account file should also be divided according to primary or major third-party paying agent:

- self-paying

- Medicare

- Medicaid

- Blue Cross

- commercial insurance

- worker's compensation

- managed care

If one third party, a specific commercial insurance carrier, for example, accounts for a significant portion of the healthcare organization's accounts, a separate classification should be created for that third party or managed-care contract.

The classifications can then be arranged on a matrix similar to the one illustrated in exhibit 12–2. Note that the matrix shows both the dollar amount and the percentage represented by each segment of the patient accounts receivable. This facilitates trend analysis and other studies of payment patterns. Because each segment has unique billing and payment characteristics, the segmentation matrix helps patient financial services managers isolate potential trouble spots and take corrective action.

The number of days of revenue uncollected is a key indicator in the analysis of each accounts receivable segment because each paying agent is likely to have a different healthcare service utilization profile.

In summary, the segmentation matrix is another tool patient financial services managers can use to expedite the collection of cash. This technique, along with improvements that suit the needs of the individual healthcare organization, should be incorporated into every healthcare organization's management information system. Patient financial services managers must overcome any resistance to building the technique into their organization's

EXHIBIT 12–2

Segmentation Matrix of Patient Accounts Receivable

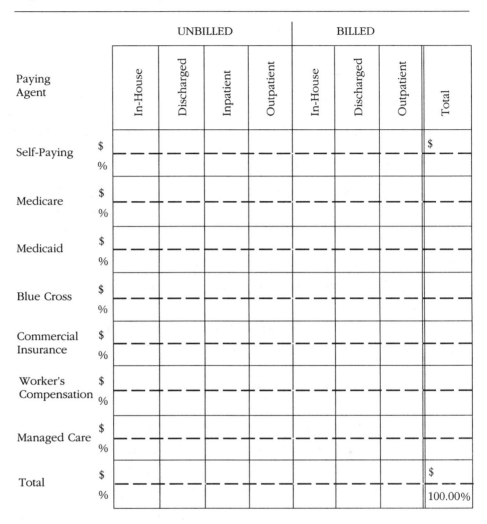

Paying Agent	UNBILLED				BILLED			
	In-House	Discharged	Inpatient	Outpatient	In-House	Discharged	Outpatient	Total
Self-Paying $ %								$
Medicare $ %								
Medicaid $ %								
Blue Cross $ %								
Commercial Insurance $ %								
Worker's Compensation $ %								
Managed Care $ %								
Total $ %								$ 100.00%

management information system by steadfastly maintaining that data processing is limited only by the imagination and ability of its designers and users. Patient financial services managers cannot perform effectively without adequate, accurate, and timely information, and segmentation analysis is an important part of that information. In the end, no one in the healthcare organization gets paid if cash is not brought in; cash is the healthcare organization's lifeblood.

Monitoring Bad Debts and Accounts Out for Collection

Whether the healthcare organization has an in-house or outside collection agency, or uses both, appropriate devices for monitoring their relative effectiveness and cost/benefit must be developed. The monitoring process should also serve as an internal audit system that protects the healthcare organization from improper handling of accounts placed for collection.

Here are ten guidelines that are essential for monitoring accounts referred to collection agencies:

1. Have a written, board-approved policy for identifying and processing accounts classified as bad debts and uncollectibles.

2. Have at least two individuals above the patient financial services manager—with one of them preferably being a board member—responsible for reviewing and approving all referrals of accounts to collection agents and all identification of accounts as uncollectible.

3. Have at least two bonded collection agents handle bad debt accounts, and have still another agent handle all accounts returned as uncollectible. (This measure is a final test of an account's actual uncollectibility.)

4. Have a written agreement with every collection agent used that stipulates that all accounts without payment activity within six months are to be returned to the healthcare organization.

5. Require the collection agent to obtain the healthcare organization's approval in writing for any compromise settlements.

6. Require that the healthcare organization's internal or external auditors perform interim audits of the accounts referred to each collection agent.

7. Require each collection agent to submit a monthly aged trial balance and progress reports on all accounts handled.

8. Require the agent to have the healthcare organization's written approval before undertaking litigation.

9. Analyze and compare the collection effectiveness and net cost of each agent at least semiannually.

10. Establish a balance sheet reserve account for all accounts referred to collection agents. The method for establishing such an account follows.

All patient accounts receivable should be reviewed monthly to determine their collectibility. Any account, regardless of age or length of time since discharge, considered to be a collection problem by the patient financial services manager should be identified and written off as a bad debt. The healthcare organization's accounting department will use the following compound journal entry to record accounts identified as bad debts and approved for collection.

Assume that Memorial Medical Center's bad debt accounts total $20,000:

Bad Debt Expense $20,000
Agency Accounts Receivable $20,000
    Reserve for Bad Debts $20,000
    Active Accounts Receivable $20,000

The debit entries record the amount to be written off as a bad debt expense in the statement of operations and establish an asset account in the statement of condition. The credit entries establish a reserve account to totally offset the agency accounts receivable asset account and remove the accounts from the active accounts receivable in the statement of condition.

To illustrate these entries further, assume that $500 is collected in cash. The following compound journal entry must be made:

Cash $500
Reserve for Bad Debts $500
    Recoveries from Bad Debts $500
    Agency Accounts Receivable $500

The debt entries increase the cash account and reduce the reserve account in the statement of condition. The credit entries reduce the bad debt expense on the statement of condition as well as the amount of agency accounts receivable.

To continue the illustration, if accounts totaling $5,000 were returned to the healthcare organization as uncollectible, the following adjusting entry removes the accounts from the statement of condition:

Reserve for Bad Debts $5,000
    Agency Accounts Receivable $5,000

A permanent file should be established for accounts removed from the healthcare organization's books because they are considered uncollectible. This file will serve as a collection record that the patient financial services department staff can check when admitting patients. The check will reveal, among other facts, whether a patient being admitted has been a collection problem for the healthcare organization in the past.

The ten guidelines and the system for handling bad debts and uncollectible accounts provide these advantages:

- They provide control over bad debt accounts and ensure additional collection efforts after the healthcare organization has exhausted its own.

- They provide for a realistic reserve for bad debts that can be adjusted and controlled monthly.

- They comprise a systematic means of exerting constant and ongoing vigilance over bad debt offenders.

- They enhance the healthcare organization's ability to identify bad debts in advance.

- They improve the cash inflow from patient accounts receivable.

Implementing Electronic Data Interchange

Another key to effective receivables management is electronic data interchange (EDI)—the exchange, among organizational entities, of computer processable data in a standard format. This standard format is not a computer "language," and there is no "incompatibility" between it and any user's existing computer software or operating system. Using an EDI standard is somewhat analogous to using International Morse Code for radio communications: one electronic standard can be used across multiple languages. Users of EDI need to translate information from their internal computer systems into the EDI standard that is being used for transmissions to and from other entities.[24]

The 835 Health Care Claim Payment/Advice is the national EDI standard for paying healthcare claims. It provides a standard for initiating payment and transmitting remittance information from one organization's computer to another's, even if the two organizations use different software and hardware. The 835 can be used to send remitttance information only, to initiate payment only, or to both initiate payment and send remittance information. It is one of a group of more than 150 standards for electronic business documents developed by the Accredited Standards Committee (ASC) X12 of the American National Standards Institute (ANSI).[25]

Some of the benefits of the 835 EDI system to the payers include the following:

- electronic remittance information and electronic fund transfer

- reduced provider inquiries

- basis for automated secondary billing

- more accurate cash management forecasting enabled by electronic fund transfer

- should eliminate the security risks related to check stock for the payer

- possibly less expensive that the use of their paper equivalents[26]

Benefits to the healthcare providers include, but are not limited to, the following:

- mail handling

- check depositing

- reconciliation of bank deposits with remittance detail

- entry of remittance information

- posting Medicare, Medicaid, and other payer payments

- patient account identification

- review and reconciliation of submitted charges with the amount paid

- generation and posting of the closing entries

- generation of patient balance bills, secondary billing, and communications to the payer about disputes or misunderstandings[27]

Automation of some of these tasks is aided by the receipt of EDI remittance information, but automation will also require additional programming to integrate the EDI message into the provider's system.[28]

Some may think that electronic claims payment may not be adopted by the payers because it might lead to a loss of float. This should not be the case. Paying a claim electronically describes *how* it is paid, not *when* it is paid. Electronic payment systems can be scheduled so that the funds move to the provider's account on an exact day planned.[29] EDI offers the potential for faster payment to the healthcare provider; therefore, it should not be ignored by any patient financial services manager. In fact, the delay of even a few days in receiving payment can pay for the system's cost.[30]

Summary

The system and procedures that this chapter describes for monitoring and controlling accounts receivable are not ends in themselves. Rather, managers should view them as the nucleus that their healthcare organization can use for evaluating and improving its present internal audit and control structure. The organization should analyze its structure at least once a year and make any adjustments dictated by changes in its socioeconomic environment.

NOTES

1. Richard L. Marrapese and William R. Titera, *Internal Control of Hospital Finance: A Guide for Management,* rev. ed. (Chicago: American Hospital Publishing, Inc., 1989), xi.

2. Institute of Internal Auditors, *Statement of Responsibilities of Internal Auditing* (Altamonte Springs, Fla: Institute of Internal Auditors, 1990).

3. L. Vann Seawell, *Hospital Financial Accounting: Theory and Practice,* 2nd ed. (Westchester, Ill.: Healthcare Financial Management Association, 1987), 122.

4. Institute of Internal Auditors, *Statement of Responsibilities of Internal Auditing.*

5. Howard J. Berman, Lewis E. Weeks, and Steven F. Kukla, *The Financial Management of Hospitals,* 7th ed. (Ann Arbor, Mich.: Health Administration Press Division of the Foundation of the American College of Healthcare Executives, 1990), 59–60.

6. Berman, Weeks, and Kukla, *The Financial Management of Hospitals,* 60.

7. Seawell, *Hospital Financial Accounting,* 123.

8. Marrapese and Titera, *Internal Control of Hospital Finance,* 1.

9. Seawell, *Hospital Financial Accounting,* 115.

10. Marrapese and Titera, *Internal Control of Hospital Finance,* 1.

11. Berman, Weeks, and Kukla, *The Financial Management of Hospitals,* 58–59.

12. L. Vann Seawell, *Introduction to Hospital Accounting,* 3rd ed. (Westchester, Ill.: Healthcare Financial Management Association, 1992), 338.

13. Vicki L. Romero and Judith B. Henry, *The CFO's Expectations for Patient Financial Services* (Westchester, Ill.: Healthcare Financial Management Association, 1991), 7.

14. Seawell, *Hospital Financial Accounting,* 131.

15. American Hospital Association et al., *National Health Care Billing Audit Guidelines* (Chicago: American Hospital Association, 1992), 6.

16. Seawell, *Hospital Financial Accounting,* 124.

17. Seawell, *Hospital Financial Accounting,* 124.

18. D. Michael Warner, Don C. Holloway, and Kyle L. Grazier, *Decision Making and Control for Health Administration: The Management of Quantitative Analysis,* 2nd ed. (Ann Arbor, Mich.: Health Administration Press, 1984), 68.

19. Warner, Holloway, and Grazier, *Decision Making and Control for Health Administration,* 75.

20. Berman, Weeks, and Kukla, *The Financial Management of Hospitals,* 347.

21. Berman, Weeks, and Kukla, *The Financial Management of Hospitals,* 348.

22. Ronald J. Hy, *Financial Management for Health Care Administrators* (New York: Quorum Books, 1989), 109.

23. Hy, *Financial Management for Health Care Administrators,* 33.

24. James J. Moynihan, *Implementation Manual for the 835 Health Care Claim Payment/Advice: Guidelines for Electronic Payment of Healthcare Claims Using the ANSI ASC X12 Electronic Data Interchange (EDI) Standard* (Westchester, Ill.: Healthcare Financial Management Association, 1992), 3.

25. Moynihan, *Implementation Manual for the 835 Health Care Claim Payment/Advice,* 3–4.

26. Moynihan, *Implementation Manual for the 835 Health Care Claim Payment/Advice,* 6.

27. Moynihan, *Implementation Manual for the 835 Health Care Claim Payment/Advice,* 7.

28. Moynihan, *Implementation Manual for the 835 Health Care Claim Payment/Advice,* 7.

29. Moynihan, *Implementation Manual for the 835 Health Care Claim Payment/Advice,* 6.

30. Robert H. Carlisle and Karen L. Hackett, *The Medicare Payment System Slowdown and Loss of PIP: How to Respond* (Oak Brook, Ill.: Healthcare Financial Management Association, 1986), 11.

Patient Financial Services' Impact on the Healthcare Organization's Marketing and Public Relations

A number of healthcare executives continue to avoid promoting their healthcare organization with marketing and public relations because they believe such tactics smack of hucksterism. Nonetheless, aggressive healthcare marketing, which includes public relations, can mean the difference between survival and failure for some healthcare organizations. Chapter 13 will describe the basis for the healthcare marketing concept as well as its mission and functions. The chapter concludes with a discussion of effective patient financial services involvement in its organization's marketing efforts.

The Marketing Concept

Most healthcare organizations have been marketing their services for years—they just never considered their tactics to *be* marketing. For example, healthcare organizations are constantly recruiting physicians, nurses, and other professionals who will assist in providing the quality of care that enhances the facility's reputation in the community. Recruiting and maintaining medical and nursing staff of this caliber is a classic example of basic healthcare marketing practices. The marketing concept is based upon a voluntary and fair exchange of values between the healthcare organization and its constituency, i.e., its medical staff, patients, and employees.

The healthcare organization needs physicians and nurses to admit and care for its patients. In exchange, the healthcare system offers these professionals admitting privileges, modern facilities with state-of-the-art equipment, parking spaces, medical offices, physician and nurse lounges, and other benefits. Often the organization's managers and administrators need to review and evaluate these exchanges. For example, physicians participating in the Utilization Review and Quality Assurance committees or some other administrative function may feel that they are contributing more to the organization than they are receiving from it. These types of situations will always occur; management must resolve them to mutual satisfaction.[1]

Healthcare Marketing's Mission

One of the primary purposes of any healthcare marketing program is to maintain and expand the healthcare organization's market share. The organization can employ at least two methods to accomplish these goals:

1. continue to negotiate a series of exchanges with existing consumers in a manner that is mutually beneficial, and

2. attract new consumers to the existing client base while at the same time protecting, and never neglecting, the longtime consumers.[2]

Healthcare Marketing's Functions

As figure 13–1 illustrates, marketing provides overall structure upon which all organizational efforts, both internal and external, must be focused to enhance market share and expand market size. Marketing includes the following functions:

- sales (direct and promotional)
- advertising
- public relations
- market research
- product development

With the advent of managed-care contracting and other similar healthcare providing arrangements, many healthcare organizations are employing

FIGURE 13–1
Marketing Organizational Structure

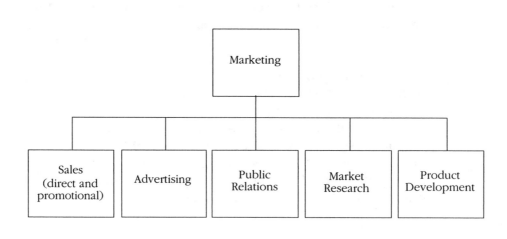

salespeople to make direct contact with major employers and other potential purchasers of healthcare services to negotiate and finalize managed-care contracts. Clearly, an effective sales staff can be a survival tactic for today's healthcare organization.

If many healthcare professionals once considered "selling" health care to be unprofessional and unethical, they viewed advertising these services in the same way. Historically, it simply was not professionally ethical for a healthcare organization to be involved in either one of these functions. This viewpoint also existed in the legal and accounting professions, but to survive in an increasingly competitive environment, lawyers and accountants eventually became more assertive in promoting their services. Similarly, escalating competition for market share in the healthcare environment has caused all healthcare providers to reexamine their positions regarding marketing and all of its ramifications.

The purpose of advertising is to attract attention, usually on a short-term basis, to a new product or service, and to periodically remind the public of the institution providing this product or service. Advertising significantly differs from public relations in that it is short-term oriented to attract and retain consumers to the product, service, or organization. Public relations, on the other hand, is long-term oriented to foster an external image and maintain lines of communication with the organization's publics.

Public relations was once considered to be the healthcare facility's eyes, ears, and mouth. It continues to be a "soft" marketing tool that emphasizes keeping the public informed about the organization. For example, announcing the hiring of a prominent specialist, the installation of state-of-the-art equipment, or the amount of charity the healthcare organization has rendered on behalf of the community are examples of public relations messages.

Market research has two primary purposes:

1. to identify unmet market needs or services, and

2. to identify the demographics and psychographics of an identified target market.

The first objective can be accomplished by informally discussing with individuals and subsequently documenting their identification of unsatisfied healthcare market needs in the community, such as a treatment center for pregnant teens. Market research's demographic and psychographic aspects require considerably more sophisticated and extensive data and analysis, which usually can be obtained readily through the use of a database market information system.

Once the healthcare provider identifies unmet market needs; analyzes market characteristics; and develops, prices, and packages the new product or service, the formal step of marketing begins: convincing the public that it needs the new product or service.

Patient Financial Services Managers' Role in Marketing

The patient financial services department should be in the forefront of its healthcare organization's marketing efforts. In most facilities, it is the personnel from this department who have most contact with the facility's primary constituents: the medical staff, employees, patients, and patients' families.

A recent survey indicated that the method and timeliness of patient billing often determined whether patients wanted to return to a particular healthcare provider. The survey also revealed that patients, frequently under strain from their illness and financial pressures, typically relieve their stress by berating the patient financial services personnel. Therefore, if these employees maintain an understanding and helpful attitude, they are an important factor of the healthcare organization's public relations and marketing program.[3]

In managing accounts receivable, patient financial services managers need to view the process as too complex to begin after a patient is discharged. Rather, the process should start with a patient's preadmission and continue until the patient pays the account or management decides to write it off as uncollectible.[4] Figure 13–2 depicts the key control points for effectively controlling patient accounts receivable. These areas are

- preadmission,
- admission,
- in-house,
- discharge, and
- postdischarge.

In addition to determining the effectiveness and efficiency of the institution's admitting, billing, and collection procedures, these control points can influence the public's perception of the facility's quality of care and its reputation within the community. The attitude of the preadmitting clerk, the admitting personnel, and the billing clerk or cashier create a lasting impression and can influence the patient's choice of one facility over another.

Preadmission

From the moment that patients and their families enter the healthcare facility, they are watching, judging, and forming impressions and opinions about the institution and its personnel's efficiency, courtesy, professionalism, and general attitude toward them. Many, if not all, patients admitted into a healthcare institution are apprehensive at best and angry at worst. They just don't want to be there! Many are frightened and resentful. Patients need to feel reassured that all will go well and that they will be served by capable, caring people from the day they are admitted to the day they are discharged. To

FIGURE 13–2
**Five Control Points for Effective Patient Financial Services Marketing
and Collections**

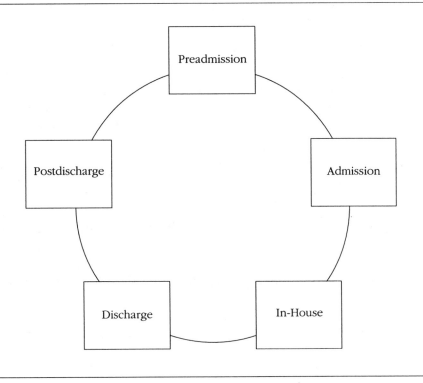

help provide this reassurance amidst the stress of entering the facility, most healthcare organizations employ a preadmission process.

The preadmission procedure, usually the first *vocal* contact between the prospective patients and the facility, helps set the tone for the patients' stay. Preadmission gives patients a first impression of the facility. If the telephone interview is conducted by someone who is courteous, patient, and understanding, and allows prospective patients enough time to ask questions about the organization's services and procedures, it should alleviate much of the patients' fear, apprehension, and resentment.

On the other hand, if the preadmission procedure is abrupt and cursory, patients may get the impression that they are going to become routine cases to be led through a maze of medical technology by technicians. If the patients perceive inefficiency, lack of caring, and tension, that is how the community will come to view the facility's operation. Regardless of how the employees perceive their organization, it is what the patients and families perceive that has the most impact on the facility's public image. It is their perception that can promote the institution's acceptance within the community.

An effective preadmission procedure does not necessarily guarantee an efficient and smooth-running admitting process, nor does it assure that all incoming patients will be completely satisfied. But the preadmission process *can* go a long way toward relieving patients' apprehensions and fostering a positive image for the healthcare organization.

Admission

Whereas the preadmission process is the first vocal contact between patients and the healthcare organization, the admission procedure is the first *visual* encounter patients and their families have with the facility's personnel. Being promptly admitted by a cheerful and courteous individual in an attractive, uncluttered, and relaxed atmosphere helps to create a lasting favorable impression upon those going through the process. The admitting process is further enhanced if patients are escorted promptly to their rooms or, in case of outpatients, to the point of service.

Beginning with the preadmission and admission functions and all throughout the time the patients are in the healthcare facility's care as either inpatients or outpatients, the degree of respect and courtesy initially extended by the patient financial services personnel will go far toward making up for any deficiencies in dietary, medical, or nursing care that the patients may perceive.

In-House

While patients are in the healthcare facility, the quality of care rendered by the organization's entire staff, not just the nursing staff, is absolutely essential to the public's positive regard of the facility as well as to the patients' perception of the total care they received.

Compassion and caring will always stay in vogue. They are the least costly and yet the most effective marketing devices any organization can use. Moreover, they help to create the kind of congenial environment within which management can obtain its marketing goals, which might include the following:

- satisfactorily meet the patient's perceived medical and emotional needs and expectations

- create a caring environment that encourages repeat visits

- promptly and efficiently collect payment for services rendered.[5]

Discharge

The admission process gave the patients and their families their first visual impression of the healthcare facility; the discharge process will be the *final* and probably the *most remembered* impression they will have after leaving the institution. Therefore, it is essential that employees identify and address any patient dissatisfaction during the patient's stay or, at the latest, during the discharge process.

Courtesy, consideration, concern, and efficient service can do much to pacify many patient complaints; the discharge point is probably the *last opportunity* that the facility's employees will have to resolve any perceived problems. If a patient or family member leaves the facility dissatisfied, the tone has been set as to how promptly the patient will pay the bill, or whether it will be paid at all.

Postdischarge

Marketing should not stop when patients leave the healthcare facility. After discharge, most patients may believe that those who rendered care have forgotten about them. Yet this is the time that patients may be most receptive to additional evidence of caring from the organization. For example, one healthcare facility's emergency services department routinely telephones the discharged patients or their families to see how each patient is feeling and whether the facility can do anything else to lessen the trauma of the emergency admission and hospital stay.

This and other types of extended caring help to create an organizational environment to which patients, families, friends, and neighbors will want to return should it become necessary. Such care, especially for emergency patients, also facilitates in the collection process.

Marketing to the Family Unit

From a marketing standpoint, the healthcare facility's staff cannot afford to neglect patients' families, including the extended family (friends, neighbors, etc.). Perhaps these individuals may require medical care and/or hospitalization in the future; their choice of facility will certainly be influenced by their perception of the quality of service and care rendered to a relative, friend, or neighbor. It is imperative, therefore, that the organization market itself to the entire family unit (see figure 13–3).

Every successful business depends upon repeat customers; it is not any different in the healthcare industry. Patient satisfaction or dissatisfaction frequently originates in the patient financial services department. The benefits accruing to the facility from satisfied patients are numerous and ongoing; however, dissatisfied patients can cause disaster, especially to the organization's cash flow.

Satisfied patients typically pay their bills promptly. Together with family and friends, they will speak highly of the healthcare facility's staff and services to everyone who asks about their hospital stay. Dissatisfied patients, on the other hand, will challenge charges, fail to make timely payments, or

FIGURE 13–3

Patient Financial Services Department's Target Markets

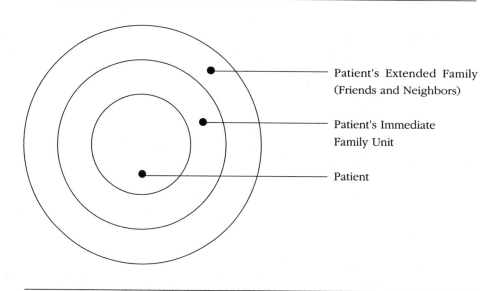

refuse to pay the bill at all. At best, they will pay reluctantly, and often with a poor report to family and friends about the facility and its quality of care.

The healthcare facility's staff and employees may perceive the organization as the best in the marketplace, its community. However, if its patients and the general public do not share in that perception, then the provider's marketing program is not achieving its goals.

NOTES

1. Allen G. Herkimer Jr., "Marketing: A Patient Account Manager's Responsibility," *The Journal of Patient Account Management,* (April–May 1990), 18–22.
2. Herkimer, "Marketing," 18–22.
3. Bernstein, Harris, and Meloy, "Focus Groups Improve Billing Practices, Patient Relations," *Healthcare Financial Management* (May 1989), 57–60.
4. Howard J. Berman, Lewis E. Weeks, and Steven F. Kukla, *The Financial Management of Hospitals,* 7th ed. (Ann Arbor, Mich.: Health Administration Press Division of the Foundation of the American College of Healthcare Executives, 1990), 348.
5. Herkimer, "Marketing," 18–22.

The Future for Patient Financial Services Managers

Most of today's patient financial services managers are in the position by happenstance.[1] Nonetheless, during 1989 they oversaw the collection of more than $231 billion for nongovernmental healthcare facilities providing general services and acute care, thus providing 90 percent of the facilities' gross revenues.[2] However, patient financial services managers can no longer depend upon happenstance to obtain and retain their job: many of their traditional functions have been eliminated, modified, or expanded in recent years due to changes in the healthcare industry and environment.

This chapter will explore future challenges in the healthcare industry that will affect these managers, and then it will identify strategies to help them retain their position. Chapter 14 concludes with a career action plan for those planning on entering the profession.

The Healthcare Industry in Transition

As stated in the Preface, a silent but steady evolution has taken place in the healthcare industry during the last decade, particularly in healthcare facilities. Reflecting this phenomenon is the fact that the word *hospital* is virtually obsolete as groups of healthcare facilities pool their resources by associating under a corporate umbrella or under a contract arrangement.[3] One of the earliest signs of this change occurred nearly ten years ago, when the Federation of American Hospitals changed its name to the Federation of American Healthcare Systems. Another sign of the times came recently, when the very conservative American Hospital Association (AHA) changed the name of its journal from *Hospitals* to *Hospitals & Health Networks*. Moreover, AHA coined the term *community care networks* to identify regional health networks.[4] In the interim, a few hospital associations, starting with California, have incorporated *healthcare system* or a similar phrase into their new name. Clearly, the healthcare industry is once again in a state of transition.

Patient Financial Services Managers' Expanding Responsibilities

The present-day patient financial services managers' position may be the best example of healthcare's silent evolution—more so than any other position in the healthcare industry. The need for a steady and increasing flow of cash is critical to every healthcare organization's survival today. If the organization cannot meet its cash needs, it may well be doomed. The patient financial services managers' role, therefore, is almost certain to expand in the future and become even more critical to the organization's viability.

Today, patient financial services managers' future increasingly depends upon their ability to exercise the imagination, initiative, and ingenuity needed to cope with the changes in the healthcare industry that have already occurred and with those that will certainly develop. These managers' challenge is to foresee changes and prepare for them intelligently. Their role is no longer limited to the collection of cash, even though that is still a key responsibility of their position.

Patient Financial Services Management: An Overview

When the author entered the healthcare industry, nearly ten years before Medicare, the position of financial services manager was then called credit manager. The title was obviously a misnomer because the position more resembled that of a bill collector. During those years healthcare providers, especially hospitals, did not give credit despite patients' expecting it.

Patients entered hospitals. Care was very seldom, if ever, refused. At discharge, patients or the responsible parties would pay what they could afford. The credit manager would then try to negotiate some form of payment program, even if it was only five or ten dollars per month. Initial billing usually required only one bill (statement) to Blue Cross or the insurance company. Follow-up billing to the patient continued sometimes for years, until the bill was paid or turned over to an attorney or collection agency. However, many healthcare providers and hospitals frowned on collection agencies, often refraining from referring any delinquent accounts to them for payment; such a payment recovery method was considered bad for public relations. In such cases, management retrospectively reviewed accounts for classification as either charity or a bad debt.

When the federal government implemented Medicare and Medicaid in 1966, the billing office staffs of most healthcare providers almost immediately doubled in size to accommodate the multiple billing requirements for Medicare's Part A and Part B, as well as the increased patient load. As a result of these programs, together with increased responsibility and involvement in the organization's cash flow, the hospital credit manager became a patient account manager.

Things have not changed much since then. There are only more ever-changing governmental regulations with attendant complications. This means that today's patient account managers and those who aspire to this profession must be prepared for more changes. We will be examining the following areas of concern in this chapter:

- position title

- position qualifications

- new responsibilities

- major opportunity areas

- other future considerations

Much of this chapter's content was obtained from a delphi survey group representing many geographical sections of the country. The group's members included the president of a management firm, a corporate director of accounts receivable, a managed-care contract administrator, an attorney who deals exclusively with healthcare organizations, and a number of practicing account managers of freestanding and/or multifacility healthcare systems.[5]

Position Title

The healthcare industry's most prevalent title for these managers' position is *patient account manager,* but a majority of the survey team believes that this title, which came into vogue in the early seventies, does not represent all the functions currently demanded of the position. Since Medicare's implementation of diagnosis-related groups and its prospective payment system, along with the healthcare industry's expanded use of electronic data processing, heightened awareness of public relations and marketing, and increased emphasis on productivity and quality improvement, the healthcare financial management environment has changed substantially.

A title more representative and descriptive of the position's present and future responsibilities, the survey team believes, is *patient financial services,* to which may then be added *director, manager, vice president,* or *assistant administrator.* Regardless of the title a healthcare organization ultimately chooses, this manager in all probability will continue to report to the healthcare organization's chief financial officer (CFO). There is, however, a new trend developing wherein the manager reports directly to the organization's treasurer, rather than to the CFO.

Position Qualifications

Many of today's patient financial services managers worked their way up within the institution or its business office. Promotion often came through attrition or seniority rather than because of skill, knowledge, or formal education. In the past, the highest level of education attained by these managers was a high school diploma, but this situation is rapidly changing. In 1990, 64.5 percent of the patient financial services managers had advanced degrees, compared with 51.2 percent in 1987.[6] The survey panel's consensus is that a bachelor's degree in business, accounting, or healthcare administration is going to be this position's minimum educational requirement. In fact, a master's degree will undoubtedly be required by the year 2000.

In addition to these traditional educational requirements, the new patient financial services managers must adopt a schedule of lifetime learning to keep current with all of the constantly and rapidly occuring governmental and technological changes. Society is now entering what Peter Drucker calls the "New Knowledge Society." In his book *The New Realities,* Drucker states that in the future, we are going to need retraining throughout our lives, and that learning process will be taking place both in school and at the workplace. In a knowledge environment, Drucker warns, change will be more rapid; new skills will constantly need to be mastered if we are to stay at the peak of our ability to contribute.[7] But the learning process does not stop here—certification and recertification programs for the position are here to stay. For example, the Healthcare Financial Management Association (HFMA) awards individuals who have passed a comprehensive examination the right to use Certified Manager of Patient Accounts (CMPA) after their name. In addition, the American Guild of Patient Account Management (AGPAM) has the Certified Patient Account Manager (CPAM) and the Certified Clinic Account Manager (CCAM) certification programs. Perhaps the time will come when these organizations agree upon one certification program for patient financial services managers.

Aside from enrolling in degree and certification programs, however, successful managers also must be able to lead people and to work in a collaborative manner throughout the organization and the industry.

New Responsibilities

Patient financial services managers of the future must have a comprehensive understanding of, and feel comfortable with, all aspects or electronic data processing used for patient accounting. This knowledge is essential if they want their employers to identify and respect them as key members of their healthcare organization's multidisciplined financial management team. They must watch trends constantly and adjust operating systems according to the community's perceived needs and benefits. They also must be good at problem solving, and always seeking and testing creative approaches to old responsibilities and new challenges.

If claims processing becomes uniform, and there's no reason to believe otherwise, the need for healthcare organizations to employ numerous reimbursement experts will decrease because all providers and payers would be sharing the same data sets.[8] Relevant clinical data, probably in the form of outcome data, would increase to both the provider and the payer. The collection, processing, and analyzing of these data will be a shared responsibility between the patient financial services and medical records departments. Those financial divisions who are not responsible for medical records, take notice.

Managed care is a relatively new responsibility for patient financial services managers; the system began in the early eighties as risk-based management, but the nineties will be the decade of managed-care contracts. It is predicted that most acute-care hospitals will have at least 75 percent to 85 percent of their inpatients covered by fixed-price (risk-based) managed-care payment systems by 1993.[9] This means that patient financial services managers must be involved during the contract negotiation process, and, more importantly, they must have the ability (and information!) to monitor, audit, and evaluate each contract from a recoupment and documentation standpoint. In other words, patient financial services managers of the future will be responsible for evaluating the cost/benefit of every managed-care contract their healthcare organization enters into. They must know how to perform a cost analysis of each contract and compare these results with the cash amount received and other benefits from the contractor. For this process to work, the managers must administer each contract as a single "product" in a "product-line" operation. This product line probably would be organized according to client type, such as employers of less than fifty people, employers of fifty to 250 people, employers of 250 to two thousand people, and employers of more than two thousand people.

In addition to knowing what the costs are during and after each managed-care contract, patient financial services managers also must know what their organization's costs are for rendering services before and during the contract negotiation process. The impact of volume changes, rate changes, and other variables typically discussed during the contract negotiation must be identified.

Why should patient financial services managers be involved in the managed-care contract negotiation process? Isn't that the CFO's and/or the chief executive officer's (CEO's) responsibility? Yes, the CFO and CEO are on the contract-negotiating team, but they're not the *whole* team. Who is in a better position than patient financial services managers to know

- what the payment pattern is for each healthcare service purchaser?

- which payers pay on time and which ones complicate the organization's claim processing?

- who is currently held responsible for the organization's cash inflow?

Since cash inflows are becoming more critical to the survival of every healthcare organization, another area of responsibility in which patient financial services managers must involve themselves is the organization's strategic planning process. This involvement must be on an organizationwide basis, as well as departmental. Most healthcare organizations have adopted, at least, a three- to five-year horizon for their strategic planning program. This goal forces the institution's management team to plan for the future, even though it may be somewhat cloudy, to help prepare the organization for changing events and markets.

Marketing and public relations are organizational activities in which patient financial services managers must involve themselves and act with knowledge and authority. It is the survey group's opinion that strategic marketing and public relations programs, along with efficient and courteous business practices, will be the chief influences upon the consumer's choice of healthcare facility, and whether they will return to the facility for repeat business.

Major Opportunity Areas

Now and in the foreseeable future, the federal and state governments will continue to be the greatest problem (and opportunity) for any healthcare provider; they will continue to change the rules, often retroactively, and to confuse both the provider and patient. To cope profitably with this area of concern, healthcare managers must know and keep up with governmental rules, playing the game decisively, authoritatively, and effectively.

Technological changes, too, may provide new management opportunities and challenges. The survey group believes that eventually all communication, especially between third-party payers and healthcare service providers, will be electronic. Any organization that fails to keep up with information and communications technology will be at a disadvantage when attempting to compete effectively with more sophisticated competitors. Moreover, many healthcare organizations will allow employees to work at home at computer workstations connected to the organization data processing network, offering an excellent opportunity for managers to implement an employee incentive program. These changes will test patient financial services managers' managerial skills while improving departmental productivity and reducing employee turnover. It's going to be a fast-moving, high-tech environment; there will be no room for laissez-faire management!

It appears certain that in the future, the healthcare organization's business office will be much smaller, yet more inviting and more efficient for admitting and discharging patients; the office will be staffed by fewer, but highly skilled and more expensive, personnel. However, to manage the organization's cash inflows effectively, patient financial services managers must have accurate and complete patient information, which is possible only if the organization has planned an efficiently operating "front-end" management information system that meets all billing requirements and regulations. This system will interface, real time, with the physician and the third-party insurer's offices.

In addition to advanced technology; fewer, yet more highly skilled personnel; and home workstations, another challenge appears on the horizon for the nation's healthcare industry: a national health insurance (NHI) program. The United States' currently pluralistic, somewhat competitive, and partially regulatory healthcare system has generated a number of higher management positions, including patient financial services managers. In fact, the government spends 18 percent of its total healthcare expenditure on administration: on collecting premiums, on detailed bills providers submit, and on fiscal intermediaries to review claims and make payments to providers.[10] A single-payer, universal-access, mandatory insurance program would eliminate the need for a number of top- and middle-management positions, most of the admitting, billing, related personnel, and much of the computer capability that is for processing billings to multiple payers.[11]

However the current universal-access and NHI debates are resolved, one result appears to be certain: less funds for healthcare providers.

Yet, another major problem/opportunity area is the healthcare provider's role in financing the cost of health care. Accounts receivable represents one of the largest assets, excluding plant assets, for most healthcare organizations—billions of dollars. For a typical healthcare organization, net patient accounts receivable may represent as much as one-half of its total assets and three-fourths of its current assets.[12] Based upon a recent study, the average daily patient census in the nation's community healthcare facilities is approximately 794,000 inpatients, which generates nearly $2.5 billion in annual revenue or $687 million per calendar day. Using these totals and estimating that the average number of day's revenue uncollected is 73, this means that the nation's 5,000-plus healthcare systems are financing the nation's health care. Collectively, their patient accounts receivable approximates $49.5 billion at any one time.[13] Moreover, very few of these organizations are charging interest for these uncollected accounts. At only a 3-percent annual interest rate, this represents approximately $1.5 billion of lost revenue, or opportunity costs, imposed annually upon these organizations. Even if the healthcare organizations could generate additional funds using the receivables as collateral, they would certainly have to pay the lender more than 3-percent interest.

Patient accounts receivable, as they are presently being managed by most healthcare organizations, are a negatively performing asset that imposes needless costs on the organization.[14] Not only are the healthcare systems losing revenue, they are also incurring administrative and collection costs. The challenge to all levels of healthcare management, then, is to discover or develop methods for obtaining better utilization of patient accounts receivable.

Other Future Considerations

There are a number of other current or possible trends that savvy patient financial services managers should be tracking, for any one of them could change the nature of the profession:

- What if capitation becomes the only or the dominant payment system for all healthcare organizations?

- What if a one-payer payment system is produced by the Clinton administration's healthcare task force?

- What if all healthcare claims were required to be processed through electronic data interchange (EDI)?

- What if all healthcare claims had to be paid to the healthcare provider through EDI?

- What if there were virtually no bad debts?

- What if there were virtually no charity cases?

- What if there was no need for special arrangements for workers' compensation and personal liability cases?

- What if the healthcare reform law achieves the Clinton task force's goal of administrative simplification, resulting in major downsizing of patient financial services staffs?

- What if there were no need for collection attorneys or agents?

- What if all patients were required to be reviewed for means testing?

- What if all of the healthcare organizations' purchasers were mega-sized health maintenance organizations or preferred provider organizations similar to California's Wellpoint, with its two-million-plus members?[15]

Finally, what if many of the patient financial services managers' functions were eliminated or modified as a result of the aforementioned trends? Certainly, these possibilities can become realities—witness the changes already in place in many countries.

What would be left for patient financial services managers to do? Admissions, cashiering, and those other "up-front" reponsibilities still may be needed, but interestingly, a recent survey indicates that a smaller proportion of patient financial services managers were responsible for outpatient registration in 1992 than in 1990, down from 50 percent to 43 percent. Fewer of these managers were responsible for emergency room registration in 1992 as well, down from 47 percent to 41 percent. These percentages are in direct contrast to the managers' increases in responsibility for outpatient and emergency room registration from 1988 to 1990.[16] A similar decline in responsibility was reported for inpatient admissions, which dipped from 57 percent in 1990 to 50 percent in 1992. Additionally, patient financial services managers reported that they had 6-percent less responsibility for ambulatory care registration, and their cashiering responsibilities were down 7 percent. According to the survey, this decline in "up-front" responsibilities was somewhat unexpected, considering the direct effect admissions and registration have on collections and public relations.[17]

As a result of this information, some questions come to mind: Who has assumed these responsibilities? Why the change? What are the patient financial services managers doing instead? The most important question is probably this: What are these managers going to do about this shift in responsibilities if it comes?

With the possibility that many of these "what-if" changes may occur, patient financial services managers must seriously examine their role in the healthcare environment of the future, which will undoubtedly include some form of managed care. There is a good chance that these mega-network groups or alliances, accountable health partnerships, or health insurance purchasing cooperatives will dominate the healthcare industry.[18] What if these huge purchasing alliances do, in fact, become the way of life? What will the patient financial services managers' role be in this managed-care environment?

The fact is that these alliances and networks have already been implemented in Florida, and they have been working relatively successfully in California for years.[19] However, what is important to keep in mind is this: patient financial services managers need to change the profession's present structure to reflect the revolutionary changes in health care. If this doesn't happen, then the big question would be: Is there really a need for patient financial services managers?

It is highly possible that the healthcare industry may revert to using someone who is responsible for managing the admission and discharge processes. This person would report to a more highly skilled individual designated as the cash and contract administrator (CCA) or assistant treasurer responsible for any and all areas of cash inflows and outflows, including cashiering. Part of the CCA's responsibility might be the negotiating, monitoring, and conducting of cost-benefit analyses for all managed-care contracts. This person would be accountable to the healthcare organization's corporate treasurer, not the CEO or CFO.

Preparing for a Successful Career

In addition to the customary qualifications and credentials, a positive attitude heads the list of requirements for a successful career in patient financial services management.

Of equal importance, however, is a commitment to the profession. Total commitment, and extending themselves beyond the normally expected levels of performance, usually results in favorable recognition for patient financial services managers, not only by the employer but by their peers as well.

EXHIBIT 14–1

Sample of a Career Action Plan for the Patient Financial Services Professional

Immediate Goals *(1 to 3 Years)*	*Intermediate Goals* *(4 to 6 Years)*	*Long-Range Goals* *(7 to 10 Years)*
1. Obtain job in the patient financial services department.	1. Become a supervisor in the patient financial services department.	1. Become director of patient financial services.
2. Complete bachelor's degree program.	2. Start master's degree program.	2. Complete master's degree program.
3. Join HFMA, AGPAM, or another professional organization.	3. Obtain CMPA, CPAM, or other certification.	3. Maintain recertification.
4. Become active in the local chapter of professional organization.	4. Become active in a national professional organization.	4. Maintain active status in professional organization.
5. Write at least one article for publication in a professional journal.	5. Conduct research or lead workshops in areas of interest.	5. Continue to write about patient financial services topics.
6. Select the type of organization in which you want to work: hospital, long-term care facility, corporation, consulting, etc.	6. Select the geographical area you want to live in.	6. Locate in an area and workplace that you will enjoy.

Being an active member in a professional association such as Healthcare Financial Management Association and/or the American Guild of Patient Account Management can enhance one's professionalism. After joining the organization(s), be visible and contribute to the local chapter's activities; again, attitude and one's degree of commitment usually result in recognition, regionally and often nationally. Experience has shown that active involvement in a professional association and in a healthcare community usually results in more gratification and recognition for the individual.

An entrepreneurial spirit is an essential attribute to the successful healthcare professional. The dynamics of the healthcare industry require innovation, creativity, and the willingness to take risks. For example, most healthcare providers have stretched their financial resources to the limit; they now need new sources of revenue. The creative, innovative people who can develop these new financial resources will be tomorrow's healthcare industry leaders.

Career planning is a must for successful patient financial services managers. Most successful careers don't just happen; they are planned, either formally or informally. The career action plan in exhibit 14–1 illustrates a ten-year approach to three stages of career development. The plan assumes that the aspiring patient financial services professional is neither active in a professional association nor has the appropriate formal education, experience, and credentials.[20] Remember, however, that the suggested plan is not "written in stone"; it should be sufficiently flexible to allow the planner to adjust to the changing environment and requirements.

All patient financial services managers owe it to themselves and their employer to maintain their professionalism: keep current with future trends in the profession, stay on the cutting edge of change with state-of-the-art management techniques and technology, and remain sufficiently flexible to effectively adjust to any and all changes in the healthcare industry.

Professionalism in management requires something else, perhaps the most important ingredient of all for success: integrity, in every activity and in every encounter. It may take some time to achieve a reputation for this most desirable and necessary attribute, but conversely, integrity can be lost or destroyed very quickly. Integrity, after it has been earned, must be cherished and protected. It is the aspiring or established manager's most valuable asset.

Finally, success in every endeavor demands persistence. Remember the words of Franklin Roosevelt, who was certainly no stranger to challenges:

> It is common sense to take a method and try it. If it fails, admit it frankly and try another. But above all, try something.[21]

Let us prepare ourselves and our staffs for what promises to be a dynamic, exciting, and rewarding future in health care.

NOTES

1. Judith Nemes, "Patient Accounts Managers' Roles Expand, but Few Recruiting, Training Programs Exist," *Modern Healthcare* (June 17, 1991), 70–72.
2. Nemes, "Patient Accounts Managers' Roles Expand, but Few Recruiting, Training Programs Exist," 70–72.
3. Howard J. Berman, Lewis E. Weeks, and Steven F. Kukla, *The Financial Management of Hospitals,* 7th ed. (Ann Arbor, Mich.: Health Administration Press Division of the Foundation of the American College of Healthcare Executives, 1990), 715.
4. Patrick W. Philbin, "From the Ground Up," *Hospitals & Health Networks* (June 5, 1993), 46.
5. Allen G. Herkimer Jr. et al., "The New Age of Patient Account Management," presented at the American Guild of Patient Account Management's Annual National Institute in San Antonio, Texas, October 31, 1990.
6. Nemes, "Patient Accounts Managers' Roles Expand, but Few Recruiting, Training Programs Exist," 70.
7. Richard A. Nenneman, "The Knowledge Society," *World Monitor* (September 1990), 79.
8. Dan Rode, "Managed Competition: Is There a Future for PFS Managers?" *Healthcare Financial Management* (May 1993), 142.
9. Russell C. Coile Jr., "Managed Care Poised to Dominate Health Delivery and Financing During This Decade," *Medical Benefits* (April 15, 1990), 2–3.
10. Thomas P. Weil, "The U. S. Healthcare System after NHI," *Hospital Topics* 69, no. 2 (Spring 1991), 36–40.
11. Weil, "The U.S. Healthcare System after NHI," 39.

12. Robert L. Newton, "Measuring Accounts Receivable Performance: A Comprehensive Method," *Healthcare Financial Management* (May 1993), 33.

13. Allen G. Herkimer Jr., "Cost of Patient Accounts Receivable," unpublished, 1993.

14. Herkimer, "Cost of Patient Accounts Receivable," 33.

15. John Herrmann, "Blue Cross of California Goes for the Gold," *Healthcare System Review* (May–June 1993), 17.

16. David Zimmerman and Bruce Nelson, "Patient Accounts Managers Prepare for Change," *Healthcare Financial Management* (May 1993), 38.

17. Zimmerman and Nelson, "Patient Accounts Managers Prepare for Change," 38–39.

18. Rode, "Managed Competition," 142.

19. Russell C. Coile Jr., "California Health Care 2001: The Outlook for America's 'Bellwether' State," *Hospital Strategy Report* 5, no. 4 (February 1993).

20. Allen G. Herkimer Jr., "Suggestions for Success in Patient Financial Services," *Patient Accounts* (May 1991), 2, 4.

21. John Bartlett, *Familiar Quotations,* edited by Emily Morison Beck et al., 15th and 125th anniversary ed. (Boston: Little, Brown, and Company, 1980), 779:7.

Glossary

Account, Contra. An asset account that adjusts the gross value of an asset to a net value. Examples include reserve for bad debts and depreciation.

Account, Control. A general ledger account (e.g., accounts receivable, accounts payable) that records all the debit and credit transactions which occur in the account, usually supported by a listing of the subsidiary accounts.

Account, Subsidiary. The individual account(s) (e.g., patient bill, vendor invoice) whose total (trial balance listing) should equal the amount in the respective general ledger control account.

Accounting, Accrual. An accounting system that requires that all revenues, expenses, and other related transactions, such as allowances, be recognized and recorded as they occur, regardless of cash flow.

Accounting, Cash. An accounting system that records only cash received and cash collected; thus, there is no accounting for accounts receivable and accounts payable.

Accounting Controls. As part of the healthcare organization's internal control system, these methods and measures exist primarily for the purposes of safeguarding the organization's assets and to assure a high degree of reliability in the information generated by the accounting process.

Accounting, Double-Entry. An accounting system in which the recording of every transaction requires a minimum of two entries or changes in the accounting records. The basic principle of double-entry accounting is that for every debit there must be an equal and offsetting credit.

Accounting, Financial. Information derived from an organization's accounting system is typically classified as either financial (general) accounting or managerial accounting. Financial accounting is concerned with reporting an organization's activities to outside groups, so its information takes the form of financial statements that summarize the activities of the entire organization.

Accounting, Fund. A system of accounting that separates an organization's monies and other assets and liabilities into self-balancing unrestricted and restricted funds to facilitate fiduciary control over each purpose of the fund.

Accounting Journals. Books of original entry for recording all of a facility's transactions; these journals usually include the general journal, cash receipts journal, cash disbursements journal, purchase journal, and payroll journal.

Accounting, Managerial. The process of developing and using accounting information in planning, controlling, and developing special reports for making decisions and formulating long-range plans.

Activity Ratios. Ratios that measure how efficiently the healthcare organization is using its assets.

Adjusted Standard Hours Required (ASHR). The result of dividing the total standard hours required by the performance factor.

Administrative Controls. Those methods and measures in the organization's internal control system that essentially focus on improving the efficiency with which the organization's employees perform activities; they also secure a high degree of compliance with established managerial policies.

A La Carte Rate. Rates prospectively established for every service a healthcare organization provides. This rate is also known at the per-service rate.

Algebraic Method. A cost-finding method employing algebraic formulas and the computer. These formulas are designed to identify costs in departments that serve each other by recognizing the relationship that exists between those departments.

All-Inclusive Rate. One rate, prospectively established, which includes all of the service a patient receives during a specific period of time, such as per patient day or per diagnosis. This rate is also known as the per-diem rate.

Allowance, Administrative. A deduction from gross revenue (similar to a sales discount) that is established by the healthcare institution's governing board and/or administration for employees, physicians, clergy, etc.

Allowance, Charity. A deduction from gross revenue (*see* **Administrative Allowance**) that is written off from the patient's bill. In most cases, the patient must be identified as a charity patient before or at the time of admission for service.

Allowance, Contractual. A deduction from gross revenue (*see* **Administrative Allowance**) that is the difference between the total amount paid by the third-party payer (Medicare, Medicaid, and, in some states, worker's compensation and Blue Cross) and the healthcare provider's total gross charge for services. This amount is written off by the provider because it has no recourse to the patient.

Asset, Capital. An asset having a life of more than one year that is not bought and sold in the ordinary course of business.

Asset, Current. An asset that is usually consumed or exhausted within one year; i.e., patient accounts receivable, cash, etc.

Asset, Fixed. An asset that usually has a useful life of more than one year; i.e., equipment, building, etc.

Audit Log. A historic record kept by a healthcare provider or payer that records a particular party's audit experience.

Average Daily Revenue Uncollected. One of the most frequently used ratios to evaluate the management of patient accounts receivable, this ratio determines the number of days' average daily revenue uncollected in the patient accounts receivable files.

Average Length of Stay (ALOS). The result of dividing the total number of patient days by the number of patient discharges for a corresponding time period.

Bad Debt. An account that management believes the debtor cannot or will not pay, even though the debtor may have the resources to pay.

Bad Debt Reserve. A contra account that makes an allowance for uncollectible accounts, thus reducing the gross total of patient accounts receivable.

Billing Audit. A process for determining whether data in a provider's health record and/or appropriate and referenced medical record correspond with services listed on a provider's bill. Providers conduct such audits either through an internal control process or by hiring an external auditor.

Billings, Patient. A macro statistic that can be used to measure the productivity of the patient financial services department. A preferred measurement, micro patient billings, would be based upon the type of billing (Medicare inpatient, Medicare outpatient, etc.), which is related to the amount of resources required to generate the billing.

Break-Even Analysis. A procedure that evaluates the price of a department's production unit and determines its break-even point as well.

Break-Even Point. A financial position at which point the total revenue equals the total expenses.

Budget. A financial plan that authorizes the costs and/or revenues a department plans to expend in performing its function for a period of time, such as one year.

Budget, Appropriation. A type of budget used primarily by government agencies and municipalities. In this approach, the user establishes fixed expenditures for each department or cost center. Expense overruns or underruns cannot be transferred to another department without formal approval.

Budget, Capital. A financial plan that projects the planned acquisition of capital or fixed assets.

Budget, Control. A target budget whose projected volume has been adjusted to the actual volume of activity, thus eliminating any differences due to volume.

Budget, Fixed or Target. A financial plan that is developed based upon a fixed volume of activity, such as number of patient days.

Budget, Fixed-Period. An approach to budgeting that identifies a period of time—for example, one month, one year, or two years—and develops a budget to cover that period of time.

Budget, Moving. A financial plan that always projects a fixed amount of time by deleting the most recent month's activity and adding another month's activity.

Budget, Operating. A financial plan that projects an organization's revenues, expenses, and profit or loss; the statement of purpose and statistical forecast expressed in financial terms.

Budget, Program or Project. A budget type that outlines costs and revenues for one specific program; for example, in-house collection of accounts.

Budget, Variable or Flexible. A financial plan that usually recognizes variable and fixed expenses and can be adjusted to the actual volume of activity.

Budget, Zero-Base. A budgeting system that requires an organization's responsibility centers to periodically justify their existence with a decision package for management that describes the center's costs, revenues, and benefits to the entire organization. Management prioritizes each decision package to meet the organization's desired total budgeted revenues and expenses.

Budgetary Control System. A management system that utilizes budgets to forecast and monitor the facility's costs and productivity.

Capital Expenditure. A fixed asset that generally has a useful life of more than one year.

Capital Expenditure Plan. As part of the organization's budgetary control system, the capital expenditure plan represents management's perception of the organization's capital needs for a long period of time—usually a minimum of three years.

Capitation Funding. A variation of prospective reimbursement whereby the organization agrees to deliver the needed products and/or services for a fixed per-capita amount per period. Healthcare maintenance organizations (HMOs) operate under such funding.

Cash Flow. The recording and forecasting of the cash that an organization collects and disburses.

Cash Flow Forecast. A document that attempts to project the amount of cash an organization will receive and disburse over a period of time.

Cash Inflow. The amount of cash that an organization receives from all sources.

Cash Outflow. The amount of cash that an organization pays out to all sources.

Chart of Accounts. A list of account titles with numerical symbols designed for compiling financial data regarding an organization's assets, liabilities, equity, revenues, and expenses.

Concurrent Audit. A billing audit that is conducted before the issuance of an interim or final bill.

Contractual Allowance. The difference between the healthcare facility's published rates and the cost deemed allowable by the third-party payer.

Contribution. The dollar difference between a service's net price and its variable cost.

Contribution Margin. The difference, expressed as a percentage, between the net price of a service and the variable cost of the service.

Core Positions or Staff. The minimum number and variety of positions with which a department can operate; these positions typically are considered to be fixed costs.

Cost-Benefit Analysis. A financial examination of the cost to produce a product or service and the financial and nonfinancial benefits derived from the product/service.

Cost Center. Term used to identify a department or an area that is responsible for an assigned group of expenses and/or revenues; also known as a responsibility center.

Cost Finding. The process of allocating the costs of a facility's nonrevenue-producing departments to each other and to the facility's revenue-producing departments. An integral part of an organization's budgetary control system, cost finding forms the basis for its rate-setting process.

Costs. *See also* **Expenses.**

Costs, Accounting. Costs determined in accordance with generally accepted accounting principles; the organization's total financial requirements are not a consideration.

Costs, Actual. Incurred expenses that can be supported by documentation.

Costs, Attainable. A type of standard cost that allows for downtime and lost time, yet it is strict enough to encourage improved productivity and to give employees a sense of achievement when they reach the standard.

Costs, Basic. A static standard cost type, thereby providing a basis for comparing actual costs. However, due to this standard's inflexibility, it cannot reflect market fluctuations or changes in costs and methods.

Costs, Direct. Costs for which a department manager is responsible and usually has the ability to control.

Costs, Economic. A healthcare facility's costs, other than operating, which might include such items as education, research, bad debts, working capital, and community health programs.

Costs, Fixed. Total departmental costs that usually do not change, regardless of changes in volume of activity (i.e., depreciation, insurance, management salaries, etc.).

Costs, Ideal. A type of standard cost, ideal costs represent the absolute minimum cost possible under the best conceivable operating conditions.

Costs, Indirect. Costs that are allocated to a using department, such as computer services, electricity, and heat, and for which the department manager has relatively little control over the amount charged.

Costs, Inflation. Costs incurred to spend at the same previous rate whose costs have increased due to the nation's inflation. Inflation costs are usually expressed as a percentage.

Costs, Operating. Costs incurred during the normal course of carrying out the day-to-day functions of a department or facility.

Costs, Opportunity. Costs or lost revenue caused if assets, goods, or services are applied to an alternative use.

Costs, Programmed. Cost that are usually fixed for the year, but are scheduled to be spent at irregular intervals; i.e., staff development programs at professional institutes, insurance premiums, etc.

Costs, Replacement. Costs incurred to replace any capital equipment.

Costs, Social. Costs that management knowingly or unknowingly imposes on general or specific segments of society as a result of its decision, such as the closing of an AIDS clinic, etc.

Costs, Standard. The average, usually annual, cost of variable-cost items, calculated by dividing the total annual cost by the total annual volume of activity. For example: total cost of office supplies divided by the total number of admissions.

Costs, Step-Variable. Costs that may change abruptly at intervals according to relevant range of volume activity.

Costs, Variable. Total departmental costs that usually change in direct proportion to the volume of the department's activity; i.e., food, office supplies, part-time salaries, etc.

Current Ratio. A liquidity ratio that determines the ratio between a facility's current assets and current liabilities.

Deduction from Gross (Patient) Revenue. The difference between the healthcare provider's gross (published) charges and the amount of cash received for payment; the result is net patient revenue (*see* **Allowances, Administrative, Contractual, and Charity.**)

Delegation of Responsibility. The process of assigning specific organizational and/or departmental functions to specific individuals; the authority guidelines to perform these functions are usually clearly defined.

Departmental Productivity. The analysis of a department's total production units generated over a period of time (i.e., month, year, etc.) divided by the number of person-hours worked and/or paid during the same period of time.

Deposits, Patient. Money given to a healthcare facility, usually at the time of admission, to be applied against the patient's total stay in the facility; more appropriately called a prepayment.

Depreciation. An accounting procedure that amortizes, as a noncash operating expense, the cost of a fixed asset over the useful life of the asset.

Depreciation, Funded. A systematic method of depositing cash in a specific fund for the express purpose of replacement and/or purchase of capital assets. The healthcare organization's monthly provision for depreciation serves as the basis for determining the amount to be deposited; i.e., 100 percent, 75 percent, 50 percent, 115 percent, etc., depending upon the amount of cash available at the time of deposit.

Diagnosis-related Groups (DRGs). A system of prospective payments to a healthcare provider, usually a healthcare facility, that is all-inclusive for the services a patient receives in the facility based upon the diagnosis; initiated by the Medicare program.

Direct Allocation. A cost-finding method that allocates the costs of the nonrevenue-producing centers only to the revenue-producing centers.

This method does not allocate any of the costs of the nonrevenue-producing centers to the other nonrevenue-producing centers, and it does not compensate for the different demand levels for nonrevenue-producing departments' services to revenue-producing departments.

Documentation. Written confirmation that serves as evidence that a transaction actually occurred.

Double Apportionment Method. Also known as the double-distribution method, this cost-finding approach recognizes that nonrevenue-producing centers render service to other nonrevenue-producing centers as well as to revenue-producing centers. Under this method, nonrevenue-producing centers are not considered permanently closed after management has allocated their costs. Instead, they are re-opened in the second part of the apportionment process to receive allocated costs from other nonrevenue-producing centers from which they have received services.

Duties, Separation of. Separation of duties and/or functions to assure that no individual or department is totally responsible for all of the related activities; i.e., cash received, cash deposited, bank reconciliation, crediting accounts receivable accounts, etc.

Elasticity. Amount of variance between the minimum and maximum number of labor hours and/or cost to provide a required service. For example, a core staff of a given size can handle a suddenly lower volume of activity (negative elasticity) or a suddenly higher volume of activity (positive elasticity) for a period of time.

Electronic Data Interchange (EDI). The exchange, among organizational entities, of computer-processable data in a standard format.

Entry Point. Location from which a patient enters a healthcare facility: inpatient admitting desk, emergency services, ambulatory admitting desk, etc.

Equity. The difference between the organization's total assets and its total liabilities.

Expectancy Levels. The level of anticipated production computed by multiplying the expected volume of activity by the sum of the normal standard time and the related P,F,&D factor.

Expense-to-Cash Ratio. The relationship between the total (direct and indirect) expense required by the provider to produce the related services or products and the amount of cash it actually received for the services.

Expenses. *See also* **Costs.**

Expenses, Committed. Sometimes called capacity expenses, committed expenses include all fixed expenses that are incurred in the operation of the plant, equipment, and basic or core staff. Examples are depreciation, ultilities, taxes, insurance, and salaries for key or core personnel.

Expenses, Planned or Budgeted. Those expenses that management predicts through the budgeting process or by estimates.

Expenses, Programmed. A fixed expense that arises periodically from management decision regarding policies. Examples of programmed expenses include insurance premiums, auditing fees, and training programs.

Expenses, Variable Noncapital and Nonsalary. Those cash outflow requirements that usually vary in direct proportion to the volume of work; i.e., patient days and outpatient visits.

External Audit. An audit conducted by an independent certified public accountant. This audit provides the public and the healthcare organization's governing board with an annual statement of opinion on the validity of the organization's fiscal-year statements. In addition, the external auditor appraises the organization's internal control systems and compares the organization's effectiveness and operations with those of similar institutions.

Fact Finding. The process of analyzing a certain system and/or procedure to determine how the system works; usually a preliminary process before decision making or systems design.

Feedback. Performance reporting (actual vs. planned) system that reports to the individual(s) responsible for managing a department or responsibility center.

Financial Analysis. The process of analyzing an organization's financial statements. Financial analysis can assist management in making rational decisions in keeping with the mission, goals, and objectives of the healthcare facility. It involves two types of comparisons: evaluating the facility's performance according to past, present, and forecasted ratio trends; and comparing the facility's ratios with those of another facility, or with a regional, state, or national industry average.

Financial Audit. An audit testing the integrity of the organization's accounting and statistical records.

Financial Ratios. Method for evaluating a facility's liquidity, leverage, activity, profitability, and profit planning, using data from a facility's financial statements.

Fiscal Intermediaries. Medicare claims agents and payers who have been approved by the Social Security Administration to act in this capacity.

Fiscal Year. An annual accounting period that need not begin on January 1 and end on December 31.

Float. An intangible and relatively uncontrollable amount of cash that the healthcare organization can use by taking advantage of cash in transit. Float represents the portion of the bank balance created by the time interval between the drawing of checks on the facility's account and the actual debiting of the account for those checks.

Flowcharting. Method used to diagram, through the use of symbols and lines, a procedure and/or system; frequently used in internal and/or external auditing. Gantt charts and PERT charts are common examples.

Full Financial Requirements. Those resources necessary for meeting current operating needs; permitting the physical plant's replacement when appropriate; and allowing for changing community health and patient needs, education and research, and all other factors necessary to the institutional provision of healthcare services.

Fund Balance. Term used in fund accounting to identify the equity of the fund.

Fund, Operating or General. An unrestricted fund used by a healthcare facility to record the receipt and disbursement of all of its cash.

Fund, Restricted. Fund that imposes a restriction on the healthcare facility, usually by the donor or grantor, as to how the fund is to be used.

Fund, Unrestricted. Fund that may be used as directed by the facility's management or governing board.

Gantt Chart. Flowcharting method, using time lines, for systematically recording and graphically illustrating tasks to be performed, the time the task is to be completed, the person responsible, etc.

General Ledger. All the asset, liability, equity, revenue, and expense accounts used by a facility; the total debit and credit balances of these must be equal.

Goals, Organizational. Usually a nonquantified ambition to be achieved by an organization, department, and/or an individual, supported by quantified objectives.

Goal-oriented. A person who is eager to accept challenges, wants definite goals, and feels a need to reach established objectives.

Health Care Financing Administration (HCFA). The federal agency that administers the financing of governmental medical programs, such as Medicare and Medicaid.

Health Maintenance Organization (HMO). A managed-care plan that offers a menu of healthcare services to its members by its preferred providers; usually, members prepay for the services to be received through monthly premiums.

Health Record. A compilation of data supporting and describing an individual's healthcare encounter, including data on diagnoses, treatment, and outcome. The health record was formerly called a medical record or a clinical record.

Humantology of Budgeting. The tempered and responsive application, by management, of a structured and individual assignment of functional responsibilities within a relevant range of authority, based upon the principles of mutual faith and trust among the working associates, and knowledgeable and active participation by these people in their endeavor to achieve the organization's established, acceptable, and attainable mission, goals, and objectives.

Imprest Fund. A fixed amount of cash set aside for a specific purpose, such as patient refunds, petty cash, and payroll, whose total is always maintained by replacing the exact amount paid out.

Incurred-but-Not-Reported (IBNR) Claims. Unknown, unreceived payment claims (liabilities) from a healthcare provider that has rendered service to a member of the provider's healthcare plan, usually a managed-care plan.

Internal Audit. An independent appraisal function established within an organization to examine and evaluate its activities as a service to the organization. The objective of internal auditing is to assist members of the organization in the effective discharge of their responsibilities. To this end, internal auditing furnishes them with analyses, appraisals, recommendations, counsel, and information concerning the activities reviewed. The audit objective includes promoting effective internal controls at reasonable cost.

Internal Control. A group of accounting systems and procedures designed to systematically and automatically serve as safeguards to protect the integrity of the organization's accounting information. It also assists the organization's management team by building automatic devices into the management information system to ensure compliance with established policies, systems, and procedures.

Job Analysis. The process of analyzing, through the use of observations, conversations, etc., one specific job to identify the function the position is performing. This process is usually required before job descriptions can be documented.

Job Description. The process of documenting the functions one specific position (job) is required to perform. In addition, the description may include such information as immediate supervisor, job code and labor grade, primary and secondary functions, and qualifications.

Journals. *See* **Accounting Journals.**

Ledger. The groups of accounts used in recording the organization's transactions—a book of secondary entry.

Leverage Ratios. Ratios that measure the equity generated by the healthcare facility compared with the financing provided by the facility's creditors. These ratios include, but are not limited to, the debt ratio, the times interest earned ratio, and the fixed-charges coverage ratio.

Liquidity Ratios. Ratios that help to identify and evaluate the healthcare facility's ability to meet its maturing short-term (current liabilities) obligations. These ratios include, but are not limited to, the following: current, quick, and acid test.

Liabilities, Current. Debts due within one year or less.

Lost Charges. Services that were rendered by the health care provider, but, for some reason or other, were never charged to the patient's account.

Manage. To handle or direct with a degree of skill or address.

Managed Care. A risk-based contract and/or plan, usually lasting for one-year intervals, between the healthcare provider and a healthcare purchaser; payment for anticipated services is usually based on monthly premiums paid (per capita) to the healthcare provider by the purchaser.

Management, Multilateral. A management style that encourages the involvement of the organization's entire staff or part of it, such as Theory Y and/or Z.

Management Planning. The process management uses to organize and to plan strategy to successfully achieve an identified mission and its set of objectives in an orderly and systematic way.

Management, Unilateral. A management style that tends to be somewhat autocratic, such as Theory X.

Management Style. The manner in which a manager chooses to organize, control, and delegate the responsibilities of a department responsibility center; Theories X, Y, and Z are the most popular methods of classifying management styles.

Margin of Safety. The percentage by which net patient revenue can decline before the healthcare organization experiences a loss.

Market Segmentation. A technique commonly used in market analysis, market segmentation divides the entire market into groups and subgroups by using relevant characteristics of the entire population. This process helps to pinpoint opportunities for improvement.

Mission Statement. The overall purpose of the organization and/or department, supported by goals and objectives.

Negotiated Rate. A rate or price that is mediated between a healthcare provider, i.e., hospital, physician, etc. and a healthcare purchaser, i.e., insurance company, HMO, employer, etc. for a list of healthcare services at a predetermined rate for an established length of time.

Net Worth. The equity of a healthcare organization, computed by subtracting total liabilities from total assets.

Noncash Expense Items. Expenses, such as depreciation (the amortization of a capital asset), that are included in a healthcare facility's statement of operations, but do not require any cash outlay during the reporting period; the cash outlay was made when the capital asset was purchased.

Nonoperating Revenue. Revenue received by a healthcare organization that is not directly related to the care and treatment of patients; e.g., interest earned, grants, etc.

Nonrevenue-producing Departments. Departments and/or responsibility centers of a healthcare provider that usually do not generate revenue for the services they produce; e.g., medical records, dietary, laundry, etc.

Nonsalary Expenses. All operating expenses that are not directly related to employees' compensation; include contract and/or purchased service labor.

Normal Task Time. The average amount of time required to perform a task; usually used as the basis for calculating a standard time.

Objective, Organizational. Generally, a quantified objective or strategy that may identify the person responsible, date to be completed, method for evaluating performance, and budget impact. The objective supports a goal.

Operational Audit. An audit that concentrates on systems in an effort to spot weaknesses. In addition to ensuring the effectiveness of the healthcare organization's operational systems, this audit also ensures the systems' conformity to management goals and objectives.

Operating Manual. A manual, usually loose-leaf, of all of the department and/or organization's standard plans.

Operating Revenue. Revenue generated by a healthcare organization for the care and/or treatment of a patient.

Organizational Chart (Structure). A graphic chart that identifies a healthcare organization's major function areas (financial services, general services, medical services, nursing services) together with their respective departments (patient financial services, dietary medical and surgical nursing, laboratory). Separate detailed organizational charts may be developed to identify individual employees.

Organization Structure. A description, usually in chart form with delegated lines of responsibility, of a healthcare organization. The structure is frequently used as the basis for establishing the organization's chart of accounts and its management reporting system.

Overhead. Expenses that a department usually cannot control, such as electricity, heat, light, and power, yet may be charged to the using department based upon some statistical and/or cost analysis.

P,F,&D Factor. A time factor that is added to the normal standard task performance time to allow for personal time, fatigue, and other delays.

Patient Days. The number of days a patient stays in the healthcare facility; usually counted from midnight census to midnight census.

Patient Financial Services. The department or division of a healthcare organization responsible for the organization, management, and control of, but not limited to, the following functions: preadmission, admission, billing, cashiering, discharging, and collection of patient accounts receivable.

Patient Service Representative (PSR). An organizational structure that assigns to one PSR the admitting, billing, collection, and other functions and communications for processing a specific patient's accounts receivable. Patients are usually assigned to specific PSRs by sections of the alphabet. For example: PSR #1, A–F; PSR #2, G–K; etc.

Per Capita. A prospective payment system that is usually a monthly payment to a healthcare provider, such as an HMO, to pay for services to be received by the contracting individual.

Per Case. An all-inclusive prospective system of payment for healthcare services that includes all the services a patient receives during the stay. *See* **Diagnosis-related Groups.**

Per Diem. An all-inclusive prospective method of payment for healthcare services that includes all services received by a patient during one patient day.

Per Service. Also known as a la carte, this prospective payment system charges the patient only for each service purchased or received; each service has a specific price.

Performance, Departmental. The total number of production units, such as billings and admissions, produced by a department for a period of time.

Performance, Employee. The total number of production units produced by one employee for a period of time.

Performance Evaluation. A comparison of the planned amount of production units expected to be produced, either by a department and/or an employee, with the actual amount of production units generated over a period of time.

Performance Factor. The result, usually expressed as a percentage, of dividing the normal productive time by the sum of the total reported productive time and the delay time (P,F,&D). Performance factors are determined by management to differentiate expected performance levels from the standard normal times. For example, the standard normal time may be ten billings per hour; a new clerk might be expected to perform at only 75 percent of this capacity.

Performance Standards. A predetermined level of productivity for a machine, employee, department, etc.

Petty Cash. A fixed amount of cash set aside as daily working cash to pay for small purchases, and not necessarily recorded in the facility's accounts payable.

Planning. The act or process of making or carrying out plans; the establishment of goals, policies, and procedures for a social or economic unit.

Policy. A general plan of action, usually approved by the organization's governing board, that guides the healthcare organization's personnel in their conduct and daily operations.

Preferred Provider. A healthcare provider that has been approved by a healthcare purchaser (HMO, managed-care plan, etc.) as a provider of healthcare services to its members.

Procedure. A systematic, usually documented, method of how a policy and related organizational plan is to be performed.

Product. A service, within a product line, that is generated by a healthcare provider; e.g., normal delivery, emergency service, etc.

Product Line. A group of related products or services that are produced by a healthcare provider; e.g., surgical services, women's health, cardiopulmonary, etc.

Production Standard. A predetermined amount of work, such as the number of billings per hour, expected to be performed by an employee for an established amount of time.

Production Unit. A quantitative measurement of work performed.

Production Unit, Macro. A quantitative measurement of service produced by a healthcare department that usually does not have any relationship to the amount of resources required to generate the service; e.g., patient day, outpatient visit, laboratory test, etc.

Production Unit, Micro. A quantitative measurement of service produced by a healthcare department that usually does have a direct relationship to the amount of resources required to generate the service. Examples: ICU patient day, thirty-minute emergency room visit, Medicare inpatient billing, CAP unit values for laboratory tests.

Productivity. The ratio of outputs (e.g., a department's services) to the amount of inputs (resources) over a specific period of time.

Profit and Loss Statement (P&L). Usually referred to as the healthcare provider's statement of operations, which reports the organization's revenue, expenses, and profit or loss for a period of time.

Profitability Ratios. Ratios measuring the organization's overall effectiveness in terms of generating profits compared with the facility's revenue and investment.

Program Evaluation and Review Technique (PERT). A flowcharting method that does not use time lines and assists in planning and scheduling the sequence of individual project tasks and in reviewing the project as a whole; occasionally referred to as the critical path method (CPM).

Programmed Expenditures. Noncapital, nonsalary cash flow requirements, such as utilities, rent and/or leases, insurance, and mortgage payments. These expenses are essential to provide the facilities and equipment necessary to perform services to patients.

Prospective Payment System. A method used to establish the amount (price) of payment a healthcare organization is going to receive before the service is rendered; e.g., per service (a la carte), per diem, per case, per capita.

Published Charges. Charges that appear on a patient's bill; the provider's gross charges.

Rate Setting. The process a healthcare organization uses to establish the gross prices it will charge all of its patients.

Ratio of Charges to Charges (RCC). A costing distribution method that systematically appropriates a healthcare facility's total charges to a user's charges and uses this ratio to distribute the facility's total expenses to the user's share of the costs.

Relative Value Unit (RVU). A micro, quantitative method for measuring the productivity of a department and/or an employee. College of American Pathologists (CAP) units are an example.

Relevant Range of Activity. The length of the volume of activity certain resources can serve before requiring additional resources. For example: three PSRs can serve five hundred admissions; for more than that, one additional PSR is required.

Resource Based Relative Value Scale (RBRVS). An example of a weighted unit of measurement, which reflects the mix of micro service-unit outputs for various departments. The RBRVS groups the inputs necessary to provide physician services into three categories: physician work, practice expenses, and opportunity costs.

Responsibility Budgeting. A method for budgeting, accounting, and reporting the revenues and/or expenses incurred by one specific department manager; usually ties in directly with the facility's organizational structure.

Retrospective Audit. A billing audit conducted after the issuance of an interim or final bill.

Retrospective Payment System. A payment system that a healthcare purchaser uses to pay a healthcare provider at the provider's actual cost of services purchased. Reconciliation of costs and interim payments is always made after the services are generated and received.

Revenue, Deferred. A current liability that records the receipt of payment for services not rendered to the purchaser.

Revenue-producing Departments. Departments of a healthcare facility that typically generate revenue for the services it produces, such as radiology, laboratory, and pharmacy.

Salary Expenses. All expenses incurred by a healthcare facility that are directedly related to the payment of services (e.g., salaries, wages, Social Security) of its full- and part-time employees; usually includes only those employees whose earnings are reported to the Internal Revenue Service on W-2 forms, and does not include contract or purchased service labor.

Self-balancing Funds. A collection of asset, liability, and equity accounts which, when summarized and totaled, can be organized into a standard statement of condition or balance sheet. These types of accounts are frequently found in a fund accounting system.

Self-paying. A patient in a healthcare facility who does not have any insurance coverage and is usually totally responsible for the payment of his/her health care; otherwise, it designates an account that has received the third-party insurance payment and has a balance due and payable by the patient.

Sensitivity Testing. An extended variation of break-even analysis, sensitivity testing is the process of taking known factors and evaluating them under changing conditions. Since price is the only variable factor in the break-even formula, it lends itself uniquely to this testing.

Span of Control. A cardinal rule of organizational structuring which states that there is a limit on the number of subordinates reporting to one supervisor. Usually, the higher a supervisor is in the organization management hierarchy, the fewer subordinates will be reporting to him/her.

Standard Cost. The amount of any specific expense-variable item per production unit.

Standard Plans. A set of organizational plans that are separated into policies, procedures, and methods to assure management's uniform application of them.

Standard Rate. This term can refer either to an average or actual charge for an individual service generated by a revenue-producing department, the average rate an employee is paid per hour, or the average cost per production unit.

Standard Task Time. The calculated amount of time required to perform a task that includes the normal task time plus a factor for P,F,&D.

Statement of Cash Flow. A report that lists all cash inflows (receipts) and cash outflows (disbursements), together with the healthcare facility's beginning and ending cash balance, for a period of time.

Statement of Condition. Sometimes known as a balance sheet, this statement lists a facility's total assets, liabilities, and equity as recorded at one specific time.

Statement of Operations. Sometimes known as an income statement and/or profit and loss statement, this statement reports a facility's total revenue, expenses, and profit or loss for a period of time.

Statement of Purpose. An element of the organization's budgetary control system, this statement is a narrative report that identifies and quantifies a department's mission, goals, and objectives; assumptions; strategy to be used to obtain these goals and objectives; required resources; and standards of acceptable or expected performance.

Statement of Source and Use of Funds. A financial statement that reports the use of funds (current assets) and the source of funds (current liabilities) from one specific time period to another; the information is typically gathered from the healthcare facility's statement of condition.

Statistical Forecast. A component of the organization's budgetary control system, this forecast forms the basis for all financial projections. Inpatient and outpatient statistics comprising the plan include admissions, discharges, preadmissions, initial billings, follow-up billings, and accounts in file.

Stepdown Method. Also known as the single-apportionment method, this approach to cost finding recognizes that services rendered by certain nonrevenue-producing centers are used by other nonrevenue-producing centers as well as by revenue-producing centers or departments. The significant feature of this method is that once the costs of a nonrevenue-producing center have been allocated to other centers, the center is considered "closed."

T Account. Named for its shape, the T account is an informal tool used in double-entry accounting to record debits and credits. It serves as the substitute for a formal ledger account and appears on analysis sheets to assist the accountant in analyzing a transaction.

Target Production Level. The result of the sum of the adjusted standard hours produced, the other scheduled staff hours, and the on-call scheduled hours.

Task-oriented. A person who simply wants to do his/her particular job and has little interest in overall results.

Theory X. As promoted by Douglas McGregor, a Theory X manager believes that the average employee has an inherent dislike for work and, if possible, will avoid it. Because of this assumption, the manager must coerce, control, direct, and threaten with punishment to get the employees to work toward the organization's goals and objectives.

Theory Y. Another theory promoted by Douglas McGregor, which states that work to an employee is as natural as play or rest. The average employee does not inherently dislike work, and may find it to be a source of satisfaction. Because work will be voluntarily performed, external control or threats by management are not the only ways for the organization to achieve its goals and objectives.

Theory Z. A theory developed by William Ouchi, in contrast with McGregor's Theory X and Y, Theory Z states that the average employee possesses simultaneously the characteristics of Theories X and Y and that the overriding challenge to the manager is to create an environment in which all employees, by consensus, produce the desired goals and objectives of the organization.

Third-Party Payer. One who pays for a service or product on behalf of another individual or subscriber. The Medicare program, for example, pays a healthcare facility for services rendered to the program's subscribers.

Time-Lag Factor. An amount of time required to occur before the desired result happens. For example: the amount of time from the day a billing is mailed to the time payment is received.

Time Value of Money. The value of money to be received or to be disbursed is directly related to the timing of its receipt or disbursement.

Trial Balance. A listing of all control and/or subsidiary accounts of healthcare organization.

Transaction. Any intra- or inter-exchange of goods or services of a healthcare organization which serves as the basis of documenting and accounting for its financial activities.

Turnover, Accounts Receivable. Number of times the gross or net accounts receivable account turns over during one year computed by dividing the facility's total gross and/or net patient revenues by the facility's gross and/or net accounts receivable account total at the end of the year.

Unbilled Charges. A situation occurring when the volume of services indicated on a bill is less than the volume identified in a provider's health record documentation. Also known as undercharges.

Unity of Command. A cardinal rule of organizational structuring which states that no subordinate should report to more than one supervisor.

Unsupported or Undocumented Charges. Also known as overcharges, this situation occurs when the volume of services indicated on a bill exceeds the total volume identified in a provider's health record documentation.

Variance, Efficiency. Difference between the planned (budgeted) amount of labor hours used to produce a projected volume of activity and actual number of labor hours used, multiplied by the position's standard hourly rate.

Variance, Rate. Difference between the planned (budgeted) dollar amount of labor and/or supply cost projected and the actual cost of the labor and/or supplies used.

Variance, Usage. A common method of analyzing the differences between budgeted and actual performance for nonsalary expenses, this variance is computed by multiplying the standard rate by the difference between the actual volume and the target volume.

Variance, Volume. A situation that occurs when expenses interact under changing conditions.

Volume of Activity. The amount of work performed over a period of time; work is expressed in either macro or micro production units.

Working Capital. Excess of current assets over current liabilities (WC = CA − CL); represents the amount of current funds required to finance the healthcare organization. *See* **Statement of Source and Use of Funds.**

Index

A
Accounting
    accrual, 36–39
    cash, 36–37
    documented proof of entries, 43
    double-entry, 34–36
    entry types, 34–36
    financial, 77
    financial, compared with managerial, 72
    financial, defined, 71–72
    functional, 142
    fund, 39–41
    managerial, *See* Managerial accounting
    period, 45
    principles of, 33–41
    process of, 45–49
    process application, 58–62
    responsibility, 42, 142, 144
    system, effective, 71
    system prerequisites, 41-43, 45
Accounts receivable
    AICPA's rules for reporting net patient, 69
    as cash flow source, 48
    control points in, 312
    cycle, 300–301
    determining opportunity costs of, 269–70
    electronic data interchange (EDI) in, 306–7
    gross, deducting allowances from, 69
    liquidity measurements, 267–70
    management of, 2, 299–307
    monitoring bad debts in, 303–6
    out for collection, 304
    payer classifications in, 300–301
    payment systems in, 301
    percentage of assets in, 299, 323
    segmentation of, 301–3
Adjusted standard hours required (ASHR), 131
American Guild of Patient Account Manage-
    ment (AGPAM), 320

American Hospital Association (AHA), 39, 42,
    186, 216, 217, 317
American Institute of Certified Public Accoun-
    tants (AICPA), 41
    Audits of Providers of Health Care Services,
    66
    Hospital Audit Guide, 67
    revised reporting requirements, 66–69
    rules for classifying bad debts, 68
    rules for classifying charity care, 68–69
    rules for reporting net patient accounts
        receivable, 69
    rules for reporting patient service
        revenues, 66–67
American National Standards Institute (ANSI),
    306
ASHR. *See* Adjusted standard hours required
Assets
    computing, 60
    capital, defined, 214
    capital, recording, 43
    current, 56, 57
    current, examples of, 57
    current, *See also* Working capital
    net current, *See* Working capital
Audit
    billing, 282, 290
    external vs. internal, 279–81
    financial vs. operational, 279
    internal, *See* Internal audit
Audits of Providers of Health Care Services, 66

B
Bad debts
    AICPA's rules for classifying, 68
    assessing patient risk of, 69
    as distinguished from charity care, 69
    from Medicare deductible and
        coinsurance, 215

and Medicare program, 183
monitoring, 303–6
as operating expense, 68
Balance sheet. *See* Statement, of condition
Berman, Howard J., 126, 150, 184, 204, 205
Blue Cross, 181, 206, 300, 301. *See also* Third-
party payers
BNA Medicare Reporter, 216
Borrowings and investments
in cash flow forecast, 232–33
recording, 232–33
Break-even analysis
break-even formula, 265–66
contribution component, 264–65
contribution margin component, 265
margin of safety, 266–67
Break-even daily census, 155–56
Budget
appropriation, 145–46
in budgetary control system, 140–41
control, *See* Control budget
defined, 137, 140
fixed-period, 145
fixed or target system, 145
flexible, *See* Variable budget
operating, 150
program or project, 146
rolling or moving, 145
system types, 145–46
target, 157
variable, *See* Variable budget
variable or flexible system, 145
zero-base, 146
See also Budgetary control system;
Budgeting
Budgetary control system
approaches to 142, 144
budget's role in, 140–41
components of, 148–52
and cost finding, 181
cycle in, 151–52
defined, 137
feedback in, 150–51
functional accounting and budgeting
in, 142
"humantology" of, 138
managing for economic results, 140
and mission, goals, and objectives, 137
multilateral approaches to, 139–40
patient financial services manager's
role in, 141–42
performance evaluation in, 150–51
performance standards, 137

responsibility accounting and budgeting
in, 142, 144
See also Budget; Budgeting
Budgeting
Classification Tree, 147
functional approach, 142
"humantology" of, 138
responsibility approach, 142, 144
See also Budget; Budgetary control system

C
Capital. *See* Working capital
Capital expenditure plan
defined, 150
developing, 150
Capital expenditures, 232
Carnegie, Andrew, 19
Cash balances
and cash flow forecast, 150
ideal, 229
Cash flow analysis
daily form in, 49
patient financial services manager's
role in, 48–49
Cash flow forecast, 48
accrual vs. cash accounting in, 228
borrowings and investments in, 232–33
and cash disbursement analysis, 239–47
and cash receipts analysis, 233–38
components, 229–33
defined, 150, 227
facilitating, 150
importance of, 48
methods, 233–41, 243–46
patient financial services manager's role in,
140–41, 247–49
from patient revenue, 229
preparations for, 227–28
purposes of, 150, 228
Cash inflows, 48
and cash flow forecast, 150
increasing, 228–29
sources of, 229–31
time-lag factor, 227
See also Revenues
Cash outflows, 48
and cash flow forecast, 150
sources of, 231–32
time-lag factor, 228
See also Costs; Expenses
Cash receipts. *See* Cash inflows
CCH Medicare and Medicaid Guide, 216
Charges

published, 182, 198
published, forced inflation of, 211
published, third-party impact on,
206–13
See also Rates
Charity care
as deduction from gross patient service
revenue, 68–69
disclosing levels of, 69
as distinguished from bad debts, 69
Chart of accounts, 42–43, 60
classifying expense items in, 91
and cost classification, 153
Chart of Accounts for Hospitals, 39, 42
Code of Federal Regulations, 213
College of American Pathologists, 220
Compound accounting entries, 35–36
Contractual allowance, 206
Control
accounting, 278
administrative, 278
entry-point, 280
exit-point, 281
internal, *See* Internal control
processing-point, 280
span of, 10
Control budget, 89
defined, 163
developing, 96–96
volume of, and actual volume, 95
Cost analysis
of patient financial services department
expenses, 85–88
of patient financial services department
production units, 86–88
Cost-benefit analysis
of departmental objectives, 14, 15
Cost centers, 184–85
Cost finding
accuracy of, 125
and actual costs, 182
algebraic method, 188
applications, 182–84
as basis for rate setting, 181
and budgetary control system, 181
case study, 190, 193, 198
cost centers in, 184–185
direct-allocation method, 185–86
double-apportionment method, 186–88
double-distribution method, *See* Cost
finding, double-apportionment method
methods, 185–88
and nonrevenue-producing centers, 185,

186, 187, 188, 189
objectives of, 184
preventing less-than-cost reimbursement,
183
and production unit selection, 189
and ratio of charges to charges as applied
to costs, 68
revenue-producing centers, 185, 186, 188,
189
"short-formula 1" approach, 188
single-apportionment method, *See* Cost
finding, stepdown method
statistical bases in, 189, 190, 193
stepdown method, 186
system prerequisites, 184–85
traditional view of, in healthcare industry,
181
and valid results, 188–89
Costs
accounting, 204
actual, and cost finding, 182
actual, defined, 78
allocating, 125
allocating, *See also* Cost finding
budgeted, and cost finding, 182
comparisons of, 108
economic, 204
historical, *See* Costs, actual
operating, *See* Operating costs
opportunity, 75, 77
social, 77–78
variables in, 108.
See also Cash outflows; Expenses
Cost variability principle, 153
Credit entry, 34

D
Debit entry, 34
Delegation of authority
and organizational structure, 30
and standard plans, 30
Delegation of responsibility, 16–19
process of, 16
symptoms of weak, 16–19
Department of Health and Human Services,
183, 213
Depreciation
allocating expense of, 190
and cash flow forecast, 232
funded, 85
as noncash item, 150
Diagnosis-related groups (DRGs)
estimating cost of, 68

history of, 217
and Medicare program, 182
monitoring, 223
number of, 217
payments, 215
and prospective rate setting, 182
Disbursements of cash. *See* Cash outflows
Drucker, Peter F., 140, 205, 320

E
Elasticity
negative, 82
positive, 82
Electronic data interchange (EDI), 306–7
Employees
goal-oriented, 141
incentive plans for, 122–25
involvement, in budgetary control system
138–39
involvement, in production standard
development, 126, 133
involvement, in production standard
selection, 121–22
performance evaluation of, 120, 122
task-oriented, 141
See also Staffing
Equity
computation of, 46
defined, 46
synonyms for, 46
Expenses
applying behavioral principles of, 88–89,
91–92, 94–102
behavioral patterns of, 80, 82–84
capacity, *See* Expenses, committed
committed, 85
committed, controlling, 85
controllable, 84
direct variable, *See* Variable expenses
fixed, *See* Fixed expenses
global management of, 78
inflation, 84
noncontrollable, 84
overhead, controlling, 84
overhead, defined, 84
planned or budgeted, 78
programmed, 85
replacement, 84–85
salary and nonsalary, 150
segmented management of, 79–80
step-variable, *See* Step-variable expenses
variable, *See* Variable expenses
See also Cash outflows: Costs

F
Federal Register, 183, 214, 215
Federation of American Healthcare Systems
(FAHS), 216, 217, 317
Feedback, 11
in budgetary control system, 150–51
Financial Accounting Standards Board (FASB),
68–69
Financial Accounting Standards Board
Statement No. 6, "Elements of Financial
Statements," 69
Financial analysis
comparisons in, 252
defined, 251
ratio types, 254–56, 258–67
Fiscal year, 45
Fixed expenses
committed, 85
controlling, 80, 88
examples of nonsalary, 80, 231
examples of salary, 80
nature of, 80, 85
programmed, 85
Float, 233
Flowchart
of billing system, 282
critical path method (CPM), 291
Gantt method, 292, 298–99
and internal control, 290–99
of procedures, 27, 28
Program Evaluation and Review Technique
(PERT), 291–97
Forms, 28–29
Funding
capitation, 301
restricted, 40
unrestricted, 40

G
Generally accepted accounting principles
(GAAP), 72
Global expense management, 78
Goals
and the budgetary control system, 137
and statement of purpose, 148
Governing board, 25, 26
Graphs
in index trend analysis, 73
of performance analysis information,
120
to represent data, 73
Gross revenue
deductions from, 39

portion provided by alternative healthcare financing systems, 62

H
Healthcare Financial Management Association (HFMA), 42, 216, 217, 320
  Principles and Practices Board, 40–41
Heath Care Financing Administration (HCFA), 183
  approved cost-finding methods, 185
  audits of Medicare bad debts, 215
  basis for provider payments, 214
  research and development department, 215
Healthcare industry
  accepted accounting costs in, 204
  future trends in, 323–25
  growth of managed-care contracting in, 321
  productivity rate, 133
  traditional view of cost finding, 181
Healthcare organizations
  and advertising, 311
  board of directors, 140
  as a business, 203–4
  chief executive officer (CEO), 140
  chief executive officer, responsibilities prescribed by JCAHO, 228
  chief financial officer's (CFO's) role, 33
  comprehensive budget of, 154
  credit extension in, 299–300
  departmental profitability evaluation, 188
  efficiency in, 122–23
  equity of, 46
  evaluating financial condition/performance, 251–54
  external environment of, 4
  financial position of, 46
  financial and statistical information in, 275
  financial viability of, 181, 203
  full financial requirements of, 203
  information system, 72
  and marketing to the family unit, 315–16
  marketing program functions, 310–11
  marketing program mission, 310
  marketing of services, 309
  and market research, 311
  medical staff, communicating with, 3
  and Medicare reimbursement regulations, 216
  need for profit in, 205

percentage of assets in accounts receivable, 299
  and planning for future growth, 214
  product-line profitability monitoring, 222–223, 225
  and public relations, 311
  and published charges, *See* Charge, published
  See also Governing board; Internal audit; Internal control
Health maintenance organizations (HMOs), 301
  allocating expenses to, 68
  and per-capita rate setting, 218
  as significant percentage of healthcare organization's revenue, 62
Hospital Audit Guide, 67
Hospitals & Health Networks, 317
"Humantology" of budgeting, 138
Hy, Ronald, J., 301

I
Imprest cash account, 239
Incentive plans of employees, 122–25
Incurred-but-not-reported (IBNR) claims, 62, 65
  monitoring, 66
Indexes, 73
Inflation, 84
Institute of Internal Auditors, 276
Internal audit
  activities, 276
  auditors' reporting pattern, 277
  auditors' responsibilities, 281–82
  defined, 276
  element of surprise in, 277
  vs. external auditing, 279–81
  instruments for, 281–82, 283–90
  and management information integrity, 275
  as a managerial tool 276
Internal control
  accounting controls, 278
  administrative controls, 278
  benefits, 277
  defined, 277
  elements in, 277–78
  fundamental principle of, 280
  influenced by department mission, 4
  and management information integrity, 275
  need for regular program review, 278–79

J
Job analysis, 19–20
Job description, 20–22
    form, contents of, 113
    purpose of, 22
Joint Commission on Accreditation of
        Healthcare Organizations (JCAHO), 228
Journal, 43, 45
    types, 45

K
Kukla, Steven F., 126, 150, 184, 204, 205

L
Ledger, 43, 45
    general, 46, 60
    types, 45
Liabilities
    current, 56
    current, defined, 255
    current, examples of, 57

M
McConkey, Dale, 16
McGregor, Douglas, 2
Managed-care contracts, 218
    costing and pricing, 182
    and gross revenue concept, 67
    growth of, 321
    monitoring, 223
    as potential liability accounts, 62, 65
Managed-care organizations, 68
Management, 1
    of accounts receivable, 2, 299–307
    decisions, impact on social costs, 83–84
    and delegation of responsibility, 16–19
    for economic results, 140
    effective, 2
    styles, 2
    of subordinates, 10
    Theory X, 2
    Theory Y, 2
    Theory Z, 2
Management planning
    components, 6–7
    defined, 7
    and job analysis, 19–20
    and job description, 20–22
    operational, 11, 14–15
    organizational design and, 8–9
Management team, 42
Managerial accounting
    characteristics of effective information

        system, 72
    defined, 72
    and expense classification, 74–78
    and financial accounting, 72
    and managerial reporting, 72–74
Managerial reporting system
    developing, 72–74
    flexibility in, 73
    functions of, 72
Medicaid, 122, 206, 318
    and provider's economic requirements,
        204
    refining reporting and disbursement
        procedures, 215–16
    required cost allocation techniques, 188
    See also Third-party payers
Medical staff, 3
Medicare, 122, 181, 206, 318
    addressing deductible and coinsurance
        bad debts, 215
    and capital-related costs, 214–15
    congressional intent of, 211–12
    and day-to-day expenses, 215
    diagnosis-related groups in, *See*
        Diagnosis-related groups
    fiscal intermediaries, 183, 184, 193, 213
    and funds for future use, 213–14
    and gross revenue concept, 67
    interim payments in, 215
    "pass-through" cost items, 183–84
    periodic interim payments (PIP), 184
    prospective payment system of, 182, 183
    Provider Reimbursement Review Board
        (PRRB), 198
    and provider's economic requirements,
        204
    and reasonable-cost reimbursement, 213
    refining reporting and disbursement
        procedures, 215–16
    reimbursement improvements, 213–15
    required cost allocation techniques, 188
    retrospective payments, examples of, 183
    See also Health Care Financing Administra-
        tion; Prospective payment system;
        Third-party payers
Methods, 29–30
    defined, 27
Mission
    and the budgetary control concept, 137
    goals and objectives in, 5–6
    influences on, 4
    issues addressed in, 4
    nature of, 4

and performance evaluation, 6
and statement of purpose, 148
Motion time measurement (MTM) studies, 125
Multilateral approach, 11, 14, 15
    to budgeting, 139–40

N
*National Health Care Billing Audit Guide
    lines,* 290
National health insurance (NHI), 323
Net worth. *See* Equity
No-Nonsense Delegation, 16
Nonrevenue-producing centers, 185, 186, 187,
    188, 189
Nonsalary variance analysis, 99–101
    types of, 99
Normal task time, 126–27

O
Objectives
    approaches to setting departmental, 11
    and the budgetary control system, 137
    and employee performance, 126
    functions of, 6
    and internal audit, 276
    and statement of purpose, 148
Operating costs
    defined, 204
    managing, 78–80
    productivity's impact on, 133
    types of, 75
Operational plan, 11, 14–15
Organizational design, 8–9
    developing, 8
    and patient service representative (PSR)
        system, 10, 13
    rules of, 10
Organizational structure
    and delegation of authority, 30
    format, 42
    as a standard plan, 25
    testing for effectiveness, 42

P
Patient financial services department
    admission procedure, 314
    audit instrument, 281–82, 283–90
    controlling expenses in, 78–80
    cost analysis, 85–88
    cost-effectiveness maximization, 153
    discharge procedure, 314–15
    fixed expenses in, 157
    functions of, 2–3

goals and objectives, 5–6
historical evaluation of, 107
ideal work environment, 1–2
and in-house patient care, 314
maximizing service reimbursement, 125
mission, 4–5
operating cost evaluation, 84–85
operating manual, 30–31
and patient service representative (PSR)
    system, 10, 13
performance evaluation of, 6
performance evaluation ratio, 112
and postdischarge care, 315
preadmission procedure, 312–14
primary goal, 2
staff turnover rate, 273
standard plans in, 25–31
traditional design, 10, 12
Patient financial services managers
    certification programs for, 320
    and employee incentive plans, 122–25
    and employee performance evaluation,
        120, 122
    expanding responsibilities of, 318
    functions of, 3
    future trends to monitor, 323–25
    historical evaluation of performance,
        107–8
    identifying and quantifying goals, 139
    identifying and quantifying objectives, 139
    involvement in budgetary control process,
        138–39
    involvement in comprehensive budget,
        140
    and maximizing service reimbursement,
        125
    and methods, 29–30
    and multilateral approach to budgeting,
        139–40
    opportunity areas for, 322–23
    and policies, 25, 26–27
    position history, 318–19
    position title, 319
    preparing for career, 325–27
    primary role, 1
    and procedures, 27–29
    qualifications of, 319–20
    role in cash flow analysis, 48–49
    role in cash flow forecasting, 140–41, 227,
        247–49
    role in cost finding, 181
    role in developing managerial reporting
        system, 72–74

role in managed-care contracts, 321–22
role in marketing, 312–15
role in organizing patient financial services
 department, 1–3
and strategic planning, 321–22
and uniform claims processing, 320
and variable budget methodology, 89
Patient service representative (PSR) position
 possible functions of, 19–20
 possible qualifications, 20
Patient service representative (PSR) system,
 10, 13
 organizational structure, 142–44
Patient service revenues
 AICPA's rules for reporting, 66–68
 and charity care, 68–69
Performance, 14
Performance evaluation, 6
 in budgetary control system, 150–51
 of department, 118, 120
 of employees, 120, 122
 precise, 108
 in productivity improvement program, 107
 and standard plans, 30
Performance factor
 calculating, 131
 function of, 131
Performance standard, 21
 and the budgetary control system, 137
 defined, 15
 departmental, 11
 individual, 11
 and job description form, 113
 and production units, 113
 and statement of purpose, 148
 See also Production standard
Personal, fatigue, and delay (P,F,&D) factor,
 129
Personal, fatigue, and delay (P,F,&D) time,
 126
PERT. *See* Program Evaluation and Review
 Technique
Planning
 management, 1–22
 operational, 11, 14–15
 standard, 25–31
Policy, 25–27
 governing board's role in, 25, 26
 patient financial services manager's role in,
 25, 26
Positions
 core, 118
 step-variable, 115

variable, 115–16
 See also Staffing
Preferred provider organizations (PPOs), 62
Procedures, 27–29
 defined, 27
 written, forms of, 27–28
Production, 14
Production standards
 approaches to developing, 125
 consistent use of, 133
 developing, 125–27, 129–31, 133
 involvement approach, 126
 predetermined approach, 125–26
 See also Performance standard
Production unit
 calculating expenses per, 86
 College of American Pathologists' relative
  value unit system, 220
 in cost allocating, 125
 cost curve, 86
 and cost finding, 189
 defined, 86, 107
 in departmental performance evaluation,
  118, 120
 in employee inventive plans, 124
 employee involvement in selecting, 115
 in employee performance evaluation, 120,
  122
 examples of, 107
 importance of, 109
 importance of consistent application, 125
 macro or gross, 109–10
 and measuring department effectiveness,
  109
 micro or weighted, 110–12
 and performance standards, 113
 and rate setting, 112, 189
 and reimbursement maximization, 125
 and relative value units (RVUs), 110–11,
  112, 189, 219
 and relative value units, computing cost
  of, 220
 selecting, 112–13
 selection criteria for, 112
 in staffing and budgetary control, 115–18
 uses, 114–18, 120, 122–25
Productivity
 defined, 107
 of employees, 107
 growth, 107
 impact on operating costs. 133
 improvement program for, 107–34
 improvement program, effective, 107–9

need for improvement in, 133
rate, in healthcare industry, 133
standard rates' impact on, 89
Product line
    defined, 222
    expenses-to-cash ratio and, 222–23
    monitoring profitability of, 222–23, 225
Prospective Payment Assessment Commission
        (ProPAC)
    functions of, 215–16
    and prospective payment system profit
        margins, 214
Prospective payment system (PPS), 301
    and gross revenue concept, 67
    healthcare facilities exempt from, 213
    and profit earning, 183
    profit margins of, 214
Prospective rate setting
    common use of, 182
    defined, 182
    and diagnosis-related groups (DRGs), 182
    and managed-care contracts, 182
Public Law 92–603, 301

Q
Quality circle, 2

R
Rate
    a la carte method, *See* Rate, per-service
        method
    all-inclusive method, *See* Rate, per-diem
        method
    per-capita method, 218
    per-case or diagnosis method, 217–18
    per-diem method, 217, 218–19
    per-diem method, advantages of, 219
    per-diem method, determining, 218
    per-diem method, disadvantages, 219
    per-diem method, and reporting revenue,
        68
    per-service method, 217, 219–20
    turnover, 260
Rate setting
    ideal policy, 223-24
    methods, 217–20
    methods, *See also* Rate
    and production units, 112
    and production unit selection, 189
    prospective, *See* Prospective rate setting
    sensitivity testing and, 220–21
    statistical bases in, 189
    traditional philosophy of, 204–5

Ratios
    accounts receivable to turnover rate, 268
    acid test, 256, 258
    activity, 260–63
    average collection period, 268
    charges to charges as applied to costs
        (RCCAC), 68
    current, 256
    debt, 259
    defined, 251
    employee turnover rate, 272
    expense-to-cash, 222–23
    fixed assets turnover, 262
    fixed-charges coverage, 260
    inventory turnover to charges, 261
    inventory turnover to purchases, 262
    leverage, 258–60
    liquidity, 255–56, 258
    patient receivables to charges, 268
    patient receivables to current and total
        assets, 269
    patient receivables to equity, 269
    profitability, 263–64
    profit margin on gross charges, 263
    profit margin on net charges, 263–64
    profit-planning, 264–67
    return on equity, 264
    return on total assets, 264
    times interest earned, 259
    total assets turnover, 263
Relevant range of activity, 82
Reporting
    external, 71
    internal, 71
Resource Based Relative Value Scale (RBRVS),
        220
Revenue. *See* Gross revenue
Revenue and expense statement. *See* State-
        ment, of operations
Revenue-producing centers, 185, 186, 188,
        189
Risk-based contracts. *See* Managed-care
        contracts
Roosevelt, Franklin D., 327

S
Salary variance analysis, 97–99
    types of, 97, 98
Seawell, L. Vann, 33, 43, 139, 183, 205, 278,
        282, 291
Segmented expense management, 79–80
Self-paying patient, 300
    subsidizing third-party patients, 206–7, 211

vs. third-party payers, 204
Sensitivity testing, 220–21
  objectives, 221
  departmental, 223
Single accounting entries, 34–35
Social Security Amendments of 1983, 217,
    301
Span of control, 10
Staff. *See* Employees; Staffing
Staffing
  elasticity factor in, 82
  relevant range of activity (RRA) method in,
      82, 117–18
  requirements, 83
  requirements, determining, 115–18, 148–50
  requirements, plateaus in, 101
  step-variable, 82–83
  variable approach in, 117
  See also Employees; Positions
Standard costs
  attainable, 154–55
  basic, 154
  calculating, 156
  defined, 154, 156
  developing, 155–56
  ideal, 154
  relationship to variable budgeting, 155
  and target budget, 157
  types, 154–55
Standard methods, 29–30
Standard plans
  benefits, 30
  categories of, 25–30
  characteristics, 25
Standard production unit time, 129–30
Standard rate
  calculating, 88
  defined, 156
  developing, 155–56
  impact on productivity, 89
  and target budget, 157
Standard variable cost concept, 88
Standard variable nonsalary rate, 95
Standard variable salary rate, 94, 120
Statement
  of cash flow, 48–49, 61
  of changes in financial position, 49, 272
  of condition, 38, 46, 270–71
  of condition, compared with statement of
      operations, 48
  of condition, formula for, 46
  income, *See* Statement, of operations
  of operations, 47–48, 272

of operations, compared with statement of
    condition, 48
of operations, formulas for, 48
profit and loss (P&L), *See* Statement, of
    operations
of purpose, defined, 148
of purpose, and operating budget, 150
of sources and applications for funds, *See*
    Statement, of changes in financial
    position
*Statement of Responsibilities of Internal
    Auditing*, 276
Statistical forecast, 148–49
  and operating budget, 150
Step-variable expenses
  controlling, 82
  defined, 173
  examples of, 82
  nature of, 82
Subordinates, 10

T
T account, 34, 60
Target budget. *See* Budget, fixed or target
    system
Target production level (TPL), 131, 133
Theory X, 2
Theory Y, 2
Theory Z, 2
Third-party payers, 300, 301
  defined, 206
  examples of, 48
  filing cost reports to, 68
  impact on published charges, 206–13
  open communication with, 3
  payment procedures case study, 207–13
  and retrospective payment, 182–84
  and retrospective settlements, 182
  vs. self-paying patients, 204
  sensitivity testing and, 220–21
Time value of money, 233
Turnover rate, 260

U
Unilateral approach, 11, 14
Unity of command, 10

V
Variable budget
  accuracy of data in, 153
  concept behind, 153
  concept, variable application of, 173
  and cost control objectives, 155

developing, 91–92, 94–95, 157–59, 161, 163, 165–66
as expense control system, 88
methodology, 89
purpose, 145, 153–54
standard costs in, 154–55
and target level of activity, 154
Variable budgetary control concept, 101
Variable control budget, 166
Variable expense
    controlling, 80
    examples of, 80
    nature of, 80, 85
    and the statistical forecast, 148
    uses of, in budgeting and control, 91
Variable expense standard, 161
Variable nonsalary expense
    calculating, 96
    defined, 232
Variable production standard, 161
Variable salary expense, 95
Variance
    analysis, 97–102
    analyzing nonsalary expense, 172–73
    analyzing salary budget, 168–70, 172
    analyzing step-variable staffing and
        expense, 174, 176–79

efficiency, 97, 98
efficiency, calculating, 169
defined, 169
elimination of, 89
rate, 97, 98, 99, 100
rate, calculating, 169, 172
rate, defined, 169
usage, 172
volume, 74, 99, 100
adjusting to, 101

W
Weeks, Lewis E., 126, 150, 184, 204, 205
Weighted average monthly cash inflow
    percentage method, 235–37
Wildavsky, Aaron, 146
Working capital
    computation of, 56
    defined, 56
    factors affecting, 56–57
    impact of inflation on, 84
    sources of, 56, 57
    uses of, 56, 57–58
Work volume
    changes, impact on productivity, 89
    impact on variable expenses, 85

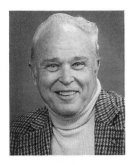

About the Author

Allen G. Herkimer Jr. is Associate Professor at Southwest Texas State University in the Department of Health Administration, where he teaches financial planning and analysis, health institution budgeting and financial planning, principles of hospital accounting, healthcare marketing, and other topics. Formerly Adjunct Professor at the Consortium of the California State University and Colleges, Dr. Herkimer also has an extensive professional background, which includes serving as Board Chairman and President of Comprehensive Health Services and Comptroller of the William W. Backus Hospital.

Currently chairing the National Task Force for the South Texas Chapter of Healthcare Financial Management Association, Dr. Herkimer regularly presents seminars and workshops in healthcare patient accounts management, healthcare marketing, and other areas. His articles on patient accounts and third-party payment have appeared in *The Journal of Patient Account Management,* the *American Journal of Medical Technology,* and many other publications.